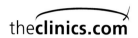

HEMATOLOGY/ ONCOLOGY CLINICS OF NORTH AMERICA

Inflammation, Hemostasis, and Blood Conservation Strategies

GUEST EDITOR
Jerrold H. Levy, MD

February 2007 • Volume 21 • Number 1

SAUNDERS

An Imprint of Elsevier, Inc.
PHILADELPHIA   LONDON   TORONTO   MONTREAL   SYDNEY   TOKYO

W.B. SAUNDERS COMPANY
A Division of Elsevier Inc.

Elsevier Inc. • 1600 John F. Kennedy Boulevard • Suite 1800 • Philadelphia, Pennsylvania 19103-2899

http://www.hemonc.theclinics.com

**HEMATOLOGY/ONCOLOGY CLINICS
OF NORTH AMERICA**
February 2007
Editor: Kerry Holland

Volume 21, Number 1
ISSN 0889-8588
ISBN-13: 978-1-4160-4322-5
ISBN-10: 1-4160-4322-5

Hematology/Oncology Clinics (ISSN 0889-8588) is published bimonthly by Elsevier Inc., 360 Park Avenue South, New York, NY 10010-1710. Months of issue are February, April, June, August, October, and December. Business and Editorial Offices: 1600 John F. Kennedy Blvd., Suite 1800, Philadelphia, PA 19103-2899. Customer Service Office: 6277 Sea Harbor Drive, Orlando, FL 32887-4800. Periodicals postage paid at New York, NY and additional mailing offices. Subscription prices are $238.00 per year (US individuals), $356.00 per year (US institutions), $119.00 per year (US students), $270.00 per year (Canadian individuals), $427.00 per year (Canadian institutions), $151.00 per year (Canadian students), $302.00 per year (international individuals), $427.00 per year (international institutions), $151.00 per year (international students). International air speed delivery is included in all *Clinics* subscription prices. All prices are subject to change without notice. **POSTMASTER:** Send address changes to *Hematology/Oncology Clinics of North America*, Elsevier Periodicals Customer Service, 6277 Sea Harbor Drive, Orlando, FL 32887-4800. Customer Service: 1-800-654-2452 (US). From outside of the US, call 1-407-345-4000.

Hematology/Oncology Clinics of North America is covered in *Index Medicus, EMBASE/Excerpta Medica*, and *BIOSIS*.

Printed in the United States of America.

SEVIER
UNDERS

Inflammation, Hemostasis, and Blood Conservation Strategies

GUEST EDITOR

JERROLD H. LEVY, MD, Professor and Deputy Chair for Research, Department of Anesthesiology, Emory University School of Medicine; Director of Cardiothoracic Anesthesiology, Cardiothoracic Anesthesiology and Critical Care, Emory Healthcare, Atlanta, Georgia

CONTRIBUTORS

GEORGE L. ADAMS, MD, Cardiology Fellow, Department of Medicine, Duke University Medical Center, Durham, North Carolina

JEREMIAH DENEVE, MD, Department of Surgery (Cardiothoracic), Cardiothoracic Research Laboratory, Carlyle Fraser Heart Center of Emory Crawford Long Hospital, Emory University, Atlanta, Georgia

GEORGE JOHN DESPOTIS, MD, Associate Professor of Anesthesiology, Department of Anesthesiology; and Associate Professor, Department of Pathology and Immunology, Washington University School of Medicine, St. Louis, Missouri

CHRISTOPHER D. HILLYER, MD, Professor, Department of Pathology and Laboratory Medicine; and Director, Transfusion Medicine Program, Emory University Hospital, Atlanta, Georgia

MAUREANE HOFFMAN, Pathology and Laboratory Medicine Service (113), Durham Veterans Affairs Medical Center; Department of Pathology, Duke University Medical Center, Durham, North Carolina

MARCIE J. HURSTING, PhD, Clinical Science Consulting, Austin, Texas

RONG JIANG, MD, PhD, Department of Surgery (Cardiothoracic), Cardiothoracic Research Laboratory, Carlyle Fraser Heart Center of Emory Crawford Long Hospital, Emory University, Atlanta, Georgia

LYNETTA J. JOBE, DVM, PhD, Department of Physiology, Mercer University College of Pharmacy and Health Sciences, Atlanta, Georgia

R. CLIVE LANDIS, PhD, Director, Edmund Cohen Laboratory for Vascular Research, University of the West Indies, Chronic Disease Research Centre, Barbados, West Indies

JEFFREY H. LAWSON, MD, PhD, Associate Professor of Surgery and Assistant Professor of Pathology; Co-Director, Center for Blood Conservation; Director of Vascular Surgery Research; and Director of Clinical Trials for Vascular Surgery, Duke University Medical Center, Durham, North Carolina

JERROLD H. LEVY, MD, Professor and Deputy Chair for Research, Department of Anesthesiology, Emory University School of Medicine; Director of Cardiothoracic Anesthesiology, Cardiothoracic Anesthesiology and Critical Care, Emory Healthcare, Atlanta, Georgia

LENNART E. LÖGDBERG, MD, PhD, Associate Professor, Department of Pathology and Laboratory Medicine, Emory University School of Medicine, Atlanta, Georgia

DOUGLAS M. LUBLIN, MD, PhD, Professor of Pathology and Immunology, Department of Pathology and Immunology, Washington University School of Medicine, St. Louis, Missouri

ROBERTO J. MANSON, MD, Surgery Fellow, Department of Surgery, Duke University Medical Center, Durham, North Carolina

DOUGALD M. MONROE, Department of Medicine, Carolina Cardiovascular Biology Center, University of North Carolina, Chapel Hill, North Carolina

JAMES MYKYTENKO, MD, Department of Surgery, Emory University School of Medicine, Atlanta, Georgia

JAMES G. REEVES, MD, Department of Surgery, Emory University School of Medicine, Atlanta, Georgia

LISA PAYNE ROJKJAER, MD, Senior Director, Clinical Development, Novartis Pharmaceuticals, East Hanover; formerly, Director, Clinical Development, Novo Nordisk Incorporated, Princeton, New Jersey

RASMUS ROJKJAER, PhD, Senior Research Director, Novo Nordisk Research US, North Brunswick, New Jersey

CHELSEA A. SHEPPARD, MD, Department of Pathology and Laboratory Medicine, Emory University School of Medicine, Atlanta, Georgia

LINDA SHORE-LESSERSON, MD, Associate Professor, Department of Anesthesiology; and Chief, Cardiothoracic Anesthesiology, Montefiore Medical Center, Bronx, New York

DAVID SINDRAM, MD, Surgery Resident, Department of Surgery, Duke University Medical Center, Durham, North Carolina

BRUCE D. SPIESS, MD, FAHA, Professor of Anesthesiology and Emergency Medicine, Department of Anesthesiology; and Director, Virginia Commonwealth University Reanimation Engineering Shock Center, Virginia Commonwealth University Medical Center, Richmond, Virginia

MARIE E. STEINER, MD, MS, Associate Professor of Pediatrics, Division of Hematology/Oncology/Blood & Marrow Transplantation; and Associate Professor of Pediatrics, Division of Pulmonary/Critical Care, University of Minnesota, Minneapolis, Minnesota

STEVEN R. STEINHUBL, MD, Associate Professor of Medicine; and Director of Cardiovascular Education and Clinical Research, Division of Cardiology, University of Kentucky, Lexington, Kentucky

KENICHI A. TANAKA, MD, MSc, Associate Professor of Anesthesiology, Department of Anesthesiology, Division of Cardiothoracic Anesthesia, The Emory Healthcare, Atlanta, Georgia

IMMANUEL TURNER, MD, Surgery Resident, Department of Surgery, Duke University Medical Center, Durham, North Carolina

JAKOB VINTEN-JOHANSEN, PhD, Professor, Department of Surgery (Cardiothoracic); and Director, Cardiothoracic Research Laboratory, Carlyle Fraser Heart Center of Emory Crawford Long Hospital, Emory University, Atlanta, Georgia

JAMES C. ZIMRING, MD, PhD, Assistant Professor, Department of Pathology and Laboratory Medicine, Emory University School of Medicine, Atlanta, Georgia

LINI ZHANG, MD, Research Assistant, Department of Anesthesiology, Washington University School of Medicine, St. Louis, Missouri

HEMATOLOGY/ONCOLOGY CLINICS
OF NORTH AMERICA

Inflammation, Hemostasis, and Blood Conservation Strategies

CONTENTS   VOLUME 21 • NUMBER 1 • FEBRUARY 2007

The authors propose that hemostasis occurs in a stepwise process, regulated by cellular components in vivo. The effectiveness of hemostasis in vivo depends not only on the procoagulant reactions but also on the fibrinolytic process. Causes of coagulopathic bleeding include consumption of coagulation factors and platelets, excessive fibrinolysis, hypothermia, and acidosis. Generation of the right amount of thrombin during the coagulation process not only may be essential for effective hemostasis but also may set the stage for effective wound healing.

Postoperative hemorrhage and thrombosis is a significant problem during the perioperative period. Understanding the complex and dynamic interplay of factors, proteins, and enzymes during coagulation is imperative to maintain balance between hemostasis and thrombosis. To improve patient outcome, each patient should be risk stratified for bleeding or thrombosis during the preoperative examination. Additional research focused on improvement in screening tools, monitoring, and therapeutic regimens for surgical patients with a coagulopathy are warranted.

Coagulation is a finely tuned sequence of reactions beginning with the interaction between tissue factor (TF) and its substrate, factor VII (FVII), and resulting in the formation of a fibrin clot localized to the site of vascular endothelial disruption. While important for fibrin clot formation, thrombin also plays a role in stabilizing the clot against premature fibrinolysis by activating thrombin activatable fibrinolysis inhibitor (TAFI) and factor XIII (FXIII), the terminal enzyme in the coagulation cascade. Despite use of antifibrinolytic agents in various types of surgery to inhibit clot lysis, thereby limiting blood loss and patient exposure to allogeneic blood products, numerous patients still require transfusions for nonsurgical bleeding. This article describes new concepts of localized hemostasis, a potential role for clot stabilization, and inhibition of fibrinolysis for control of bleeding.

Regulation of Thrombin Activity—Pharmacologic and Structural Aspects

Kenichi A. Tanaka and Jerrold H. Levy

Thrombin is an essential serine protease for survival. Since the discovery of heparin in the early twentieth century, significant advances have been made in the understanding of thrombin structure and function in coagulation system. Endogenous anticoagulant proteins in blood tightly regulate thrombin generation, but additional anticoagulant agents may be necessary to suppress excessive thrombin formation or defective anticoagulant proteins. Despite the availability of an array of anticoagulant agents based on chemical and biological engineering technologies, anticoagulation therapy remains a challenge for clinicians in terms of balancing bleeding and thrombosis. The aim of this article is to review endogenous serine protease inhibitors and novel antithrombotic agents in relation to pharmacologic regulation of thrombin.

Platelet Inhibitors and Monitoring Platelet Function: Implications for Bleeding

Linda Shore-Lesserson

Cardiovascular disease is prevalent in our medical and surgical patient population. Patients who have atherosclerotic heart disease suffer from endothelial disorders that predispose them to plaque and thrombus formation in diseased arteries. As our knowledge of platelet physiology improves, we can understand the contribution of platelet activation to arterial disease and we can specifically inhibit that activation with platelet-inhibitory drugs. The recent increase in the number of coronary interventional procedures performed has spawned the increasing use of antiplatelet medication as prophylaxis against thrombus formation in the instrumented artery.

Heparin-induced Thrombocytopenia, a Prothrombotic Disease

Jerrold H. Levy and Marcie J. Hursting

Heparin-induced thrombocytopenia (HIT) is a serious, yet treatable prothrombotic disease that develops in approximately 0.5% to 5% of heparin-treated patients and dramatically increases their risk of thrombosis (odds ratio, 37). The antibodies that mediate HIT (ie, heparin-platelet factor 4 antibodies) occur more frequently than the overt disease itself, and, even in the absence of thrombocytopenia, are associated with increased thrombotic morbidity and mortality. HIT should be suspected whenever the platelet count drops more than 50% from baseline (or to $<150 \times 10^9$/L) beginning 5 to 14 days after starting heparin (or sooner if there was prior heparin exposure) or new thrombosis occurs during, or soon after heparin treatment, with other causes excluded. When HIT is strongly suspected, with or without complicating thrombosis, heparins should be discontinued, and a fast-acting, nonheparin alternative anticoagulant such as argatroban should be initiated immediately. With prompt recognition, diagnosis, and treatment of HIT, the clinical outcomes and health economic burdens of this prothrombotic disease are improved significantly.

Anti-inflammatory Strategies and Hemostatic Agents: Old Drugs, New Ideas
Jerrold H. Levy

Hemostatic abnormalities occur following injury associated with both cardiac and noncardiac surgery. These changes are part of inflammatory pathways with signaling mechanisms that link these diverse pathways. The inflammatory response to surgery is exacerbated by allogeneic blood transfusion by enhancing intrinsic inflammatory activity and directly increasing plasma levels of inflammatory mediators. Surgical patients can be preventively treated with pharmacologic agents to modulate inflammatory responses. Multiple studies have reported preventive pharmacologic therapies to reduce bleeding and the need for allogeneic transfusions in surgery. Strategies for cardiac surgical patients during cardiopulmonary bypass include administration of either lysine analogs, such as epsilon aminocaproic acid and tranexamic acid, or the serine protease inhibitor aprotinin.

Protease Activated Receptors: Clinical Relevance to Hemostasis and Inflammation
R. Clive Landis

The protease-activated receptors (PARs) are a unique family of vascular receptors that confer on cells an ability to sense, and respond to, local changes in the proteolytic environment. They are activated by serine proteases of the blood coagulation cascade, notably thrombin, and are linked to thrombotic and inflammatory effector pathways. In surgery with cardiopulmonary bypass (CPB), thrombin is generated in large quantities in the extracorporeal circuit and can exert systemic effects by way of platelet and endothelial PAR1. Aprotinin (Trasylol), a serine protease inhibitor used in cardiac surgery, preserves platelet function, and attenuates the inflammatory response by protecting the PAR 1 receptor on platelets and endothelium.

Platelets as Mediators of Inflammation

Steven R. Steinhubl

An expanding body of evidence continues to build on the central role of inflammation in the progression and clinical manifestations of atherosclerosis. Platelets, long thought to play only a reactionary role at the time of endothelial disruption, are now recognized as important mediators of the inflammatory process. Platelet activation, which is modulated by both inflammatory and hemostatic factors, can lead to the release of hundreds of proteins–many with known proinflammatory functions. Although compelling evidence is lacking that antiplatelet therapies directly lower markers of inflammation, there are intriguing, although preliminary, data suggesting that markers of inflammation predict the clinical benefit of antiplatelet therapies.

Inflammation, Proinflammatory Mediators and Myocardial Ischemia–reperfusion Injury

Jakob Vinten-Johansen, Rong Jiang, James G. Reeves, James Mykytenko, Jeremiah Deneve, and Lynetta J. Jobe

Ischemic myocardium must be reperfused to terminate the ischemic event; otherwise the entire myocardium involved in the area at risk will not survive. However, there is a cost to reperfusion that may offset the intended clinical benefits of minimizing infarct size, postischemic endothelial and microvascular damage, blood flow defects, and contractile dysfunction. There are many contributors to this reperfusion injury. Targeting only one factor in the complex web of reperfusion injury may not be effective because the untargeted mechanisms induce injury. An integrated strategy of reducing reperfusion injury in the catheterization laboratory involves controlling both the conditions and the composition of the reperfusate to target the broadest array of mechanisms of injury. Mechanical interventions such as gradually restoring blood flow or applying postconditioning may be used independently in or conjunction with various cardioprotective pharmaceuticals in an integrated strategy of reperfusion therapeutics to reduce postischemic injury.

Transfusion Risks and Transfusion-related Pro-inflammatory Responses

George John Despotis, Lini Zhang, and Douglas M. Lublin

Despite improvements in blood screening and administration techniques, serious adverse events related to transfusion continue to occur, albeit at a much lower incidence. In addition to the development and implementation of new screening and blood purification/modification techniques and implementation of an optimal blood management program, the incidence and consequences of transfusion reactions can be reduced by a basic understanding of transfusion-related complications. Although acute hemolytic transfusion reactions, transfusion-associated anaphylaxis and sepsis, and transfusion-associated acute lung injury occur infrequently, diligence in administration of blood and monitoring for development of respective signs/symptoms can minimize the severity of these potentially life-threatening complications. In addition, emerging blood-banking techniques such as psoralen-UV inactivation of pathogens and use of patient identification systems may attenuate the incidence of adverse events related to transfusion. With respect to optimizing blood management by means of an effective blood management program involving pharmacologic and nonpharmacologic strategies, the ability to reduce use of blood products and to decrease operative time or re-exploration rates has important implications for disease prevention, blood inventory and costs, and overall health care costs.

Transfusion-related Acute Lung Injury
Chelsea A. Sheppard, Lennart F. Lögdberg, James C. Zimring, and Christopher D. Hillyer

With the success of reducing the risk of transfusion-transmitted infectious diseases, noninfectious serious hazards of transfusion have come to the forefront with respect to transfusion safety. Transfusion-related acute lung injury has emerged as a dominant noninfectious serious hazard of transfusion. Improved understanding of its pathophysiology is needed to improve clinical strategies to deal with the risk. Such understanding, in turn, will depend on the continued progress in development of good model systems, in vitro and in vivo, for experimental studies. As the pathologic mechanisms are elucidated, a universal definition and strategies for the prevention and/or mitigation may become more tangible. This article reviews the clinical manifestations, evolving definition, incidence, pathophysiology, animal modeling, donor screening, and deferral algorithms as they relate to transfusion-related acute lung injury.

Transfusion Algorithms and How They Apply to Blood Conservation: The High-risk Cardiac Surgical Patient
Marie E. Steiner and George John Despotis

Considerable blood product support is administered to the cardiac surgery population. Due to the multifactorial etiology of bleeding in the cardiac bypass patient, blood products frequently and empirically are infused to correct bleeding, with varying success. Several studies have demonstrated the benefit of algorithm-guided transfusion in reducing blood loss, transfusion exposure, or rate of surgical re-exploration for bleeding. Some transfusion algorithms also incorporate laboratory-based decision points in their guidelines. Despite published success with standardized transfusion practices, generalized change in blood use has not been realized, and it is evident that current laboratory-guided

HEMATOLOGY/ONCOLOGY CLINICS
OF NORTH AMERICA

HEMATOLOGY/ONCOLOGY CLINICS
OF NORTH AMERICA

Preface

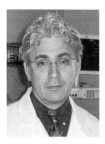

Jerrold H. Levy, MD

Guest Editor

I nflammation, as part of normal host protective systems, serves to limit injury in patients as a host surveillance mechanism. Different stimuli activate inflammatory pathways with signaling mechanisms that link these diverse pathways. Inflammatory responses can also result from allogeneic blood transfusions that contain protein and cellular components. These responses range from hypersensitivity to adverse organ system dysfunction. Thus, the role of blood conservation in managing hospitalized patients, especially critically ill patients, is increasingly being investigated and appreciated.

Hemostatic abnormalities occur in patients after a broad spectrum of injury, as part of pathophysiologic processes (ie, atherosclerosis, infections), or subsequent to traumatic or surgical interventions. Hemostatic activation is critically linked to inflammatory responses by a network of humoral and cellular components including proteases of the clotting and fibrinolytic cascades. Hemostatic initiation, thrombin generation, contact activation, and other pathways amplify inflammatory responses to produce collectively end-organ damage as part of host defense mechanisms.

Cross talk between activation of inflammation and hemostasis occurs, where cytokines and other inflammatory mediators activate coagulation proteases to modulate inflammation through specific cell receptors including protease-activated receptors. Strategies directed at inhibiting coagulation activation have been reported in experimental and early clinical studies and include inhibiting tissue factor–mediated activation of coagulation or restoration of physiologic anticoagulant pathways by recombinant human activated protein C or antithrombin. In disseminated intravascular coagulation, overactivation of thrombin, clotting, or both leads to bleeding complications; depletion of coagulation proteins and platelets and endothelial dysfunction produce

0889-8588/07/$ – see front matter
doi:10.1016/j.hoc.2006.11.014

microvascular dysfunction and a thrombotic state. These sequelae can occur to varying degrees in our critically ill patients.

Surgical patients often receive transfusions with multiple blood products. They have a unique circumstance as they can be preventively treated with pharmacologic agents to better modulate inflammatory responses and downstream responses. Multiple studies have reported preventive pharmacologic therapies to reduce bleeding and the need for allogeneic transfusions in surgery. Strategies for cardiac surgical patients during cardiopulmonary bypass (CPB) include administration of the lysine analogs including epsilon aminocaproic acid, tranexamic acid, or aprotinin (Trasylol). Novel therapies are also under investigation that involve recombinant approaches.

In September 2005, a group of multidisciplinary physicians and scientists in the areas of hematology, inflammation, cardiology, surgery, anesthesiology, neurology, critical care, and transfusion medicine representing multiorganizational specialties met at Emory University to review topics in inflammation, hemostasis, and blood conservation strategies. The proceedings from this meeting are presented here. Part of the purpose of the meeting was also to understand inflammation and bleeding, understand the role of transfusions and other therapies, and strategize solutions to the growing issues involving blood management and health care quality and delivery.

National medical and regulatory organizations have developed guidelines for blood transfusions, but these guidelines remain inconsistent and unenforceable. The way blood is used in the surgical setting is normally left to the discretion of individual physicians. However, transfusion practices vary based on knowledge level and overall interest. Further, these variances may affect procedures that routinely involve a significant amount of blood loss. Thus, establishing scientifically based guidelines to guide blood management within the health care system is an important undertaking.

The Inflammation, Hemostasis and Blood Conservation Strategies forum also reviewed the latest science surrounding the management of surgical bleeding. Although guidelines for transfusion are not clearly defined, blood needs to be used judiciously, especially in procedures that involve significant blood loss such as cardiac surgery and orthopedic procedures. Discussion at the event centered on three key topics: the risks of blood transfusion, the potential benefits of anti-inflammatory strategies and blood-sparing agents, and the overall need for better blood management strategies to improve the overall quality of patient outcomes.

My colleague, Robert J. Bachman, who is Chief Operating Officer, Emory University Hospital, summarized the importance of the Inflammation, Hemostasis and Blood Conservation Strategies forum. "Blood management is on the minds of people at every level of the hospital. It is critical that physicians and institutions give more attention to managing blood as an essential component of improving patient care, and delivering quality services in the context of modern healthcare administration."

The chapters included in this edition of *Hematology/Oncology Clinics of North America* represent important aspects from the meeting related to our current understanding of hemostasis and links to inflammation by thrombin signaling, platelet activation, and overall issues related to ischemia–reperfusion injury. The chapters review therapeutic issues in treating these patients; three important chapters regarding blood issues address current transfusion risks; transfusion-related acute lung injury, an increasingly recognized problem associated with transfusion therapy; and transfusion algorithms and rational approaches to administering blood. Finally, one of the most important chapters is a novel review of blood and transfusions by Bruce Spiess, an insightful crusader of blood conservation and, like me, a believer of multimodal perspectives essential to blood conservation.

To all the participants who made this meeting possible, I thank you for your outstanding efforts, and your important contributions to science and clinical care. This meeting was supported by unrestricted educational grants from Bayer, Novo Nordisk, Eisai, and Zymogenetics.

Jerrold H. Levy, MD
Department of Anesthesiology
Emory University School of Medicine
1364 Clifton Road N.E.
Atlanta, GA 30322, USA

and
Cardiothoracic Anesthesiology and Critical Care
Emory Healthcare
1364 Clifton Road N.E.
Atlanta, GA 30322, USA

E-mail address: jerrold.levy@emoryhealthcare.org

Hematol Oncol Clin N Am 21 (2007) 1–11

HEMATOLOGY/ONCOLOGY CLINICS
OF NORTH AMERICA

Coagulation 2006: A Modern View of Hemostasis

Maureane Hoffman[a,b,*], Dougald M. Monroe[c]

[a]Pathology and Laboratory Medicine Service (113), Durham Veterans Affairs Medical Center, 508 Fulton Street, Durham, NC 27705, USA
[b]Department of Pathology, Duke University Medical Center, Durham, NC 27710, USA
[c]Department of Medicine, Carolina Cardiovascular Biology Center, CB#7035, University of North Carolina, Chapel Hill, NC 27514-7035, USA

HOW WELL DO WE REALLY UNDERSTAND COAGULATION?

In the 1960s two groups proposed a waterfall or cascade model of coagulation composed of a sequential series of steps in which activation of one clotting factor led to the activation of another, finally leading to a burst of thrombin generation [1,2]. Each clotting factor was believed to exist as a proenzyme that could be converted to an active enzyme.

The original cascade models were subsequently modified to include the observation that some procoagulants were cofactors and did not possess enzymatic activity. The coagulation process is now often outlined in a Y-shaped scheme, with distinct intrinsic and extrinsic pathways initiated by factor XII (FXII) and FVIIa/tissue factor (TF), respectively, as outlined in Fig. 1. The pathways converge on a common pathway at the level of the FXa/Fva (prothrombinase) complex. The coagulation complexes are generally noted to require phospholipid and calcium for their activity. This scheme was not actually proposed as a literal model of the hemostatic process in vivo. The lack of any other clear and predictive concept of physiologic hemostasis, however, has meant that most physicians and students of coagulation viewed the cascade as a model of physiology. This view has been reinforced by the fact that screening tests of the adequacy of the extrinsic pathway (prothrombin time [PT]) and the intrinsic pathway (activated partial thromboplastin time [aPTT]) are often treated as though they are predictive of clinical bleeding.

This work was supported by grant RO1 HL48320 from the National Institutes of Health and by the United States Department of Veteran's Affairs (MH).

*Corresponding author. Pathology and Laboratory Medicine Service (113), Durham Veterans Affairs Medical Center, 508 Fulton Street, Durham, NC 27705.
E-mail address: maureane.hoffman@med.va.gov (M. Hoffman).

0889-8588/07/$ – see front matter
doi:10.1016/j.hoc.2006.11.004

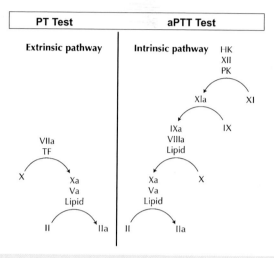

Fig. 1. The extrinsic and intrinsic pathways in the cascade model of coagulation. These two pathways are conceived as each leading to formation of the factor Xa/Va complex, which generates thrombin. *Lipid* indicates that the reaction requires a phospholipid surface. These pathways are assayed clinically using the prothrombin time (PT) and activated partial thromboplastin time (aPTT), respectively. HK, high molecular weight kininogen; PK, prekallikrein.

Although the cascade concept of coagulation was treated as though it were a model of coagulation in vivo, many people recognized that the intrinsic and extrinsic systems could not operate in vivo as independent and redundant pathways as implied by this model. It was clear that even though deficiencies of each of the factors in the intrinsic pathway could have equally long aPTT values, they had dramatically different risks of hemorrhage. Deficiencies of FXII are not associated with significant hemorrhage, deficiencies of FXI might or might not be associated with hemorrhage, but deficiencies of factors VIII and IX are consistently associated with hemorrhage.

The key observation that the FVIIa/TF complex activated not only FX but also FIX [3], suggested that the pathways were linked. Other important observations led to the conclusion that activity of the FVIIa/TF complex is the major initiating event in hemostasis in vivo [4,5]. It was still not clear why an intact extrinsic pathway could not compensate for the lack of FIX or VIII in hemophilia, however.

CAN AN EMPHASIS ON THE ROLE OF CELLS IMPROVE OUR UNDERSTANDING OF COAGULATION?

It was recognized from the earliest studies of coagulation that cells were important participants in the coagulation process. Of course, it is clear that normal hemostasis is not possible in the absence of platelets. In addition, TF is an integral membrane protein and thus its activity is normally associated with cells. Because different cells express different levels of pro- and anticoagulant proteins and have different complements of receptors for components of hemostasis, it is logical that simply representing the cells involved in coagulation as phospholipid vesicles may overlook the important contributions of cells in directing hemostasis in vivo. The authors' studies in a cell-based experimental model of coagulation [6–8] and the existing literature led us to propose [9] that hemostasis actually occurs in a step-wise process, regulated by cellular components in vivo, as outlined in the following sections.

Step 1: Initiation of Coagulation on TF-bearing Cells

The goal of hemostasis it to produce a platelet and fibrin plug to seal a site of injury or rupture in the blood vessel wall. This process is initiated when TF-bearing cells are exposed to blood at a site of injury.

TF is a transmembrane protein that acts as a receptor and cofactor for FVII. Once bound to TF, zymogen FVII is rapidly converted to FVIIa through mechanisms not yet completely understood but possibly involving FXa or noncoagulation proteases. The resulting FVIIa/TF complex catalyzes activation of FX and activation of FIX. The factors Xa and IXa formed on the TF-bearing cells have distinct and separate functions in initiating blood coagulation [7]. The FXa formed on the TF-bearing cell interacts with its cofactor Va to form prothrombinase complexes and generates a small amount of thrombin on the TF cells (Fig. 2A). By contrast, the FIXa activated by FVIIa/TF does not act on the TF-bearing cell and does not play a significant role in the initiation phase of coagulation. If an injury has occurred and platelets have adhered near the site of the TF-bearing cells, the FIXa can diffuse to the surface of nearby activated platelets. It can then bind to a specific platelet surface receptor [10], interact with its cofactor, FVIIIa, and activate FX directly on the platelet surface.

Most of the coagulation factors can leave the vasculature and their activation peptides are found in the lymph [11]. It is likely, therefore, that most (extravascular) TF is bound to FVIIa even in the absence of an injury, and that low levels of FIXa, FXa, and thrombin are produced on TF-bearing cells at all times. This process is kept separated from key components of hemostasis by an intact vessel wall, however. The very large components of the coagulation process are platelets and FVIII bound to multimeric von Willebrand factor (vWF). These components normally only come into contact with the extravascular compartment when an injury disrupts the vessel wall. Platelets and FVIII-vWF then leave the vascular space and adhere to collagen and other matrix components at the site of injury.

Step 2: Amplification of the Procoagulant Signal by Thrombin Generated on the TF-bearing Cell

Binding of platelets to collagen or by way of vWF leads to partial platelet activation. The coagulation process is most effectively initiated, however, when enough thrombin is generated on or near the TF-bearing cells to trigger full activation of platelets and activation of coagulation cofactors on the platelet surface in the amplification step (as illustrated in Fig. 2B). Although this amount of thrombin may not be sufficient to clot fibrinogen, it is sufficient to initiate

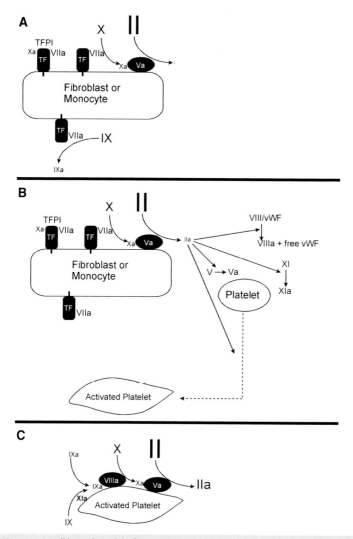

Fig. 2. Steps in a cell-based model of coagulation. (A) Initiation occurs on the TF-bearing cell as activated FX combines with its cofactor, FVa, to activate small amounts of thrombin. (B) The small amount of thrombin generated on the TF-bearing cell amplifies the procoagulant response by activating cofactors, factor XI, and platelets. (C) The large burst of thrombin required for effective hemostasis is formed on the platelet surface during the propagation phase.

events that prime the clotting system for a subsequent burst of platelet surface thrombin generation. Experiments using a cell-based model have shown that minute amounts of thrombin are formed in the vicinity of TF-bearing cells exposed to plasma concentrations of procoagulants, even in the absence of platelets. The small amounts of FVa required for prothrombinase assembly on TF-bearing cells are activated by FXa [12] or by noncoagulation proteases produced by the cells [13] or are released from platelet that adhere nearby. The small amounts of thrombin generated on the TF-bearing cells are responsible for [8,14]: (1) activating platelets, (2) activating FV, (3) activating FVIII and dissociating FVIII from VWF, and (4) activating FXI. The activity of the FXa formed by the FVIIa/TF complex is restricted to the TF-bearing cell, because FXa that dissociates from the cell surface is rapidly inhibited by TFPI or AT in the fluid phase. In contrast to FXa, FIXa can diffuse to adjacent platelet surfaces because it is not inhibited by TFPI and is inhibited much more slowly by AT than is FXa.

Step 3: Propagation of Thrombin Generation on the Platelet Surface

Platelets play a major role in localizing clotting reactions to the site of injury because they adhere and aggregate at the sites of injury where TF is also exposed. They provide the primary surface for generation of the burst of thrombin needed for effective hemostasis during the propagation phase of coagulation (Fig. 2C). Platelet localization and activation are mediated by vWF, thrombin, platelet receptors, and vessel wall components, such as collagen [15].

Once platelets are activated, the cofactors Va and VIIIa are rapidly localized on the platelet surface [6]. As noted above, the FIXa formed by the FVIIa/TF complex can diffuse through the fluid phase and also bind to the surface of activated platelets. Likewise, FXI also binds to platelet surfaces and is activated by the priming amount of thrombin [14,16], bypassing the need for FXIIa. The platelet-bound FXIa can activate more FIX to IXa. Once the platelet tenase complex is assembled, FX from the plasma is activated to FXa on the platelet surface. FXa then associates with FVa to support a burst of thrombin generation of sufficient magnitude to produce a stable fibrin clot.

The large amount of thrombin generated on the platelet surface is responsible for stabilizing the hemostatic clot in more ways than just promoting fibrin polymerization. In fact, most of the thrombin generated during the hemostatic process is produced after the initial fibrin clot is formed. The platelet-produced thrombin also stabilizes the clot by: (1) activating FXIII [17], (2) activating TAFI [18], (3) cleaving the platelet PAR-4 receptor [19], and (4) being incorporated into the structure of the clot.

The role of FXI in hemostasis has been a point of some controversy, because even severe FXI deficiency does not result in a hemorrhagic tendency comparable to that seen in severe FVIII or IX deficiency. This discrepancy can be explained if FXI is viewed as an enhancer or booster of thrombin generation. FXIa activates additional FIXa on the platelet surface to supplement FIXa/FVIIIa complex formation and enhance platelet surface FXa and thrombin generation. FXI thus is not essential for platelet-surface thrombin generation, as are FIX and FVIII, and its deficiency does not compromise hemostasis to the degree seen in FIX and FVIII deficiency.

Our knowledge of the platelet contribution to thrombin generation continues to evolve. There is evidence that there is more than one population of activated platelets, one of which has been referred to as COAT (COllagen And Thrombin stimulated) platelets [20]. These platelets have enhanced thrombin-generating ability because of enhanced binding of both tenase and prothrombinase component [21,22]. The in vivo relevance of these findings is not yet clear, but it may be that the greatest procoagulant activity is generated on platelets that have bound to collagen matrix and also been exposed to thrombin. Once the exposed collagen matrix is covered by a platelet/fibrin layer, additional platelets that accumulate are not activated to the COAT state, thus tending to damp down the procoagulant signal as the area of the wound is occluded by a hemostatic clot.

Although each step of the cell-based model has been depicted as an isolated set of reactions, including initiation, amplification, and propagation, they should be viewed as an overlapping continuum of events. For example, thrombin produced on the platelet surface early in the propagation phase may initially cleave substrates on the platelet surface and continue to amplify the procoagulant response, in addition to leaving the platelet and promoting fibrin assembly.

The cell-based model of coagulation shows us that the extrinsic and intrinsic pathways are not redundant. Let us consider the extrinsic pathway to consist of the FVIIa/TF complex working with the FXa/Va complex and the intrinsic pathway to consist of FXIa working with the complexes of factors VIIIa/IXa and factors Xa/Va as illustrated in Fig. 3 (from Ref. [23]). The extrinsic pathway operates on the TF-bearing cell to initiate and amplify coagulation. By contrast, the intrinsic pathway operates on the activated platelet surface to produce the burst of thrombin that causes formation and stabilization of the fibrin clot.

FIBRINOLYSIS

Even as the fibrin clot is being formed in the body, the fibrinolytic system is being initiated to disrupt it. The final effector of the fibrinolytic system is plasmin, which cleaves fibrin into soluble degradation products. Plasmin is produced from the inactive precursor plasminogen by the action of two plasminogen activators: urokinase-type plasminogen activator (uPA) and tissue-type plasminogen activator (tPA). The PAs are in turn regulated by plasminogen activator inhibitors (PAIs). Plasminogen is found at a much higher plasma concentration than the PAs. The availability of the two PAs in the plasma therefore generally determines the extent of plasmin formation. tPA release from endothelial cells is provoked by thrombin and venous occlusion [24]. tPA and plasminogen both bind to the evolving fibrin polymer. Once plasminogen is activated to plasmin it cleaves fibrin at specific lysine and arginine residues, resulting in dissolution of the fibrin clot.

Thrombin-activatable inhibitor of fibrinolysis (TAFI) is a zymogen that can be activated (TAFIa) by thrombin or plasmin [18]. As fibrin is degraded by plasmin, C-terminal lysines are exposed that enhance activation of additional plasminogen to plasmin. TAFIa removes the C-terminal lysines from fibrin and thereby inhibits the cofactor activity of fibrin for plasminogen activation.

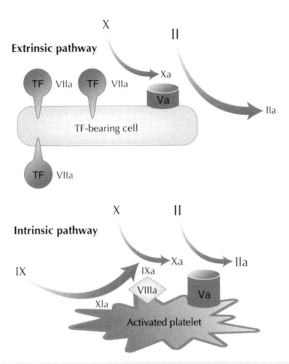

Fig. 3. The extrinsic and intrinsic pathways in the cell-based model of coagulation. The role of the cell-based extrinsic pathway (*top*) is to act on the TF-bearing cell to generate the small amounts of thrombin (factor IIa) involved in initiating coagulation. The role of the cell-based intrinsic pathway (*bottom*) is to act on the platelet surface to generate the burst of thrombin needed to form a stable fibrin clot. TF, tissue factor.

Fibrinolysis is essential for removal of clots during the process of wound healing and for removing intravascular clots that might otherwise be manifest as thrombosis. Intravascular deposition of fibrin is also associated with the development of atherosclerosis. An effective fibrinolytic system therefore tends to protect against the chronic process of atherosclerotic vascular disease and the acute process of thrombosis. Conversely, defects of fibrinolysis increase the risk for atherothrombotic disease. For example, elevated levels of plasminogen activator inhibitor-1, an inhibitor of fibrinolysis, are associated with an increased risk for atherosclerosis and thrombosis [25] as are decreased levels of plasminogen [26]. The effectiveness of hemostasis in vivo depends not only on the procoagulant reactions but also on the fibrinolytic process.

WHAT DOES ALL THIS MEAN FOR CLINICAL LABORATORY TESTING?

It should be clear from the preceding discussion that our commonly used clinical coagulation tests do not really reflect the complexity of hemostasis in vivo.

That does not mean that the PT and aPTT are useless. We just need to understand what they can and cannot tell us. These screening coagulation tests are abnormal when there is a deficiency of one or more of the soluble coagulation factors. They do not tell us what the risk for clinical bleeding will be. Two patients who have identical aPTT values can have drastically different risks of hemorrhage. All of our common coagulation tests including the PT, aPTT, thrombin clotting time, fibrinogen levels, and coagulation factor levels tell us something about the plasma level of soluble factors required for hemostasis. Their clinical implications must be evaluated by the ordering physician. Just because the PT and aPTT are within the normal range it does not follow that the patient is at no risk for bleeding. Conversely, a mild elevation in these clotting times does not mean that the patient is at risk for bleeding after an invasive procedure.

Many whole blood coagulation tests are jockeying for position as a means of evaluating overall hemostatic status in selected clinical settings. Although whole blood tests have the advantage that they may reflect the contributions of platelets to the hemostatic process, they still do not reflect the contributions of the TF-bearing cells and local tissue conditions. Any laboratory test requires skilled interpretation and clinical correlation in evaluating the true risk for bleeding.

WHAT CAUSES BLEEDING IN PREVIOUSLY NORMAL PATIENTS?

Many patients who experience significant hemorrhage do not have an underlying bleeding tendency that can be identified before a bleeding episode. Bleeding following surgical or accidental trauma or during a medical illness is often associated with the development of an acquired coagulopathy. The hallmark of coagulopathy is microvascular bleeding, which means oozing from cut surfaces and minor sites of trauma, such as needle sticks. Microvascular bleeding can lead to massive blood loss.

Causes of coagulopathic bleeding include consumption of coagulation factors and platelets, excessive fibrinolysis, hypothermia, and acidosis.

Consumption of Coagulation Components

We normally think of disseminated intravascular coagulation (DIC) when we talk of consumption. Clotting factors and platelets can also be consumed during appropriate physiologic attempts at hemostasis, however. In this case it is appropriate to replace the depleted factors with transfusion therapy.

DIC can be much more complicated to manage [27]. The mainstay of treatment is to treat the underlying disorder, such as sepsis. In early or mild/compensated DIC administration of low-dose heparin may be considered to control the procoagulant response to inflammation, infection, or malignancy. In more severe or advanced DIC, however, replacement therapy may be necessary to treat the bleeding tendency associated with depletion of coagulation factors and platelets.

Excessive Fibrinolysis

The process of fibrinolysis is initiated whenever coagulation is initiated. When attempts at hemostasis are unsuccessful, a significant amount of fibrinolytic activity may still be generated and thwart subsequent efforts at hemostasis. Fibrinolytic inhibitors have thus proven to be useful in some circumstances.

Hypothermia

Many patients become hypothermic during medical illness or following surgical or accidental trauma [28]. Hypothermia can directly interfere with the hemostatic process by slowing the activity of coagulation enzymes. Less well recognized is the finding that platelet adhesion and aggregation is impaired even in mild hypothermia [29]. In hypothermic coagulopathic patients, raising the core temperature can have a beneficial effect on bleeding by improving platelet function and coagulation enzyme activity.

Acidosis

Acidosis can have an even more profound effect on procoagulant function than hypothermia, although the two metabolic abnormalities often coexist. A drop in the pH from 7.4 to 7.2 reduces the activity of each of the coagulation proteases by more than half [30]. Acidosis should be considered as a possible contributor to coagulopathic bleeding in medical and surgical patients.

WHAT HAPPENS AFTER THE BLEEDING STOPS?

Once hemostasis is completed the process of wound healing can begin. The hemostatic plug must be stable enough to maintain hemostasis, yet be removed as the tissue defect is permanently closed. Fibrinolysis is accomplished by the action of plasmin, probably in concert with other leukocyte proteases. The neutrophils that initially accumulate at a site of injury are replaced over the course of a few days with macrophages that engulf and degrade cellular debris and components of the fibrin clot. The macrophages also secrete cytokines and growth factors that facilitate the migration of fibroblasts and endothelial cells into the wound site. In the case of a skin wound, the dermis is replaced by highly cellular and vascular granulation tissue, while the surface epithelium proliferates and migrates from the margins to cover the surface of the wound. Many of the activities involved in wound healing are influenced by thrombin. Thrombin plays a major role in platelet activation and degranulation. Several key cytokines modulating wound healing are released from activated platelets, including transforming growth factor beta (TGFβ1) and platelet-derived growth factor (PDGF). The amount and rate of thrombin generated during hemostasis influences the initial structure of the fibrin clot—the framework on which cell migration takes place. In addition, thrombin has chemotactic and mitogenic activities for macrophages, fibroblasts, smooth muscle cells and endothelial cells. Generation of the right amount of thrombin during the coagulation process not only may be essential for effective hemostasis but also may set the stage for effective wound healing.

References

[1] Macfarlane RG. An enzyme cascade in the blood clotting mechanism, and its function as a biological amplifier. Nature 1964;202:498–9.

[2] Davie EW, Ratnoff OD. Waterfall sequence for intrinsic blood clotting. Science 1964;145: 1310–2.

[3] Østerud B, Rapaport SI. Activation of factor IX by the reaction product of tissue factor and factor VII: additional pathway for initiating blood coagulation. Proc Natl Acad Sci U S A 1977;74:5260–4.

[4] Nemerson Y, Esnouf MP. Activation of a proteolytic system by a membrane lipoprotein: mechanism of action of tissue factor. Proc Natl Acad Sci U S A 1973;70:310–4.

[5] Nemerson Y. The tissue factor pathway of blood coagulation. Semin Hematol 1992;29: 170–6.

[6] Monroe DM, Roberts HR, Hoffman M. Platelet procoagulant complex assembly in a tissue factor-initiated system. Br J Haematol 1994;88:364–71.

[7] Hoffman M, Monroe DM, Oliver JA, et al. Factors IXa and Xa play distinct roles in tissue factor-dependent initiation of coagulation. Blood 1995;86:1794–801.

[8] Monroe DM, Hoffman M, Roberts HR. Transmission of a procoagulant signal from tissue factor-bearing cell to platelets. Blood Coagul Fibrinolysis 1996;7:459–64.

[9] Hoffman M, Monroe DM 3rd. A cell-based model of hemostasis. Thromb Haemost 2001;85:958–65.

[10] Rawala-Sheikh R, Ahmad SS, Monroe DM, et al. Role of gamma-carboxyglutamic acid residues in the binding of factor IXa to platelets and in factor-X activation. Blood 1992;79: 398–405.

[11] Le D, Borgs P, Toneff T, et al. Hemostatic factors in rabbit limb lymph: relationship to mechanisms regulating extravascular coagulation. Am J Physiol 1998;274:H769–76.

[12] Monkovic DD, Tracy PB. Activation of human factor V by factor Xa and thrombin. Biochemistry 1990;29:1118–28.

[13] Allen DH, Tracy PB. Human coagulation factor V is activated to the functional cofactor by elastase and cathepsin G expressed at the monocyte surface. J Biol Chem 1995;270: 1408–15.

[14] Oliver J, Monroe D, Roberts H, et al. Thrombin activates factor XI on activated platelets in the absence of factor XII. Arterioscler Thromb Vasc Biol 1999;19:170–7.

[15] Falati S, Gross P, Merrill-Skoloff G, et al. Real-time in vivo imaging of platelets, tissue factor and fibrin during arterial thrombus formation in the mouse. Nat Med 2002;8:1175–81.

[16] Baglia FA, Walsh PN. Prothrombin is a cofactor for the binding of factor XI to the platelet surface and for platelet-mediated factor XI activation by thrombin. Biochemistry 1998;37:2271–81.

[17] Lorand L. Factor XIII: structure, activation, and interactions with fibrinogen and fibrin. Ann N Y Acad Sci 2001;936:291–311.

[18] Bajzar L, Manuel R, Nesheim ME. Purification and characterization of TAFI, a thrombin-activatable fibrinolysis inhibitor. J Biol Chem 1995;270:14477–84.

[19] Ofosu FA. Protease activated receptors 1 and 4 govern the responses of human platelets to thrombin. Transfus Apher Sci 2003;28:265–8.

[20] Alberio L, Safa O, Clemetson KJ, et al. Surface expression and functional characterization of alpha-granule factor V in human platelets: effects of ionophore A23187, thrombin, collagen, and convulxin. Blood 2000;95:1694–702.

[21] Dale GL, Friese P, Batar P, et al. Stimulated platelets use serotonin to enhance their retention of procoagulant proteins on the cell surface. Nature 2002;415:175–9.

[22] Kempton CL, Hoffman M, Roberts HR, et al. Platelet heterogeneity: variation in coagulation complexes on platelet subpopulations. Arterioscler Thromb Vasc Biol 2005;25:861–6.

[23] Hoffman M, Monroe DM. Rethinking the coagulation cascade. Curr Hematol Rep 2005;4: 391–6.

[24] Szymanski LM, Pate RR, Durstine JL. Effects of maximal exercise and venous occlusion on fibrinolytic activity in physically active and inactive men. J Appl Physiol 1994;77:2305–10.

[25] Huber K, Christ G, Wojta J, et al. Plasminogen activator inhibitor type-1 in cardiovascular disease. Status report 2001. Thromb Res 2001;103(Suppl 1):S7–19.

[26] Xiao Q, Danton MJ, Witte DP, et al. Plasminogen deficiency accelerates vessel wall disease in mice predisposed to atherosclerosis. Proc Natl Acad Sci U S A 1997;94:10335–40.

[27] Mueller MM, Bomke B, Seifried E. Fresh frozen plasma in patients with disseminated intra-vascular coagulation or in patients with liver diseases. Thromb Res 2002;107(Suppl 1): S9–17.

[28] Eddy VA, Morris JA Jr, Cullinane DC. Hypothermia, coagulopathy, and acidosis. Surg Clin North Am 2000;80:845–54.

[29] Wolberg AS, Meng ZH, Monroe DM 3rd, et al. A systematic evaluation of the effect of tem-perature on coagulation enzyme activity and platelet function. J Trauma 2004;56:1221–8.

[30] Meng ZH, Wolberg AS, Monroe DM 3rd, et al. The effect of temperature and pH on the ac-tivity of factor VIIa: implications for the efficacy of high-dose factor VIIa in hypothermic and acidotic patients. J Trauma 2003;55:886–91.

Hematol Oncol Clin N Am 21 (2007) 13–24

HEMATOLOGY/ONCOLOGY CLINICS
OF NORTH AMERICA

The Balance of Thrombosis and Hemorrhage in Surgery

George L. Adams, MD[a], Roberto J. Manson, MD[b],
Immanuel Turner, MD[b], David Sindram, MD[b],
Jeffrey H. Lawson, MD, PhD[b,c,*]

[a]Department of Medicine, Duke University Medical Center, Box 2622, MSRB, Research Drive,
Durham, NC 27710, USA
[b]Department of Surgery, Duke University Medical Center, Box 2622, MSRB, Research Drive,
Durham, NC 27710, USA
[c]Department of Pathology, Duke University Medical Center, Box 2622, MSRB, Research Drive,
Durham, NC 27710, USA

Understanding the biology of hemostasis and thrombosis is critical to the diagnosis, management, and stabilization of the postoperative patient with hemorrhage or thromboembolism. A surgeon's goal is to maintain balance between perioperative hemostasis and pathologic thrombosis to prevent adverse events. However, bleeding and clotting remains a significant perioperative complication. The Duke series of death and complications occurring from 2001 to 2003 estimated that 55% of the complications were related to hemorrhage or thrombosis resulting in 67 deaths—27% related to bleeding and 31% associated with thrombosis (unpublished data).

Blood coagulation is a physiologic defense mechanism that maintains the integrity of the mammalian circulatory system in response to vascular damage. It is a dynamic mechanism that involves a balance between coagulation and fibrinolysis to prevent hemorrhage or thrombosis. The cascade of events in response to injury, whether traumatic or surgical, is a complex series of linked events that require the interaction of both cellular elements and blood plasma proteins. This interaction at a cellular level determines which way the balance will lean: hemorrhage versus appropriate hemostasis versus pathologic thrombosis.

CELL-BASED MODEL OF COAGULATION

The hemostatic mechanism has been described as a cascade of enzymatic reactions resulting in the formation of thrombin, which converts fibrinogen to fibrin and forms the basis of a blood clot [1,2]. Although based on a sequence

*Corresponding author. Department of Surgery, Duke University Medical Center, Box 2622, MSRB, Research Drive, Durham, NC 27710. E-mail address: lawso006@mc.duke.edu (J.H. Lawson).

0889-8588/07/$ – see front matter
doi:10.1016/j.hoc.2006.11.013

of reactions, the regulation of blood coagulation is dynamic and more complex than this model suggests. Accordingly, a cell-based model of coagulation [3] establishes a physiologic, integrated, and functional view of complex biochemical events occurring on cellular surfaces on which a vascular insult occurs. The evolving structural-functional scheme of coagulation can be divided into three phases: initiation, amplification, and propagation.

Normally, the endothelial cells supported by a subendothelial matrix, line the vascular space and provide a barrier between the circulating blood and the extravascular tissue. The luminal surface is nonthrombogenic secondary to the constitutive expression of heparin sulfate, proteoglycans, thrombomodulin, and nonadherent phospholipids as well as the release of nitric oxide, prostacyclin, and tissue plasminogen activator into the vascular space.

The initiation phase is triggered by physical (trauma or surgery) or molecular signals, which convert the resting endothelium into a focus of procoagulant activity. After activation, heparin sulfate proteoglycans are removed from the endothelial surface resulting in decreased antiprotease activity from antithrombin III. In addition, down-regulation of thrombomodulin occurs on the cell surface, which, under normal circumstances, binds thrombin resulting in a complex that activates Protein C. Activated protein C functions to proteolytically degrade the cofactors Va and VIIIa. Thus, when antithrombin III and thrombomodulin are down-regulated, the potential for increased coagulation occurs.

Initiation continues on intact cells or cellular fragments bearing the transmembrane glycoprotein tissue factor (Fig. 1) [4]. Results of in vitro and in vivo studies have shown tissue factor activity can be induced by a number of growth factors including fibroblast growth factor, platelet-derived growth factor, interleukin-1, and tumor necrosis factor [5–7]. Tissue factor binds coagulation zymogen factor (f) VII. Activated (f) VII converts fIX and fX to their active enzyme forms. Activated fX (Xa) then converts prothrombin (fII) to thrombin (IIa) and activates factor V (fV) to factor Va (fVa), thus enhancing the local procoagulant environment.

Instrumental to the initiation phase is the change in phospholipid endothelial cell membrane composition resulting in more acidic phospholipid head groups. These acidic groups attract negatively charged rafts promoting the assembly of enzymatic complexes on the cell surface. The localization of clotting factors to the point of vascular damage propagates the clotting response. Therefore, the formation of an appropriate cellular environment, which includes the appearance of tissue factor, alteration in composition of phospholipids, down-regulation of thrombomodulin on the cell surface, and removal of endogenous heparins are important in the initiation of the coagulation enzymatic cascade.

During the amplification phase, bioamplification occurs with surface-bound thrombin-activating platelets as well as activation of fV, fXI, and fVIII. Of note, fVIII is activated by cleaving it from von Willebrand factor. fXIa generates additional fIXa, the action of which is accelerated by fVIIIa, whereas fVa accelerates and amplifies the action of fXa.

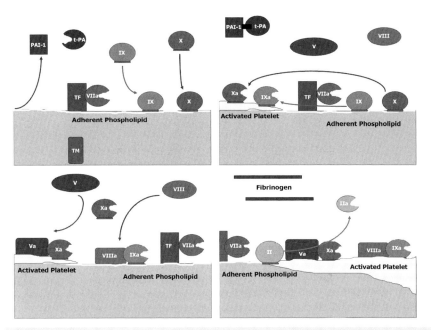

Fig. 1. Cell-based model of coagulation: Initiation phase (see text for details).

In the propagation phase, fX is further activated by the binding of fIX to activated platelets as well as thrombin generation from fXa and fVa attaching to the membrane surface. Thrombin has multiple hemostatic roles including activation of platelets through G protein–coupled protease-activated receptors [8], conversion of soluble fibrinogen into a tridimensional network of fibrin, and the constriction of endothelium-denuded cells. The multimeric protein, von Willebrand factor, promotes thrombus growth via platelet glycoprotein Ib by acting as a bridge for the initial tethering and translocation of platelets to subendothelial collagen. In addition, it induces the surface expression of platelet glycoprotein IIb/IIIa resulting in stable adhesion and subsequent aggregation of activated platelets to newly formed and polymerizing fibrin strands [9].

REGULATION OF COAGULATION

Regulation of coagulation and thrombin and fibrin generation occur through a series of processes: termination, elimination, and stabilization. Termination of coagulation is regulated by at least four plasma proteins: tissue factor pathway inhibitor (TFPI), antithrombin III, protein C, and protein S. Endothelial cells and platelets release TFPI, which inhibits TF, fVIIIa, and fXa. Antithrombin III inhibits thrombin, fIXa, fXa, fXIa, and the fVIIa-TF complex. Protein C is a vitamin K–dependent inhibitor of fVa and fVIIIa, activated by the thrombin/thrombomodulin complex. Protein S is a cofactor in protein C–mediated fVa and fVIIIa inhibition. Also, protease nexin II released by platelets is an inhibitor of soluble-phase fXIa [10].

Elimination of fibrin deposits (fibrinolysis) begins at the thrombin surface. Fibrin attracts plasminogen and tissue plasminogen activator (t-PA) to its lysine residues, whereas single-chain urokinase plasminogen activator (scu-PA) binds to plasminogen. Tissue plasminogen activator converts plasminogen to plasmin while plasminogen converts scu-PA to urokinase-tissue plasminogen activator (u-PA), producing additional plasmin from plasminogen. As the plasmin concentrations increase, fibrin is degraded into soluble fragments, D-dimers. The regional control of fibrinolysis is essential to disruption of a local thrombus. Fibrinolysis is normally regulated to a clot-specific region; however, trauma and surgery may cause systemic plasmin activation resulting in systemic fibrinolysis.

Coagulation stabilization counteracts fibrinolysis through thrombin-activated fXIIIa, thrombin-activatable fibrinolysis inhibitor (TAFI), plasminogen activator inhibitor type 1 (PAI-1), and alpha-2 antiplasmin. fXIIIa converts fibrin into a tight-knit aggregate. TAFI, activated by TAFIa, removes lysine residues from fibrin, impairing fibrin's capacity to bind plasminogen and t-PA. PAI-1 is a rapid and irreversible inhibitor of t-PA and u-PA. And alpha-2 antiplasmin is a high-affinity plasmin inhibitor.

As seen throughout this cell-based hemostatic process, platelets derived from megakaryocytes play an integral role. Under normal endothelial conditions, platelets are inhibited by nitric oxide and prostacyclin. In the absence of normal endothelial tissue, the platelets adhere to the subendothelial matrix either directly by collagen or via glycoprotein receptors. The shear of blood flow activates the platelets and serves as a focus for clot propagation.

Although the cell-based model of coagulation along with regulation thrombin and fibrin generation outline the components of this complex system, it is critical to understand its limitation in emphasizing the interdependence of the different systems on each other. The hemostatic response is dynamic not only involving the components and interactions listed above but also in conjunction with different physiologic environments. In the setting of human physiology and stress, competing biochemical pathways often appear to push and pull against each other. The hemostatic "life in balance" involves the two ends of the spectrum clotting to death (stroke, myocardial infarction, thrombosis) and bleeding to death (trauma, major surgery, hemophilia) and the necessity of keeping patients as close to the center of this balance as possible. However, when surgical stress, trauma, or illness pushes one of the competing pathways out of balance, it can result in pathologic events leading to hemorrhage or thrombosis (Fig. 2). There are few studies available that have attempted to look at the interdependence of these pathways in vivo and even fewer to characterize how these events may proceed during surgery and trauma.

PERIOPERATIVE BLEEDING

Perioperative bleeding has two main causes: surgical bleeding and nonsurgical bleeding. Surgical bleeding results from failure to control bleeding from the operative site. Signs include expanding hematoma and saturated dressings. Meticulous technique and patience contribute to minimizing surgical bleeding in the

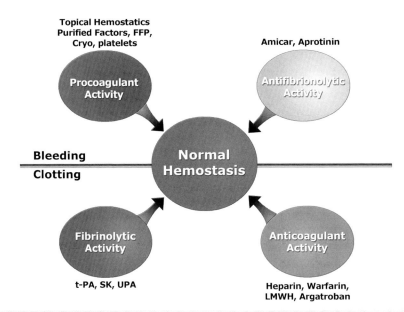

Fig. 2. Interdependence and management of pro- and anticoagulant systems that contribute to the balance of normal hemostasis.

high-risk patient. Nonsurgical bleeding is caused by failure of hemostatic pathways. This often manifests itself as generalized oozing. Signs include petechiae, purpura, and oozing from venipuncture sites, urinary catheters, and nasogastric tubes. Management of perioperative bleeding requires understanding and identifying patients at risk, recognition of hemostatic changes related to blood loss/injury/surgical procedures, institution of blood-based or pharmacologic interventions, and evaluation and understanding the results of coagulation tests for both acute and monitoring purposes. Cardiac surgery patients may also have additional issues that may contribute to bleeding that are different than those after noncardiac surgery.

PREOPERATIVE SCREENING

Identifying patients at risk for bleeding should ideally occur during the preoperative screening process. This process should focus on identifying defects in hemostasis that can be corrected preoperatively, guide management of uncorrectable hemostatic defects before surgery, and help manage unpreventable bleeding. The key to minimizing perioperative blood loss is identifying patients at significant risk through a thorough history and physical examination. A history of previous bleeding associated with dental procedures, prior surgery, routine childhood and adolescent trauma, childbirth, or a family history significant for bleeding identifies those with increased risk. Furthermore, a drug history and current medication list, including over-the-counter medications, should be explored to identify agents that affect the clotting cascade (ie, Plavix [clopidogrel], aspirin, nonsteroidal anti-inflammatory drugs [NSAIDS], and Coumadin). Objectively, bruising, petechiae, bleeding from the nose or gums, hematuria, melena, or other signs of bleeding indicate increased risk of surgical bleeding and should be documented.

Screening laboratory tests should be ordered on an individual basis depending on the patient's clinical status, bleeding history, and type of surgery planned. Four levels of increasing concern that determine the extent of preoperative laboratory testing have been devised (Table 1) [11]. Level I includes patients with a negative screening history undergoing minor surgery (ie, uncomplicated dental extraction, excisional biopsy); no screening tests are recommended. Level II includes patients with a negative screening history, contains prior surgical tests of hemostasis, and patients having major surgery (ie, cholecystectomy or bowel resection); a partial thromboplastin time (PTT) and platelet count are recommended. These level II screening tests should eliminate the risk of life-threatening bleeding that could result from an unsuspected acquired anticoagulant or thrombocytopenia. Level III includes patients whose bleeding history raises concern for defective hemostasis or who are having a procedure that may impair hemostasis (ie, cardiac surgery in which the pump oxygenator may damage the platelets, prostatectomy in which hemostasis must be maintained on raw surfaces bathed in urokinase, and central nervous system surgery in which minimal bleeding could be hazardous). Laboratory tests should screen for the following: 1) adequacy of formation of hemostatic plugs (platelet count plus a bleeding time), 2) adequacy of blood

Table 1
Preoperative hemostatic evaluation

Levels	History/Physical	Tests
Level I	• Negative history and physical examination • Minor procedure	No further testing required
Level II	• Negative history and physical examination • Major procedure	aPTT and platelet count are indicated to screen for occult disorders
Level III	• Suspicious history • Procedure with high risk of bleeding	aPTT, platelet count, PT, and BT
Level IV	• History strongly suggestive of a major hemostatic defect	BT after aspirin to rule out vWD, specific factor assays for factors VIII and IX (mild hemophilia A and B may present with a normal aPTT), and thrombin time to rule out dysfibrinogenemia.

Abbreviations: aPTT, activated partial thromboplastin time; BT, bleeding time; PT, prothrombin time; vWD, von Willebrand disease.

coagulation reactions (PTT and thromboplastin time), and 3) size and stability of the fibrin clot (plasma clotted with $CaCl_2$ screening for fibrinolysis and fXIII deficiency). Level IV includes patients whose history is very suspicious or certain of a hemostatic abnormality regardless of type of surgery. Initial screening tests should include the same tests performed for the level III patient. If results are negative, additional tests should include the following:

1) Bleeding time after administration of 600 mg of aspirin to uncover von Willebrand's disease or qualitative platelet disorder [12]. If the surgery is urgent, platelet aggregation tests using adenosine diphosphate, collagen, epinephrine, and arachidonic acid and a ristocetin cofactor assay should be performed.
2) Specific fVIII and fIX levels to uncover hemophilia.
3) Thrombin time to uncover dysfibrinogenemia or a weak heparinlike anticoagulant.

Consulting a hematologist should be considered for both level III and IV patients.

Medications that affect coagulation or platelet function such, as aspirin, NSAIDS, unfractionated heparin, and low-molecular-weight heparin should be discontinued before surgery in the majority of cases. Aspirin should be preferably stopped at least 7 days before surgery, whereas NSAIDS require only 2 days, allowing for new platelets unaffected by cyclooxygenase inhibition to develop [13]. For patients taking Coumadin, a goal International Normalized Ratio (INR) is arbitrarily chosen at < 2 for minor surgical procedures and should be stopped and to allow an INR ≤1.5 for major procedures. Coumadin should be restarted postoperatively when hemostasis is achieved. If anticoagulation is required preoperatively (ie, atrial fibrillation), unfractionated heparin or low-molecular-weight heparin should be used. Of note, the half-life of low-molecular-weight heparin is longer than that of unfractionated heparin requiring the medication to be stopped within 12 hours and 4 hours of surgery, respectively. Although perioperative bleeding is a major concern, the risk of venous thromboembolism postoperatively is far greater. Given the focus on postoperative hemorrhage, adequate thromboprophylaxis is overlooked when in essence it results in higher morbidity and mortality perioperatively.

TYPE OF SURGERY VERSUS HEMOSTASIS

Surgery requires a fine balance between bleeding and clotting to optimize patient outcome. The challenge perioperatively is that the pendulum swings toward bleeding during surgery, toward clotting immediately postoperatively, and back toward bleeding in recovery. To minimize the magnitude of the pendulum's swing, factors identified during the perioperative examination as well as the surgery being performed should be taken into account. Surgery affects the coagulation system in several ways including inducing a hyperadrenergic state [14], release of tissue plasminogen activator (TPA) resulting in hyperfibrinolysis, and consumption of coagulation factors, platelets, and physiologic anticoagulants secondary to bleeding and hemodilution from crystalloid infusion. Depending on the type of surgery, such as trauma, cardiopulmonary bypass, liver transplantation, or orthopedic surgery (described in the following paragraphs), the coagulation system is affected differently, resulting in individualized treatment strategies.

Trauma

Massive trauma releases a storm of inflammatory mediators resulting in hemostatic imbalance. Accordingly, hemorrhage is the second leading cause of death after traumatic injury [15]. The coagulopathy of trauma is a form of nonsurgical bleeding from mucosal lesions, serosal surfaces, and wound and vascular access sites after identifiable vascular bleeding has been controlled surgically. Cosgriff and colleagues [16] identified four major risk factors for the development of this associated coagulopathy: low pH, causing a reduction in coagulation factors; core temperature, effecting platelet/von Willebrand factor/glycoprotein interactions; systolic blood pressure <70 mm Hg usually secondary to hypovolemia; and injury severity score. Trauma to the brain, bone, and amniotic fluids can be directly associated with direct intravascular coagulation and consumption of clotting factors.

Cardiopulmonary Bypass

In the case of cardiopulmonary bypass (CPB), activation of the coagulation cascade occurs with extensive contact between blood and artificial surfaces. Contact activation as well as elevated levels of tissue plasminogen activator, PAI-1, tissue factor, and prothrombinase activity also triggers this hyperfibrinolytic state during CPB surgery [17,18]. Some studies show a 30% to 50% reduction in platelet count, packed cell volume (PCV), and levels of hemostatic factors after going "on pump." Platelet destruction occurs in the CPB circuit secondary to abnormal shear stress and causes further platelet dysfunction through alpha granule release and platelet microparticle generation.

Liver Transplantation

With orthotopic liver transplantation, there is a reduction in coagulation factors secondary to an intrinsic coagulopathy, which increases the likelihood of bleeding. Specifically, a reduction in TPA results in increased fibrinolytic potential, thrombocytopenia, and qualitative platelet dysfunction [19]. This process escalates with reperfusion of the donor liver inducing release of TPA, resulting in hyperfibrinolysis [20,21]. Similar physiologic events can be seen with aneurysm repair related to the mesenteric ischemia and in prostatectomies caused by urokinase release. Recently, recombinant factor VII has been successful in treating bleeding complications after liver transplantation. In fact, this agent has been shown to reduce transfusion requirements [22,23] and improve clot formation without affecting fibrinolysis [24].

Orthopedic Surgery

Orthopedic procedures, especially those involving the hip, pelvis, and spine, are associated with significant blood loss [25]. As blood is replaced by transfusions, blood loss may be exacerbated by the development of a coagulopathy related to the dilution of normal coagulation factors, alterations in acid–base status, hypothermia, or disseminated intravascular coagulation. Treatment of the coagulopathy includes reversal or elimination of the precipitating event.

On the other hand, the balance is tipped toward a hyperthrombotic state after orthopedic surgery by reasons not clearly defined. In fact, the incidence of thromboembolic disease, deep venous thrombosis, and pulmonary embolism, in patients who underwent total hip or total knee arthroplasties and patients who have sustained a fracture of the proximal end of the femur has ranged from 32% to 88% in the Western population [26–28]. Accordingly, thromboprophylaxis recommendations for initiation and duration of treatment as well as antithrombotic agents of choice have been reported for hip arthroplasty, knee arthroplasty and arthroscopy, spine surgery, neurosurgery, and trauma [29].

POSTOPERATIVE RECOGNITION OF BLEEDING

Postoperatively, patient's have an increased risk of bleeding. Attention should be placed on objective findings indicative of bleeding such as vital signs (hypotension, tachycardia, and hypothermia), depressed central venous pressure, reduction in urine output, and abnormal capillary refill. With regard to laboratory values, decreasing hematocrit levels should be investigated objectively with careful attention placed on intraoperatively placed drains looking for malposition of kinks. Only after no identifiable source is found, hemodilution may be rationalized. In addition, coagulation studies such as prothrombin time (PT), INR, PTT, and platelet count should be performed to evaluate for factor deficiency or inhibitors and thrombophilia or thrombosis. Technical causes of bleeding and coagulopathy may and often do exist in combination. It may be difficult to address the technical cause before stabilizing the coagulopathy. Thus, control of technical causes of bleeding and reversal of coagulopathy should be pursued simultaneously.

MANAGEMENT OF POSTOPERATIVE BLEEDING

Management of postoperative bleeding (see Fig. 2) requires restoration of clotting parameters to normal by means of medications, blood products/clotting factors, normothermia, and treatment of sepsis. The most commonly used blood products include platelets, fresh frozen plasma, and cryoprecipitate; platelet counts should be kept above 50,000, fresh frozen plasma should be transfused for PT prolongation with a goal of INR less than 1.5, and cryoprecipitate should be considered if the fibrinogen level is less than 0.8 g/dL [30].

Pharmacologic interventions include the use of aprotinin, lysine analogs, desmopressin (DDAVP), and recombinant factor VIIa. Aprotinin is a bovine serine protease inhibitor that inhibits plasmin resulting in antifibrinolytic activity. However, at higher doses (200-250 KIU/mL), inhibition of serine proteases such as kallikrein reduce contact factor-dependent fibrinolysis and bradykinin production [31]. Aprotinin also has been shown to significantly reduce bleeding in cardiac surgery in multiple, placebo-controlled, randomized studies [32]. Allergic reactions with repeated exposure are possible considering bovine origin of the molecule. Accordingly, a test dose should always be administered.

Lysine analogs include epsilon aminocaproic acid and tranexamic acid. Both analogs competitively inhibit plasmin binding to fibrin. In comparison with aprotinin, tranexamic acid has a decreased antiplasmin response and does not invoke an immune response, because it is not an animal product [33,34].

DDAVP is a vasopressin analog. It has no vasoconstrictor activity, improves platelet function, and increases von Willebrand factor (vWF) plasma concentrations through stimulated release from the Weibel-Palade bodies in the endothelium [35]. DDAVP derives the most benefit in patients with vWF deficiency and those with functional platelet disorders, including aspirin therapy.

Recombinant factor VIIa is a novel treatment for hemophiliacs as well as traumatic injury or surgery resulting in significant bleeding. In fact, in a liver transplantation series, injection of factor VIIa reduced the number of blood transfusions by one third [36].

Bleeding after massive transfusion can occur because of hypothermia, dilutional coagulopathy, platelet dysfunction, fibrinolysis, or hypofibrinogenemia. Transfusion of 15 to 20 units of blood products causes dilutional thrombocytopenia, and both antiplatelet agents (eg, clopidogrel, Plavix) and other anticoagulants are contributing factors to bleeding [37]. Tests for platelet dysfunction are not readily available. In the actively bleeding patients, higher fibrinogen levels should be considered, and PT and PTT levels are affected by fibrinogen levels. Furthermore, a core body temperature less than 35°C may inhibit clotting mechanisms requiring active rewarming [37].

Hemorrhage or thrombosis monitoring should start in the operating room. Routine laboratory checks for extensive surgeries include PT and PTT, complete blood count (CBC), and fibrinogen levels to help with intraoperative assessment of hemostatic function. However, surgeons are not able to make real time decisions based on these tests because they are not "point of care," limited by the time lag for results. Recently, "point-of-care" tests, including activated clotting time (ACT) and thromboelastogram (TEG), guide anticoagulation therapy intraoperatively. The ACT measures the anticoagulation effect of heparin through detection of fibrin (clot) formation. TEG monitors hemostasis by measuring the viscoelastic properties of blood as it is induced to clot but is limited by run to run variation and opinions of interpretation [38].

SUMMARY

Postoperative hemorrhage and thrombosis is a significant problem during the perioperative period. Understanding the complex and dynamic interplay of factors, proteins, and enzymes during coagulation is imperative to maintain balance between hemostasis and thrombosis. To improve patient outcome, each patient should be risk stratified for bleeding or thrombosis during the preoperative examination. Additional research focused on improvement in screening tools, monitoring, and therapeutic regimens for surgical patients with a coagulopathy are warranted.

References

[1] Davie EW, Ratnoff OD. Waterfall sequence of intrinsic blood clotting. Science 1964;145: 1310–2.

[2] Macfarlane RG. An enzyme cascade in the blood clotting mechanism, and its function as a biological amplifier. Nature 1964;202:4998–9.

[3] Becker RC. Cell-based models of coagulation: a paradigm in evolution. J Thromb Thrombolysis 2005;20(1):65–8.

[4] Giesen PL, Rauch U, Bohrmann B, et al. Blood-borne tissue factor: another view of thrombosis. Proc Natl Acad Sci U S A 1999;96:2311–5.

[5] Hartzell S, Ryder K, Lanahan A, et al. A growth factor-responsive gene of murine BALB/c 3T3 cells encodes a protein homologous to human tissue factor. Mol Cell Biol 1989;9: 2567–73.

[6] Bevilacqua MP, Pober JS, Majeau GR, et al. Interleukin 1 (IL-1) induces biosynthesis and cell surface expression of procoagulant activity in human vascular endothelial cells. J Exp Med 1984;160:618–23.

[7] Scarpati EM, Sadler JE. Regulation of endothelial cell coagulant properties. Modulation of tissue factor, plasminogen activator inhibitors, and thrombomodulin by phorbol 12-myristate 13-acetate and tumor necrosis factor. J Biol Chem 1989;264:20705–13.

[8] De Cristofaro R, De Candia E. Thrombin domains: structure, function and interaction with platelet receptors. J Thromb Thrombolysis 2003;15:151–63.

[9] Savage B, Sixma JJ, Ruggeri ZM. Functional self-association of von Willebrand factor during platelet adhesion under flow. Proc Nat Acad Sci U S A 2002;99:425–30.

[10] Walsh PN. Roles of platelets and factor XI in the initiation of blood coagulation and thrombin. Thromb Haemost 2001;86:75–82.

[11] Rapaport SI. Preoperative hemostatic evaluation: which tests, if any? Blood 1983;61(2): 229–31.

[12] Stuart MJ, Miller ML, Davey FR, et al. The post-aspirin bleeding time: a screening test for evaluating haemostatic disorders. Br J Haematol 1979;43:649–59.

[13] Colman RW, Bagdasarian A, Talama RC. Williams trait. Human kininogen deficiency with diminished levels of plasminogen proactivator and prekallikrein associated with abnormalities of the Hageman factor-dependent pathways. J Clin Invest 1975;56:1650–62.

[14] Koh MB, Hunt BJ. The management of perioperative bleeding. Blood Rev 2003;17: 179–85.

[15] Counts RB, Haisch C, Simon T, et al. Hemostasis in massively transfused trauma patients. Ann Surg 1979;190:91–9.

[16] Cosgriff N, Sauaia A, Kenny-Moynihan M, et al. Predicting life-threatening coagulopathy in the massively transfused trauma patient: hypothermoa and acidosis revisited. Journal of Trauma-Injury Infection and Critical Care 1997;42:857–61.

[17] Hunt BJ, Parrat RN, Segal H, et al. Activation of coagulation. Ann Thorac Surg 1998;65: 712–8.

[18] Jaggers JJ, Neal MC, Smith PK, et al. Infant cardiopulmonary bypass: a procoagulant state. Ann Thorac Surg 1999;68:513–20.

[19] Lewis JH, Bontempo FA, Awad SA, et al. Liver transplantation: intraoperative changes in coagulation factors in 100 first transplants. Hepatology 1989;9:710–4.

[20] Dzik WH, Arkin CF, Jenkins RL, et al. Fibrinolysis during liver transplantation in humans: role of tissue plasminogen activator. Blood 1998;71:1090–5.

[21] Porte RJ, Bontempo FA, Knot FA, et al. Systemic effects of tissue plasminogen activator associated with fibrinolysis and its relation to thrombin generation in orthotopic liver transplantation. Transplantation 1989;47:978–84.

[22] Gala B, Quintela J, Aguirrezabalaga J, et al. Benefits of recombinant activated factor VII in complicated liver transplantation. Transplantation Proc 2005;37:3919–21.
[23] Herman H, Karina M, de Wolf J, et al. Reduced transfusion requirements by recombinant factor VIIa in orthotopic liver transplantation: a pilot study. Transplantation 2001;71: 402–5.
[24] Linsman T, Leebeek F, Meijer K, et al. Recombinant factor VIIa improves clot formation but not fibrinolytic potential in patients with cirrhosis and during liver transplantation. Hepatology 2002;35:616–21.
[25] Guay J, Haig M, Lortie L, et al. Predicting blood loss in surgery for idiopathic scoliosis. Can J Anaesth 1994;41:775–81.
[26] Clark MT, Green JS, Harper WM, et al. Screening for deep-venous thrombosis after hip and knee replacement without prophylaxis. J Bone Joint Surg Br 1997;79:787–91.
[27] Culver D, Crawford JS, Gardiner JH, et al. Venous thrombosis after fractures of the upper end of the femur. A study of incidence and site. J Bone Joint Surg Br 1970;52:61–9.
[28] Kelsey JL, Wood PH, Charnley J. Prediction of thromboemolism following total hip replacement. Clin Orthop Relat Res 1976;114:247–58.
[29] Geerts WH, Pineo GF, Heit JA, et al. Prevention of venous thromboembolism: the seventh ACCP conference on antithrombotic and thrombolytic therapy. Chest 2004;126: 338S–400S.
[30] Blood Transfusion Task Force. Transfusion guidelines for massive blood loss. Clin Lab Haematol 1988;8:265–73.
[31] Levy JH. Hemostatic agents. Transfusion 2004;44:58S–62S.
[32] Sedrakyan A, Treasure T, Elefteriades JA. Effect of aprotinin on clinical outcomes in coronary artery bypass graft surgery: a systematic review and meta-analysis of randomized clinical trials. J Thorac Cardiovasc Surg 2004;128:442–8.
[33] Katsaros D, Petricevic M, Wooodhall DD, et al. Tranexamic acid reduces post-bypass blood loss. Ann Thorac Surg 1996;61:1131–5.
[34] Menichetti A, Tritapep L, Ruvolo G, et al. Changes in coagulation patterns, blood loss and blood use after cardiopulmonary bypass: aprotinin vs tranexamic acid vs EACA. J Cardiovasc Surg 1996;37:401–7.
[35] Weinstein M, Ware AJ. Changes in von Willebrand factor during cardiac surgery effect of desmopressin acetate. Blood 1988;71:648–55.
[36] Hendriks HG, Meijer K, de Wolf JT, et al. Reduced transfusion requirements by recombinant factor VIIa in orthotopic liver transplantation. Transplantation 2001;7:402–5.
[37] Levy JH. Massive transfusion coagulopathy. Semin Hematol 2006;43:S59–63.
[38] McCrath DJ, Cerboni E, Frumento RJ, et al. Thromboelastography maximum amplitude predicts postoperative thrombotic complications including myocardial infarction. Anesth Analg 2005;100:1576–83.

Hematol Oncol Clin N Am 21 (2007) 25–32

HEMATOLOGY/ONCOLOGY CLINICS
OF NORTH AMERICA

Clot Stabilization for the Prevention of Bleeding

Lisa Payne Rojkjaer, MD[a],*, Rasmus Rojkjaer, PhD[b]

[a]Clinical Development, Novartis Pharmaceuticals, One Health Plaza, East Hanover, New Jersey 07936-1080, USA
[b]Novo Nordisk Research US, 685 Highway Route 1, North Brunswick, NJ 08902, USA

Hemorrhage continues to cause considerable morbidity and mortality. Trauma and surgery can cause disruption of blood vessels and the microvasculature, acquired coagulation factor deficiencies, and severe bleeding. The acquired functional deficiencies of crucial coagulation pathway components may occur because of:

1. Hemodilution
2. Transient consumptive loss caused by massive coagulation
3. Intravascular coagulation and hyperactivation of fibrinolysis
4. Loss of coagulation function caused by extrinsic factors such as hypothermia and acidosis

Regardless of the etiology of bleeding, treatment requires rapid diagnostic evaluation and restoration of the impaired pathways. Traditional therapies for bleeding disorders replace missing coagulation factors or blood components in the patient. Both transfusion therapy and topical hemostatic reagents are used in specific medical applications. Overall demand for blood products is increasing, however, placing a growing burden on blood banks in terms of collection, supply, and cost [1–3]. Further, allogeneic blood transfusions are not innocuous, but continue to carry the risk of hemolytic and nonhemolytic transfusion reactions and other immunological adverse events, such as transfusion-related acute lung injury (TRALI), pathogen transmission, and even cancer recurrence [4–6]. In trauma, red blood cell transfusions have been associated with increased infection rates and multiorgan failure [7,8]. Thus, there is a great need for innovation toward prevention and control of bleeding that may be used in conjunction with or even as an alternative to transfusions.

The hemostatic clot is the physical entity that prevents excessive blood loss following vascular damage. The balance between clot formation and degradation at the site of vascular injury is essential in preventing excessive bleeding. The series of cellular interactions and enzymatic reactions that are triggered by

*Corresponding author. E-mail address: lisa.rojkjaer@novartis.com (L.P. Rojkjaer).

0889-8588/07/$ – see front matter
doi:10.1016/j.hoc.2006.11.001

vascular injury culminate in a final product, an insoluble fibrin clot that is resistant to premature dissolution. Recent focus has demonstrated stabilizing the hemostatic clot may be important in providing hemostasis, and the factors that are involved in both the localization and stabilization of hemostatic process to the site of vascular injury may constitute reasonable therapeutic targets for developing novel interventions. This article explores the mechanics of clot formation and stabilization, with a special emphasis on the role of coagulation factor XIII (FXIII).

LOCALIZED HEMOSTASIS

To understand the context in which coagulation factors interact to achieve hemostasis, it is important to consider the function of the vasculature and platelets. Under normal physiological conditions, the protective monolayer of endothelial cells that line the lumen of blood vessels is devoid of exposed hemostatic activators, such as tissue factor (TF) [9]. In fact, the uninterrupted endothelium synthesizes several anticoagulant molecules, such as:

1. Tissue factor pathway inhibitor, which inhibits activation of coagulation [10]
2. Tissue plasminogen activator (tPA), the major physiological activator of the fibrinolytic system [11]
3. Thrombomodulin, a regulator of the anticoagulant pathway [12]
4. Endothelial surface heparanoids that enhance inhibition of clotting factors by antithrombin [13]
5. Ecto-ADP, a suppressor of platelet activation [14]

On vascular damage and disruption of the endothelial cell layer, however, TF and extracellular matrix proteins including collagen are exposed to the flowing blood. Platelet glycoprotein (GP) Ib-mediated binding to von Willebrand factor (vWF) immobilized on collagen causes platelets to roll on the injured vessel wall. Subsequent platelet adhesion and activation are mediated by GPIIb/IIIa (integrin $\alpha_{IIb}\beta_3$) binding to immobilized vWF [15–18] and direct binding of collagen to platelet integrin $\alpha_2\beta_1$ and GPVI [19,20]. Simultaneously, exposure of functional TF to circulating plasma proteins triggers local thrombin generation, leading to additional stimulation of the adherent platelet through interaction with the protease-activated receptors (PAR)-1 and -4 [21] and GPIb [22]. Recent literature has begun to outline the key importance of accompanying platelet stimulation by TF-derived thrombin and collagen [23]. Dual activation of platelets by the collagen and thrombin receptors results in forming a subpopulation of platelets, the so-called coated platelets, also known as COAT platelets, an abbreviation for collagen and thrombin-activated platelets [24]. The coated platelets express high levels of FXIIIa coupled, α-granule derived, procoagulant proteins such as factor V, fibrinogen/fibrin, vWF, fibronectin, α_2-antiplasmin, and thrombospondin on their surfaces [25,26]. Also, binding of plasma procoagulant protein factors VIII, IX, and X are increased on the factor V-expressing platelet subpopulation (ie, the coated platelets), and the increased binding correlates with increased factor Xa and thrombin generation [27]. Finally, the authors recently reported the only example of an exogenous protein being incorporated into coated platelets [28]. The authors found that recombinant activated factor VIIa (rFVIIa) preferentially bound to coated platelets, while minimal rFVIIa was found on platelets activated with ADP, thrombin, or by means of glycoprotein (GP) VI alone, demonstrating the coated platelet may be targeted pharmacologically. Taken together, these data indicate that the most intense hemostatic activity occurs where coated platelets are formed (ie, at the interface between the flowing blood and the denuded endothelial layer). This mechanism may ensure the most intense procoagulant activity is produced at the site of vascular injury where immediate hemostasis is needed. As added platelets are recruited to the forming hemostatic clot, an intervening layer of platelets will prevent interaction with collagen and down-regulate the formation of the potent hemostatic-coated platelet subpopulation and the subsequent production of procoagulants at the site where the clot is desired.

CLOT STABILIZATION

By enhancing activation of procoagulants only at the site where a clot is desired, the coated platelets become important in ensuring stabilization of the hemostatic clot. The activity of procoagulant complexes produces a burst of thrombin generation that results in fibrin polymerization. However, the clot architecture, its mechanical strength, and resistance to fibrinolysis [29,30] depend not only on thrombin's ability to clot fibrinogen, but also on activation of secondary thrombin substrates such as FXIII and the thrombin-activatable fibrinolysis inhibitor (TAFI).

TAFI is a carboxypeptidase B-like proenzyme synthesized in the liver as a single chain glycoprotein zymogen with a molecular weight (MW) of approximately 60,000 Da [31–34]. Thrombin-activated TAFI (TAFIa) is proposed to play a key role in the interaction between the procoagulant and fibrinolytic systems. Effective fibrinolysis results from forming a ternary complex between tPA, plasminogen, and C-terminal lysine residues on fibrin. Plasminogen bound to fibrin is converted more effectively to plasmin, thereby localizing the lytic activity to the area of the clot. Plasmin degradation of fibrin generates additional C-terminal lysine residues by amplifying the system locally. The ability of TAFIa to cleave C-terminal lysines on fibrin results in down-regulation of fibrinolysis by reducing the number of plasminogen and tPA binding sites [35–39]. In factor VIII-deficient plasma, it has been shown that reduced TAFI activation results in premature clot lysis and that normal resistance to fibrinolysis could be restored by adding FVIII or recombinant factor VIIa [37,40,41], indicating that patients who have hemophilia not only have a clot formation deficiency but also accelerated clot degradation because of diminished TAFI activation. In contrast to hemophilia, however, in plasma from liver transplantation and cirrhosis patients, TAFI deficiency was not associated with increased fibrinolysis [42], suggesting that functional consequences of reduced TAFI activation is limited to conditions with severely reduced thrombin formation (such as hemophilia).

FXIII, a plasma protransglutaminase, is the terminal enzyme in the coagulation cascade, and it functions to cross-link the fibrin clot, thereby stabilizing it against premature fibrinolysis [43]. FXIII circulates in plasma as a heterotetramer with an MW of approximately 340,000 Da [44]. Hematopoietic cells constitute the principal site for biosynthesis of the FXIII A subunit. The FXIII B subunit is synthesized primarily by hepatocytes [45]. The B subunits of FXIII function as carrier proteins, stabilizing the A subunits in circulation and regulating nonproteolytic activation of FXIII [46,47]. Limited proteolysis by thrombin converts zymogen FXIII to the FXIIIa enzyme, which stabilizes the clot by catalyzing fibrin cross-linking. Although fibrin is the main substrate for FXIIIa, the molecule further contributes to the generation of a stable clot that is resistant to fibrinolysis by incorporating antifibrinolytic proteins such as α2-antiplasmin into the forming clot [43]. Maintaining a sufficient plasma level of FXIII is essential for normal hemostasis. Patients who have congenital FXIII deficiency have a bleeding tendency of varying severity, the major morbidity being secondary to intracranial hemorrhage (ICH), which is more frequent in FXIII deficiency than in other congenital bleeding disorders [48].

CLINICAL ASPECTS OF CLOT FORMATION AND STABILIZATION

The balance between coagulation and fibrinolysis often is perturbed by surgery. In liver transplantation, increased fibrinolytic activity caused by impaired clearance of profibrinolytic factors (eg, tPA), impaired synthesis of fibrinolytic inhibitors (PAI-1), platelet dysfunction, and coagulation factor deficiencies (cirrhosis) contribute to nonsurgical bleeding. Cardiopulmonary bypass-associated hemostatic defects include thrombocytopenia and platelet dysfunction (by means of hypothermia, selective activation of PAR1, and internalization of the receptor after exposure to thrombin generated in the bypass circuit, or alteration in platelet surface receptors), decreased coagulation factor levels (by means of consumption and/or hemodilution), and increased fibrinolytic activity (caused by endothelial activation and release of tPA).

Despite use of current pharmacological strategies to limit blood loss and prevent fibrinolysis, many patients still may be transfused during cardiac surgery, necessitating the development of novel strategies (eg, promoting clot stabilization) and biologic agents to reduce bleeding and improve outcomes.

New insights about FXIII are challenging the previous notion that acquired coagulation factor deficiencies that occur during surgery are not of a degree requiring specific replacement therapy. In the setting of congenital FXIII deficiency, a rare autosomal recessive bleeding disorder, it generally has been accepted that plasma FXIII levels of 5% are sufficient to maintain hemostasis [49]. Although patients who have congenital FXIII deficiency are at risk of moderate-to-severe bleeding with FXIII levels less than 4%, patients with FXIII levels as high as 53% recently have been reported to have experienced bleeding episodes [50]. Also, in the neurosurgical setting without an underlying bleeding disorder, FXIII levels less than 60% are associated with a sixfold higher risk of developing a postoperative hematoma following intracranial surgery [51]. Significant decreases in the plasma FXIII activity levels also have been reported in liver transplantation [52], in children undergoing cardiac surgery [53,54], and in general surgery patients who developed unexpected intraoperative bleeding [55].

FXIII levels have been described to decrease by approximately 40% to 60% during cardiopulmonary bypass (CPB)-assisted cardiac surgery [56]. Shainoff and colleagues [57] followed the plasma FXIII level in 19 patients undergoing routine coronary artery bypass grafting (CABG) surgery and found a significant inverse correlation with postoperative chest tube drainage volumes. Interesting, the reported FXIII levels (nadir of <45% of normal) were lower than what would be expected from hemodilution, suggesting that FXIII consumption participated in generating the acquired FXIII deficiency. Chandler and colleagues [58] analyzed the relationship between blood loss, various hemostatic factors (including the FXIII A subunit), and clot strength in 34 patients undergoing CABG surgery. Peri- and postoperative clot strengths as measured by thromboelastography (TEG) were found to be dependent on the platelet count and fibrinogen concentration, and maximum clot strength significantly increased following the ex vivo addition of FXIII. On average, FXIII levels dropped to 64% and clot strength to 77% of baseline values after 45 minutes on CPB and remained below baseline during the postoperative period. Postoperative blood loss (assessed by chest tube drainage) was correlated significantly with platelet count, FXIII A subunit levels, and clot strength measured at completing surgery. Because the platelet is the primary source of plasma FXIII A subunit [59], decreased platelet counts during surgery could potentiate FXIII deficiency beyond hemodilution or consumption. In another report, Blome and colleagues [56] confirmed a significant drop in the plasma FXIII concentration during CPB but failed to associate FXIII activity levels with the extent of postoperative bleeding. Smaller chest tube drainage volumes and the fact that all patients in this study received full dose Aprotinin may explain the apparent discrepancy.

The hypothesis that acquired FXIII deficiency predisposes cardiac surgery patients to hemorrhage has been investigated in two small controlled clinical studies. In the first study, postoperative FXIII administration was reported to reduce blood loss and transfusions in patients undergoing uncomplicated CABG surgery [60]. Twenty-two consecutive patients were assigned prospectively (in a nonblinded fashion) to either a control group or a group receiving plasma-derived FXIII; all patients received Aprotinin before and during CPB. Compared with baseline (preoperative) values, FXIII levels fell postoperatively to a mean of 54%. In the group that received FXIII, the mean plasma level rose to 103%, and on postoperative day 1 and 2 chest tube drainage was significantly lower compared with the control group. Transfusion of packed red blood cells (pRBCs) and fresh frozen plasma (FFP), although not significantly decreased, were reduced in the FXIII group. The second clinical study was a prospective, randomized, double-blinded study of multiple doses of FXIII administered immediately after administration of protamine [61]. Again, the FXIII level fell from preoperative normal values to subnormal values after CPB. FXIII administration reduced postoperative blood loss and the extent of blood transfusion after coronary surgery; however, administration was only efficacious if FXIII plasma levels were below the normal level. In this study, patients did not receive Aprotinin.

Recent years have provided significant scientific progress in understanding the mechanisms that control hemostasis. Especially, the increasing knowledge of the factors that play an important role in localizing and stabilizing the hemostatic clot may provide insights that can be utilized for developing novel therapeutic strategies to combat hemorrhage, a persistent and significant medical challenge.

References

[1] Amin M, Fergusson D, Aziz A, et al. The cost of allogeneic red blood cells—a systematic review. Transfus Med 2003;13(5):275–85.

[2] Sullivan MT, McCullough J, Schreiber GB, et al. Blood collection and transfusion in the United States in 1997. Transfusion 2002;42(10):1253–60.

[3] Varney SJ, Guest JF. The annual cost of blood transfusions in the UK. Transfus Med 2003;13(4):205–18.

[4] Kleinman S, Chan P, Robillard P. Risks associated with transfusion of cellular blood components in Canada. Transfus Med Rev 2003;17(2):120–62.

[5] Schreiber GB, Busch MP, Kleinman SH, et al. The risk of transfusion-transmitted viral infections. The Retrovirus Epidemiology Donor Study. N Engl J Med 1996;334(26):1685–90.

[6] Vamvakas EC. Transfusion-associated cancer recurrence and postoperative infection: meta-analysis of randomized, controlled clinical trials. Transfusion 1996;36(2):175–86.

[7] Goodnough LT, Shander A, Brecher ME. Transfusion medicine: looking to the future. Lancet 2003;361(9352):161–9.

[8] Hebert PC, Wells G, Blajchman MA, et al. A multicenter, randomized, controlled clinical trial of transfusion requirements in critical care. Transfusion Requirements in Critical Care Investigators, Canadian Critical Care Trials Group. N Engl J Med 1999;340(6):409–17.

[9] Drake TA, Morrissey JH, Edgington TS. Selective cellular expression of tissue factor in human tissues. Implications for disorders of hemostasis and thrombosis. Am J Pathol 1989;134(5):1087–97.

[10] Rao LV, Rapaport SI. Studies of a mechanism inhibiting the initiation of the extrinsic pathway of coagulation. Blood 1987;69(2):645–51.

[11] Levin EG, Santell L, Osborn KG. The expression of endothelial tissue plasminogen activator in vivo: a function defined by vessel size and anatomic location. J Cell Sci 1997;110(Pt 2):139–48.

[12] Dahlback B. Progress in the understanding of the protein C anticoagulant pathway. Int J Hematol 2004;79(2):109–16.

[13] Kojima T, Leone CW, Marchildon GA, et al. Isolation and characterization of heparin sulfate proteoglycans produced by cloned rat microvascular endothelial cells. J Biol Chem 1992;267(7):4859–69.

[14] Gayle III RB, Maliszewski CR, Gimpel SD, et al. Inhibition of platelet function by recombinant soluble ecto-ADPase/CD39. J Clin Invest 1998;101(9):1851–9.

[15] Matsui H, Sugimoto M, Mizuno T, et al. Distinct and concerted functions of von Willebrand factor and fibrinogen in mural thrombus growth under high shear flow. Blood 2002;100(10):3604–10.

[16] Mistry N, Cranmer SL, Yuan Y, et al. Cytoskeletal regulation of the platelet glycoprotein Ib/V/IX-von Willebrand factor interaction. Blood 2000;96(10):3480–9.

[17] Savage B, Sixma JJ, Ruggeri ZM. Functional self-association of von Willebrand factor during platelet adhesion under flow. Proc Natl Acad Sci U S A 2002;99(1):425–30.

[18] Savage B, Cattaneo M, Ruggeri ZM. Mechanisms of platelet aggregation. Curr Opin Hematol 2001;8(5):270–6.

[19] Clemetson KJ, Clemetson JM. Platelet collagen receptors. Thromb Haemost 2001;86(1): 189–97.

[20] Polgar J, Clemetson JM, Kehrel BE, et al. Platelet activation and signal transduction by con-vulxin, a C-type lectin from crotalus durissus terrificus (tropical rattlesnake) venom via the p62/GPVI collagen receptor. J Biol Chem 1997;272(21):13576–83.

[21] Coughlin SR. Protease-activated receptors and platelet function. Thromb Haemost 1999;82(2):353–6.

[22] Dormann D, Clemetson KJ, Kehrel BE. The GPIb thrombin-binding site is essential for throm-bin-induced platelet procoagulant activity. Blood 2000;96(7):2469–78.

[23] Dale GL. Coated-platelets: an emerging component of the procoagulant response. J Thromb Haemost 2005;3(10):2185–92.

[24] Szasz R, Dale GL. COAT platelets. Curr Opin Hematol 2003;10(5):351–5.

[25] Alberio L, Safa O, Clemetson KJ, et al. Surface expression and functional characterization of alpha-granule factor V in human platelets: effects of ionophore A23187, thrombin, col-lagen, and convulxin. Blood 2000;95(5):1694–702.

[26] Dale GL, Friese P, Batar P, et al. Stimulated platelets use serotonin to enhance their retention of procoagulant proteins on the cell surface. Nature 2002;415(6868): 175–9.

[27] Kempton CL, Hoffman M, Roberts HR, et al. Platelet heterogeneity: variation in coagulation complexes on platelet subpopulations. Arterioscler Thromb Vasc Biol 2005;25(4):861–6.

[28] Kjalke M, Rojkjaer R. Colocalization of recombinant human factor VIIa with its substrates on highly procoagulant COAT-platelets. J Thromb Haemost 2003;1(Suppl 1):P1265.

[29] Collet JP, Park D, Lesty C, et al. Influence of fibrin network conformation and fibrin fiber di-ameter on fibrinolysis speed: dynamic and structural approaches by confocal microscopy. Arterioscler Thromb Vasc Biol 2000;20(5):1354–61.

[30] He S, Cao H, Antovic A, et al. Modifications of flow measurement to determine fibrin gel permeability and the preliminary use in research and clinical materials. Blood Coagul Fibrinolysis 2005;16(1):61–7.

[31] Campbell W, Okada H. An arginine specific carboxypeptidase generated in blood during coagulation or inflammation which is unrelated to carboxypeptidase N or its subunits. Biochem Biophys Res Commun 1989;162(3):933–9.

[32] Eaton DL, Malloy BE, Tsai SP, et al. Isolation, molecular cloning, and partial character-ization of a novel carboxypeptidase B from human plasma. J Biol Chem 1991;266(32): 21833–8.

[33] Hendriks D, Scharpe S, van Sande M, et al. Characterisation of a carboxypeptidase in human serum distinct from carboxypeptidase N. J Clin Chem Clin Biochem 1989;27(5): 277–85.

[34] Hendriks D, Wang W, Scharpe S, et al. Purification and characterization of a new arginine carboxypeptidase in human serum. Biochim Biophys Acta 1990;1034(1):86–92.

[35] Bajzar L, Morser J, Nesheim M. TAFI, or plasma procarboxypeptidase B, couples the coag-ulation and fibrinolytic cascades through the thrombin–thrombomodulin complex. J Biol Chem 1996;271(28):16603–8.

[36] Bajzar L, Nesheim M. The effect of activated protein C on fibrinolysis in cell-free plasma can be attributed specifically to attenuation of prothrombin activation. J Biol Chem 1993;268(12):8608–16.

[37] Broze GJ Jr, Higuchi DA. Coagulation-dependent inhibition of fibrinolysis: role of carboxy-peptidase-U and the premature lysis of clots from hemophilic plasma. Blood 1996;88(10): 3815–23.

[38] Collen D, Lijnen HR. Fibrin-specific fibrinolysis. Ann N Y Acad Sci 1992;667:259–71.

[39] Redlitz A, Tan AK, Eaton DL, et al. Plasma carboxypeptidases as regulators of the plasmin-ogen system. J Clin Invest 1995;96(5):2534–8.

[40] Lisman T, Mosnier LO, Lambert T, et al. Inhibition of fibrinolysis by recombinant factor VIIa in plasma from patients with severe hemophilia A. Blood 2002;99(1):175–9.

[41] Mosnier LO, Lisman T, van den Berg HM, et al. The defective down-regulation of fibrinolysis in haemophilia A can be restored by increasing the TAFI plasma concentration. Thromb Haemost 2001;86(4):1035–9.
[42] Lisman T, Leebeek FW, Meijer K, et al. Recombinant factor VIIa improves clot formation but not fibrolytic potential in patients with cirrhosis and during liver transplantation. Hepatology 2002;35(3):616–21.
[43] Lorand L. Factor XIII: structure, activation, and interactions with fibrinogen and fibrin. Ann N Y Acad Sci 2001;936:291–311.
[44] Meyer M. [Molecular biology of haemostasis: fibrinogen, factor XIII]. Hamostaseologie 2004;24(2):108–15 [in German].
[45] Adany R, Antal M. Three different cell types can synthesize factor XIII subunit A in the human liver. Thromb Haemost 1996;76(1):74–9.
[46] Lorand L, Gray AJ, Brown K, et al. Dissociation of the subunit structure of fibrin-stabilizing factor during activation of the zymogen. Biochem Biophys Res Commun 1974;56(4):914–22.
[47] Mary A, Achyuthan KE, Greenberg CS. b-Chains prevent the proteolytic inactivation of the a-chains of plasma factor XIII. Biochim Biophys Acta 1988;966(3):328–35.
[48] Lim BC, Ariens RA, Carter AM, et al. Genetic regulation of fibrin structure and function: complex gene–environment interactions may modulate vascular risk. Lancet 2003;361(9367): 1424–31.
[49] Walls WD, Losowsky MS. Plasma fibrin-stabilizing factor activity in acquired disease. Br J Haematol 1968;15(3):327.
[50] Seitz R, Duckert F, Lopaciuk S, et al. ETRO working party on factor XIII questionnaire on congenital factor XIII deficiency in Europe: status and perspectives. Study Group. Semin Thromb Hemost 1996;22(5):415–8.
[51] Gerlach R, Tolle F, Raabe A, et al. Increased risk for postoperative hemorrhage after intracranial surgery in patients with decreased factor XIII activity: implications of a prospective study. Stroke 2002;33(6):1618–23.
[52] Himmelreich G, Muller C, Isenberg C, et al. Factor XIII activity during orthotopic liver transplantation. Semin Thromb Hemost 1993;19(3):243–5.
[53] Schroth M, Meissner U, Cesnjevar R, et al. Plasmatic [corrected] factor XIII reduces severe pleural effusion in children after open-heart surgery. Pediatr Cardiol 2006;27(1):56–60.
[54] Wozniak G, Noll T, Akinturk H, et al. Factor XIII prevents development of myocardial edema in children undergoing surgery for congenital heart disease. Ann N Y Acad Sci 2001;936: 617–20.
[55] Wettstein P, Haeberli A, Stutz M, et al. Decreased factor XIII availability for thrombin and early loss of clot firmness in patients with unexplained intraoperative bleeding. Anesth Analg 2004;99(5):1564–9.
[56] Blome M, Isgro F, Kiessling AH, et al. Relationship between factor XIII activity, fibrinogen, haemostasis screening tests, and postoperative bleeding in cardiopulmonary bypass surgery. Thromb Haemost 2005;93(6):1101–7.
[57] Shainoff JR, Estafanous FG, Yared JP, et al. Low factor XIIIA levels are associated with increased blood loss after coronary artery bypass grafting. J Thorac Cardiovasc Surg 1994;108(3):437–45.
[58] Chandler WL, Patel MA, Gravelle L, et al. Factor XIIIA and clot strength after cardiopulmonary bypass. Blood Coagul Fibrinolysis 2001;12(2):101–8.
[59] Inbal A, Muszbek L, Lubetsky A, et al. Platelets but not monocytes contribute to the plasma levels of factor XIII subunit A in patients undergoing autologous peripheral blood stem cell transplantation. Blood Coagul Fibrinolysis 2004;15(3):249–53.
[60] Godje O, Haushofer M, Lamm P, et al. The effect of factor XIII on bleeding in coronary surgery. Thorac Cardiovasc Surg 1998;46(5):263–7.
[61] Godje O, Gallmeier U, Schelian M, et al. Coagulation factor XIII reduces postoperative bleeding after coronary surgery with extracorporeal circulation. Thorac Cardiovasc Surg 2006;54(1):26–33.

Hematol Oncol Clin N Am 21 (2007) 33–50

HEMATOLOGY/ONCOLOGY CLINICS
OF NORTH AMERICA

ELSEVIER
SAUNDERS

Regulation of Thrombin Activity—Pharmacologic and Structural Aspects

Kenichi A. Tanaka, MD, MSc[a,*], Jerrold H. Levy, MD[b,c]

[a]Department of Anesthesiology, Division of Cardiothoracic Anesthesia, Emory Healthcare, 1364 Clifton Road N.E., Atlanta, GA 30322, USA
[b]Department of Anesthesiology, Emory University School of Medicine, 1364 Clifton Road N.E., Atlanta, GA 30322, USA
[c]Cardiothoracic Anesthesiology and Critical Care, Emory Healthcare, 1364 Clifton Road N.E., Atlanta, GA 30322, USA

A t the site of vascular injury, thrombin is generated through a series of reactions among protease and cellular components of coagulation (please see the article by Monroe and Hoffman elsewhere in this issue). Thrombin generation is critical in achieving adequate hemostasis, yet it needs to be down-regulated to prevent propagation of clotting beyond damaged vascular lesion. The latter is achieved by endogenous anticoagulants, namely antithrombin (AT), heparin cofactor II (HCII), proteins C and S, endothelial thrombomodulin, and tissue factor pathway inhibitor. The disruption of balance between procoagulant and anticoagulant responses can be observed in various pathologic settings. Systemic activation of coagulation is seen in severe sepsis as disseminated intravascular coagulation. Thrombotic stroke, myocardial infarction, and deep venous thrombosis result from more regional vascular thromboses. Since the early twentieth century, anticoagulation therapy has been conducted with unfractionated heparin and Coumadin derivatives [1]. Because of increased awareness of heparin-induced thrombocytopenia, however, attention has been focused on the limitations of conventional anticoagulant therapy, and novel anticoagulation therapy has been rapidly introduced during the last decade. The aim of this article is to review endogenous serine protease inhibitors (serpins) and novel antithrombotic agents in relation to pharmacologic regulation and structural interactions.

THROMBIN STRUCTURE

Thrombin is an essential protease in blood coagulation and inflammation. Its zymogen precursor, prothrombin (72 kd), circulates in plasma at 90 µg/mL

*Corresponding author. E-mail address: kenichi.tanaka@emoryhealthcare.org (K.A. Tanaka).

0889-8588/07/$ – see front matter
doi:10.1016/j.hoc.2006.11.008

(1.4 μM) [2]. When activated by factors Xa-Va (prothrombinase; see the article by Hoffman elsewhere in this issue), thrombin (36.7 kd) becomes a trypsin-like serine protease composed of two covalently linked polypeptide chains (A and B). The B chain is the main functional structure, which accommodates the active site and exosites I and II (Fig. 1). The enzymatic function of thrombin is catalyzed by its active site, which lies in the cleft in the center of the molecule, surrounded by the insertion loops: the 60-loop (hydrophobic) and the γ-loop (hydrophilic) (see Fig. 1). Thrombin preferentially cleaves the carboxyl-terminus of arginine residue of substrate, and catalytic site interactions with natural substrates are regulated by exosite interactions that confer enzymatic specificity of thrombin [3–5].

ANTITHROMBIN

AT (58 kd) is a serpin that is synthesized in the liver and circulated in the plasma. The normal concentration of human AT is approximately 140 μg/mL (2.4 μM) [6], and plasma half-life is 60 to 70 minutes [7]. The plasma AT level is well above the concentration of prothrombin (1.5 μM), from which approximately 0.36 μM is converted to thrombin after clot formation [8,9]. In circulation, heparan sulfate lining the vascular endothelium serves as a physiologic activator of AT. In clinical practice, the anticoagulant activity of AT is exploited by using unfractionated heparin (hereinafter called heparin), which is the mainstay anticoagulant in many clinical situations including thrombotic stroke, coronary interventions, cardiopulmonary bypass, and treatment of pulmonary emboli. The AT-mediated inhibition of thrombin is enhanced 1000 to 10,000 fold in the presence of heparin. Heparin binding to AT by way of heparin's pentasaccharide sequence induces major conformational changes in the

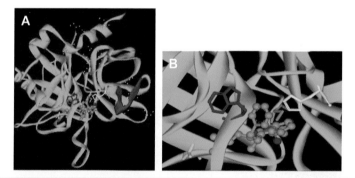

Fig. 1. (A) The structure of α-thrombin (*green*) in complex with Phe-Pro-Arg-chlormethylketone (FPRck in element color) at the catalytic domain. The exosite I and exosite II regions are indicated in white dots (3-o'clock position) and in gray dots (12-o'clock position). (B) The magnified view of the catalytic domain of of α-thrombin (*green*). Also indicated are Ser195 (*orange*) and His57 (*yellow*) in the catalytic center, negatively charged Asp189 (*turquoise*), aromatic Trp215 (*red*), the hydrophobic 60-loop (*magenta*), and the γ-loop (*gray*). Data obtained from Protein Data Bank (PDB) (*1abj*) and processed with the ViewerLite 5.0 (Accelrys, Inc., San Diego, California).

AT structure (reviewed recently by Huntington and colleagues [10]) (Fig. 2A). In addition, negatively charged sulfated heparin chain also interacts with the exosite II of thrombin. After forming a Michaelis complex with thrombin, AT inserts its reactive center loop, flips into itself, and denatures thrombin's catalytic domain [11]. This irreversible nature of thrombin inhibition by AT is different from direct thrombin inhibitors (DTIs), which only temporarily block thrombin's catalytic activity.

There are several issues in AT-mediated heparin anticoagulation. First, AT deficiency renders anticoagulation less effective. AT is essential for normal fetal development because homozygous AT deficiency in mice is lethal in utero [12]. Clinically, individuals who have heterozygous congenital AT deficiency retain 40% to 50% of normal AT activity and may present with deep venous thromboses [13]. The prevalence of AT deficiency is 1 in 2000 to 5000, and AT is inherited as an autosomal dominant trait. Congenital AT deficiency may result from decreased synthesis (type I) and dysfunctional enzyme (type II), but acquired deficiency is more frequently encountered in clinical practice. Pregnancy, hepatic dysfunction, nephrotic syndrome, and sepsis are known conditions with low AT levels. The use of estrogen, L-asparaginase, and heparin reduce AT levels. Heparin-associated AT deficiency (<60%) is observed in 10% to 20% of patients presenting for cardiac surgery, and this is particularly common in individuals who have preoperative heparin therapy over 4 days [14–16]. Second, the heparin-AT complex is large, and clot-bound thrombin is not efficiently inhibited during heparin anticoagulation [17]. In contrast, clot-bound thrombin is blocked with HCII and low molecular weight DTIs

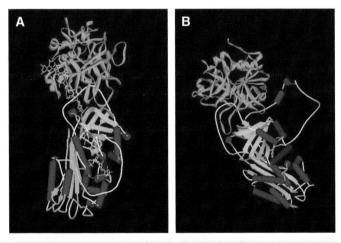

Fig. 2. (A) Complex of α-thrombin (*green*), AT (*schematic model*), and heparin (*yellow*). The central reactive loop of AT is inserted in the catalytic domain of thrombin. Heparin is attached the exosite II of thrombin molecule. Data were processed from Protein Data Bank (PDB) (*1tb6*). (B) Complex of α-thrombin (*green*) and HCII (*schematic model*). The central reactive loop of AT is inserted in the catalytic domain of thrombin. Data processed from PDB (*1jmo*).

[18]. Third, heparin itself may activate platelets, and the development of anti-body against heparin-platelet factor 4 complex may lead to heparin-induced thrombocytopenia and thromboses [19–21].

Despite these shortfalls, heparin is a potent anticoagulant with advantages of relative safety, rapid reversibility (ie, protamine), and low cost [22]. It is likely that heparin will remain the standard in certain clinical settings (eg, cardiopul-monary bypass), but a less antigenic heparin derivative may be developed in the future. Several heparin fractions and pentasaccharides are currently avail-able (eg, low molecular weight heparins, fondaparinux) that have inhibitory specificity toward factor Xa (reviewed elsewhere) [1]. The management of con-genital and acquired AT deficiency may also benefit from the recombinant technology [23,24]. The recombinant human AT (ATryn, GTC Biotherapeu-tics, Framingham, Massachusetts) is currently being evaluated in several phase II trials [24,25]. Conventionally, plasma levels of AT have been replenished with fresh frozen plasma or human plasma-derived AT concentrate (Throm-bate III, Talecris, Research Triangle Park, North Carolina). The availability of recombinant AT avoids potential donor shortages and represents a potential unlimited supply; however, regulatory agencies seem reluctant to approve a transgenic protein. The efficacy and indication of recombinant human AT should be elucidated from the results of continuing trials.

HEPARIN COFACTOR II

HCII (62 kd) is also a serpin synthesized in the liver. Its plasma concentration, 80 µg/mL (1.2 µM), is approximately half that of AT, and its half-life is 2.5 days. At the molecular level, its structure is similar to AT (see Fig. 2B). Re-cent structural analyses revealed that activation of HCII is achieved by the allosteric mechanism common to heparin and dermatan sulfate [26]. Glycos-aminoglycan (GAG) activation of HCII extrudes the N-terminal acidic tail from the body of protein, and the displaced tail interacts with exosite I of thrombin. Subsequently, thrombin is approximated to and inactivated by the reactive center loop of HCII. The interaction between thrombin and the N-ter-minus of HCII is important because HCII mutant with N-terminal tail deletion has poor reactivity with thrombin [27]. Nevertheless, the distributions and physiologic roles of AT and HCII differ in vivo. HCII is associated with mono-cyte and macrophages in the tissue of healing wound, whereas AT is associated with mast cells [28]. HCII, but not AT, binds to chondroitin sulfate and derma-tan sulfate on the surface of monocyte/macrophages [29,30].

The catalytic activity of HCII is enhanced by heparin and dermatan, whereas AT is not activated by dermatan. The substrate specificity of these ser-pins further highlights distinct functional roles: AT inhibits coagulation factors (IIa, Xa, IXa, XIa, XIIa, and VIIa) [31–34], whereas HCII inhibits only throm-bin and noncoagulant proteins such as cathepsin G and chymotrypsin [35,36].

For regulation of intravascular coagulation, AT is a dominant protease inhib-itor [37,38]. There are only a few clinical reports of congenital HCII deficiency associated with morbidity [39,40]. HCII knockout mice survive the gestational period, and their phenotype is grossly normal, whereas AT knockout leads to intrauterine death [12,41]. Thrombotic risk, however, may be increased after vascular injury. HCII knockout mice had increased thrombotic occlusion of the carotid artery after the photochemically induced endothelial injury [41]. Clinically, higher HCII activity (>80%), but not AT activity, was associated with reduced incidence of in-stent stenosis after coronary intervention [42].

Tanaka and colleagues [43] recently compared heparin with dermatan disulfate, a synthetic anticoagulant derived from 6-O-sulfation of the native dermatan sulfate (Intimatan, Celsus Laboratories, Cincinatti, Ohio). In the proposed therapeutic range (10–100 μg/mL) [44], Intimatan caused a concentration-dependent increase in partial thromboplastin time. The effects of heparin, Intimatan, and both agents in combination were also evaluated using thrombin generation assay (Appendix 1) with varied levels of endogenous AT, HCII, or both. With decreasing levels of AT and HCII, heparin and Intimatan, respectively, became less effective in thrombin inhibition. It was noted, however, that heparin's dependence on AT was much more pronounced than Intimatan's dependence on HCII (Fig. 3). Possible reasons why Intimatan exerted some thrombin inhibition without HCII may be its higher charge density (4, 6-O-disulfate) and AT-mediated thrombin inhibition. The invertebrate-derived dermatan with 4- or 6-O-sulfate residues also had weak antithrombotic activity by way of AT in HCII knockout mice [38]. In the absence of both AT and HCII, anticoagulant effects of Intimatan are negligible. When both AT and HCII are reduced to 20% to 60% of normal, addition of Intimatan to heparin is more effective than heparin or Intimatan alone [43]. Because these low levels of AT or HCII are clinically observed [45], the use of dermatan disulfate may represent an alternative anticoagulation by HCII-mediated thrombin inhibition. Further, the derivatives of dermatan sulfate do not have cross-reactivity with heparin-PF4 antibody, and therefore may be used as a heparin alternative in patients who have heparin-induced thrombocytopenia [46].

THROMBOMODULIN

Thrombomodulin is a membrane-bound glycoprotein lining vascular endothelial surfaces. It is composed of an N-terminal lectin-like domain, six epidermal growth factor (EGF)-like domains, chondroitin sulfate, transmembrane, and a cytoplasmic domain, totaling 557 amino acids. EGF domains 5 and 6 are important for thrombin binding by way of exosite I, and chondroitin sulfate supports thrombin binding by way of exosite II. Other domains are important for physiologic functions: EGF domain 4 for protein C activation, EGF domain 3 for activation of procarboxypeptidase B (precursor of thrombin activatable fibrinolysis inhibitor [TAFI]), and lectin-like domain for anti-inflammation [47,48].

The physiologic importance of thrombomodulin is exemplified by the embryonic lethality or severe juvenile thromboses in mice that have disrupted thrombomodulin encoding gene (transmembrane) forms in the vascular system [49,50]. Endothelial thrombomodulin serves a key role in switching thrombin's

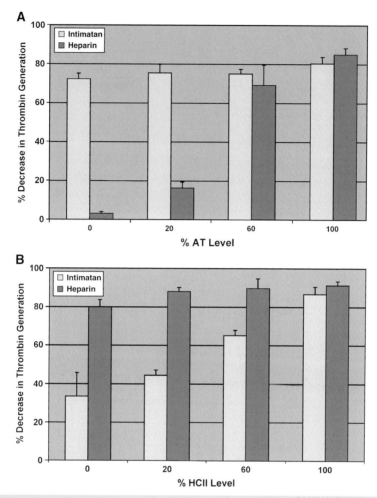

Fig. 3. (A) The effects of heparin and Intimatan on thrombin generation in platelet-poor plasma with progressively depleted AT levels (n = 6). Anticoagulant effects of heparin are dependent on AT levels, whereas Intimatan is minimally affected. (B) The effects of heparin and Intimatan on thrombin generation in platelet-poor plasma with progressively depleted HCII levels (n = 6). There is minimal effect of HCII levels on heparin anticoagulation. Anticoagulant effects of Intimatan are affected by reduced HCII levels, but Intimatan has residual anticoagulant effects in the absence of HCII.

substrate specificity to protein C and pro-TAFI from procoagulant substrates, platelet protease activated receptors (PARs) (please see the article by Landis and colleagues elsewhere in this issue), fibrinogen, and factors V, VIII, and XIII. Activated protein C (APC) exerts negative feedback on thrombin formation, and APC and TAFI exert anti-inflammatory effects [51,52]. In particular, the anti-inflammatory signaling mechanisms through the endothelial protein C receptor have important physiologic and cytoprotective roles [53–57].

In the microcirculation, endogenous thrombomodulin is present at up to 500 nM (~31.3 µg/mL) [58]. The expression of endothelial thrombomodulin is reduced by the protease cleavage of bound thrombomodulin and by the cytokine-mediated down-regulation of its synthesis (eg, tumor necrosis factor α). The levels of plasma-soluble thrombomodulin have been used as a surrogate marker for endothelial damages in proinflammatory diseases including coronary disease, cardiopulmonary bypass, and sepsis/disseminated intravascular coagulation [59–61]. The consequences of reduced thrombomodulin are decreased protein C activation and reduced scavenging of thrombin, which may lead to microvascular thromboses and organ dysfunction. Improved outcomes in the recent clinical trials of APC (Xigris, Eli Lilly, Indianapolis, Indiana) underlie the importance of regulating thrombin generation by way of thrombomodulin–protein C pathway [62,63]. Alternatively, restoring protein C activation may be achieved by supplementing functional thrombomodulin in subsets of septic patients who have disseminated intravascular coagulation [61,64,65]. Recombinant human soluble thrombomodulin (rhsTM; Asahi Kasei, Oh-hito, Japan) has been undergoing clinical trials for this indication in Japan [66]. In North America, rhsTM is currently undergoing a phase II study. According to published clinical trials (phase I/II), therapeutic levels of rhsTM were achieved with intravenous or subcutaneous administration (half-life of 48 to 72 hours) and reduced the incidence of deep venous thromboses in patients undergoing the unilateral hip replacement [67,68].

Separately from the clinical study, Tanaka and colleagues [69] investigated the contribution of protein C system to anticoagulation using soluble thrombomodulin in nonhuman primates with a thrombogenic device in the chronic arteriovenous (A-V) shunt (Appendix 2). The bolus injections of rhsTM at 0.1, 1, or 5 mg/kg achieved a dose-dependent reduction of platelet and fibrin deposition in the A-V shunt graft. In the subgroup of animals that received the 1-mg/kg dose of rhsTM, the protein C–blocking monoclonal antibody (HPC4) was also administered to test whether inhibition of APC generation would reduce antithrombotic activity of rhsTM. Contrary to the hypothesis, it was shown that thrombus formation was inhibited during the first 60 to 80 minutes without APC. These findings may be explained by the changes in plasma APC levels as follows. The deployment of the thrombogenic device in the shunt increases systemic APC levels up to 500%. With increasing dose of rhsTM, systemic increases of APC were inhibited, suggesting rhsTM-mediated rapid scavenging of thrombin. In agreement, it has been reported that rhsTM relays bound thrombin to AT [70]. The current study suggests that rhsTM functions as a DTI at the dose (>1 mg/kg) used for the experiment [69]. These findings do not completely contradict the working concept of the thrombomodulin–protein C pathway. Systemic levels of APC do not necessarily reflect localized protein C activation. It is possible that rhsTM locally supported APC generation when protein C was present and suppressed systemic leakage of thrombin. It is noteworthy that conventional anticoagulants are known to reduce protein C levels or APC activity, but rhsTM is capable of generating APC. In this regard, rhsTM represents a novel way to regulate thrombin. Failures of sepsis outcomes studies with thrombin inhibition may be due to suppressing thrombin's regulatory function to induce anti-inflammatory proteins, APC, and TAFI [71]. Additional clinical studies are necessary to elucidate pharmacologic roles and indications of rhsTM.

DIRECT THROMBIN INHIBITORS

DTIs are classified into two types (Table 1): catalytic-site inhibitors and bivalent inhibitors. The former includes argatroban and melagatran (active metabolite of ximelagatran). Argatroban is a prototypical active-site inhibitor developed by Okamoto and colleagues [72]. They initially set out to modify tosyl-arginine-methylester (TAME), a synthetic thrombin substrate introduced by Sol Sherry's group for amidolytic determination of thrombin [73]. TAME is composed of arginine with a tosyl residue at the amino-terminus and a methyl residue at the carboxy-terminus (Fig. 4A, B) and has a weak inhibitory effect on thrombin. With insertion of an oxygen atom on the tosyl group, TAME became less susceptible to amidolysis by thrombin. Okamoto and colleagues [72] continued modification of arginine derivatives and eventually reached the 805th synthetic chemical, MD805, currently known as argatroban. Argatroban's chemical structure is based on arginine, with quinoline at the amino-terminus and piperidinecarboxylic acid at the carboxy-terminus (see Fig. 4A). Argatroban competitively blocks catalytic action of thrombin by way of multiple binding mechanisms, including hydrogen bond (Gly216), negatively charged aspartic acid (Asp189), aromatic ring binding region (Trp215), and hydrophobic carboxamide-binding region (Leu99, Tyr60A, Trp60D) [74].

The bivalent inhibitors bind to exosite I and the active site. Hirudin, a medicinal leech–derived enzyme, is a prototypical drug. The binding of hirudin to thrombin is only slowly reversible [75]. The long half-life (60 minutes by intravenous route) may be problematic, particularly in patients who have renal insufficiency [76]. Bivalirudin is a designer molecule modeled after hirudin (see Fig. 4C). The carboxy-terminus of bivalirudin is similar to hirudin's carboxy-terminal dodecapeptide, DGDFEEIPEEYL, which binds to exosite I. The amino-terminus of bivalirudin is an FPRP moiety, with glycine chains that connect to the carboxy-terminus [77]. The importance of bivalent binding to thrombin is exemplified in the following study of baboon A-V shunt models (see Appendix 2). Kelly and colleagues [78] compared three synthetic peptides: D-Phe-Pro-Arg (FPR), carboxy-terminal dodecapeptide (hirugen), and bivalirudin (hirulog-1) using in vitro and in vivo nonhuman primate vascular graft models. The order of in vitro inhibition of thrombin catalytic activity was bivalirudin (0.001 μM)>FPR (61 μM)>>dodecapeptide (>2000 μM). Thrombin-induced platelet aggregation was most potently inhibited by bivalirudin (0.025 μM), whereas FPR and dodecapeptide inhibited aggregation at higher concentration (both at ~30 μM). In collagen-coated vascular graft, platelet and fibrin depositions

Table 1
Thrombin inhibitors

	Lepirudin (Refludan)	Bivalirudin (Angiomax)	Argatroban	Ximelagatran (Exanta)	Drotrecogin alfa (Xigris)	Soluble thrombomodulin
Mechanism of action	Blocks thrombin[a]	Blocks thrombin[a]	Blocks thrombin[b]	Blocks thrombin[b]	Inhibits Va and VIIIa	Protein C activation
Indication	HIT/HITT	PCI	HIT/HITT, PCI	DVT prophylaxis[c]	Severe sepsis	DVT prophylaxis[d]
Half life	1.3 h	25 min	40–50 min	3–4 h	13 min	3–4 d
Elimination	Renal	Plasma/renal	Hepatic	Renal	Plasma	Renal (>50%)
Monitoring	APTT, ACT, ECT	APTT, ACT, ECT	APTT, ACT, ECT	Not monitored	Not monitored	APTT
Comments	Anti-hirudin antibodies[e]	—	Prolong PT/INR	Prodrug of melagatran[f]	May prolong APTT	—

Abbreviations: APTT, activated partial thromboplastin time; ACT, activated clotting time; DVT, deep venous thrombosis; ECT, ecarin clotting time; HIT, heparin-induced thrombocytopenia; HITT, heparin-induced thrombocytopenia and thromboses; PCI, percutaneous coronary intervention; PT/INR, prothrombin time/international normalized ratio.

[a]Lepirudin and bivalirudin block catalytic site and exosite I of thrombin.
[b]Argatroban blocks catalytic site of thrombin.
[c]In European countries.
[d]Phase II trial.
[e]Antibody may increase anticoagulant effect, but allergic reaction is rare.
[f]Elevation of hepatic enzymes may be observed.

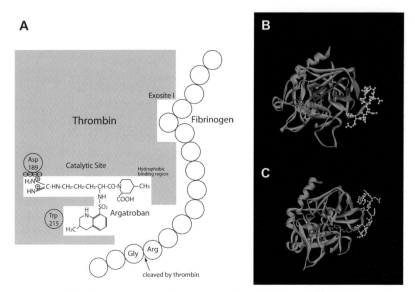

Fig. 4. (A) Schematic description of the catalytic domain of α-thrombin. (B) Stereo view of α-thrombin (green) in complex with argatroban (element color) at the catalytic domain, and hirudin carboxy-terminal dodecapeptide (yellow) on the exosite I. Also indicated are the Ser195 (orange) in the catalytic center, negatively charged Asp189 (turquoise), aromatic Trp215 (red), and the hydrophobic 60-loop (magenta). Data processed from Protein Data Bank (PDB) (1dwc). (C) Complex of α-thrombin (green) and hirulog-3. The amino-terminus (element color) of hirulog is inserted in the catalytic domain of thrombin, and argatroban and hirudin-like carboxy-terminal domain (yellow) is attached to the exosite I of thrombin. Data processed from PDB (1abi).

were dose-dependently reduced by bivalirudin with 25 to 100 nmol/kg/min infusion, but FPR was at least tenfold less effective. There was minimal thrombus inhibition with dodecapeptide even at a concentration tenfold higher than that of bivalirudin. Hence, the short half-life of bivalirudin (25 minutes) may be explained, in part, by the weak anticoagulant effects of FPR and dodecapeptide after the Pro-Arg bond in the amino-terminus of bivalirudin is cleaved by thrombin [79]. Another in vitro experiment suggests, however, that the binding of bivalirudin to thrombin is reversible at a dissociation rate 0.8 s^{-1}, whereas cleavage of FPRP by thrombin is at 0.01 s^{-1}; therefore, major dissociation does not seem to involve thrombin cleavage of bivalirudin [77].

The reversible nature of thrombin inhibition with DTIs is distinct from serpin irreversible AT inhibition. It may be considered favorable for reducing bleeding risks, particularly because there is no antidote for DTIs. This reversible inhibition may be problematic in the settings of protracted thrombin formation and stasis. During cardiac surgery, blood retained in the pleural space may clot because blood is exposed to a large amount of tissue factor, and thrombin initially blocked with DTI eventually dissociates and cleaves fibrinogen and platelets [77]. Therefore, it is unlikely that DTIs will completely replace heparin anticoagulation in certain clinical settings unless therapeutic monitoring is further improved and antidotes are developed.

The catalytic-site direct inhibitor and bivalent inhibitor may differ with respect to the efficacy of thrombin inhibition. Generally, increases in the prothrombin time (international normalized ratio [INR]) are more prolonged with catalytic-site inhibitors than with bivalent inhibitors and are in the order argatroban>melagatran>bivalirudin>lepirudin. Warkentin and colleagues [80] hypothesized that inhibition of factor Xa by argatroban and melagatran would prolonged INR, but anti-Xa effects were observed at levels higher than clinical concentrations. These investigators concluded that the higher therapeutic (molar) concentration of argatroban interferes with INR. Binding bivalirudin and lepirudin to exosite I appears to confer more specificity toward thrombin; that is, FPRCK (Phe-Pro-Arg-chlormethylketone) blocks thrombin and factor Xa. Bivalirudin and lepirudin have lower therapeutic concentrations than argatroban and melagatran. On the contrary, the blockade of exosite I per se does not confer in vivo antithrombotic effects, and additional catalytic site blockade seems to be necessary [78,81].

The armamentarium of different classes of DTIs allows clinicians to choose agents depending on the type of interventions and on the underlying condition (eg, renal failure, hepatic dysfunction). Additional human trials of DTIs should reveal their pharmacologic activity and define their clinical indications. Melagatran, however, has been removed from the marketplace.

THROMBIN MUTANTS

Because of its potent roles in platelet activation and fibrinogen cleavage, thrombin is generally viewed as a procoagulant enzyme. Nevertheless, thrombin's catalytic activity toward protein C can be viewed as its anticoagulant function. Hanson and colleagues [82] tested this hypothesis by infusing a sufficiently low dose of thrombin to elicit its anticoagulant function mediated by APC and endothelial thrombomodulin. Using the nonhuman primates with the thrombogenic device in the chronic A-V shunt (see Appendix 2), they showed that intravenous infusion of α-thrombin, 1 to 2 U/kg/min for 1 hour, increased circulating APC levels from 5 ng/mL to 250 to 500 ng/mL. Although other thrombosis markers (thrombin-AT, fibrinopeptide A, D-dimer) were elevated after thrombin infusion, the lower thrombin dose (1 U/kg/min) (1) did not deplete circulating platelets, fibrinogen, or protein C; (2) halved platelet-rich thrombi in arterial graft, and (3) reduced venous graft thrombus by over 85%. Antithrombotic effects of thrombin infusion were blocked by infusing a protein C–blocking monoclonal antibody, leading to shunt occlusion, increased loss of platelets and fibrinogen, and elevated plasma coagulation markers.

Recently, the same investigators reported a similar study with the use of a thrombin mutant that retains specificity for protein C but reduced activity toward PAR-1 and fibrinogen cleavage. The mutant thrombin has double mutations at Trp215Ala and Glu217Ala (W215A/E217A), which induce a 20,000-fold decrease in fibrinogen cleavage [83,84]. Up to 0.45 mg/kg of intravenous injection of W215A/E217A seemed to be safe, and there was a dose-dependent prolongation of activated partial thromboplastin time and platelet deposition in the A-V shunt graft [85]. The anticoagulant systemic APC levels were comparable or higher than the therapeutic dose of APC, 0.45 mg/kg, administered intravenously [63,86].

There are other experimental modifications of thrombin that convert thrombin to an anticoagulant protein. The prothrombin mutant R157A/R268A, which produces a stable form of meizothrombin in vivo, was shown to be antithrombotic using the FeCl$_3$-induced carotid injury model in mice [87]. Anhydrothrombin is prepared by conversion of the active site Ser195 of thrombin to dehydroalanine using phenylmethylsulphonylfluoride under alkaline condition [88]. In vitro assays showed that anhydrothrombin prolongs activated partial thromboplastin time and inhibits thrombin-induced and shear-related platelet aggregation [89]. The in vitro and in vivo studies of modified or mutant thrombin elucidate critical interactions among its catalytic domain, exosites, and substrates (eg, fibrinogen) [3,4,83]. It is likely that recombinant thrombin with such modifications may find therapeutic and diagnostic uses in the near future [85].

SUMMARY

Since the discovery of heparin in the early twentieth century, significant advances have been made in the understanding of coagulation systems. Development of an array of anticoagulant agents resulted from chemical and biomedical engineering technologies. Genetic sequence information (eg, single nucleotide polymorphism) from thrombophilic or hypocoagulable individuals may allow clinicians to diagnose and classify such conditions, and genetic alteration of mice provides critical information on in vivo function of coagulation factors. Thrombin is an essential serine protease for survival and self-preservation. Its ancient origin from complement C1 indicates that it has key roles in coagulation and inflammation [90]. Through understanding its wide-spectrum physiologic functions, receptor system, and signaling mechanisms, it is hoped that in the near future, it will be possible to modulate thrombin activity without harming the overall balance of coagulation and immunity [51,91].

APPENDIX 1

THROMBIN GENERATION ASSAY

The method for the automated estimation of endogenous thrombin potential by using a commercially available fluorogenic substrate (Z-Gly-Gly-Arg-AMC) has been described elsewhere [92]. Briefly, for the thrombin generation assay, 80 µL of plasma and 20 µL of the thrombin-generation trigger were added to wells of a 96-well microtiter plate (Microfluor2; Labsystems, Vantaa, Finland), followed by 20 μL of substrate/CaCl$_2$ buffer. The reaction was monitored with a microplate fluorometer (Fluoroskan Ascent; Labsystems) set at 390 nm (excitation wavelength) and 460 nm (emission wavelength). Fluorescence was recorded every 20 seconds for 90 minutes, and the acquired data were automatically processed by commercially available Thrombinoscope software (Synapse BV, Maastricht, Netherlands), that displayed the reaction progress and calculated thrombin generation (peak thrombin level).

APPENDIX 2

EXTERIORIZED CHRONIC FEMORAL ARTERIOVENOUS SHUNT MODELS OF THROMBUS FORMATION

Mmeasurements were obtained for acute thrombotic responses of native non-anticoagulated blood under well-controlled conditions of flow and geometry using a thrombogenic device (containing proximal vascular-graft and distal stasis-chamber) interposed in an exteriorized chronic arteriovenous (A-V) femoral shunt of silicone rubber tubing [82,85]. Blood flowing through the shunts was subject to all of the physiologic clearance/inhibition mechanisms. In vivo platelet hemostatic function was evaluated by determinations of template bleeding time, and coagulation was assessed by activated partial thromboplastin times. These shunt models are efficient, reproducible, and predictive of vascular thrombus formation.

The thrombogenic device in chronic exteriorized A-V femoral shunts induces the formation of arterial-type platelet-rich and venous-type fibrin-rich

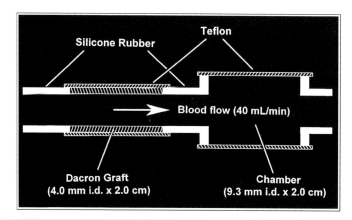

Fig. 5. Thrombogenic device used to induce thrombus formation. The device consists of a 2-cm segment of Dacron vascular graft (4.0-mm interior diameter), followed by a 2-cm Teflon chamber (9.3 mm interior diameter). The device was interposed into a chronic femoral A-V shunt in baboons. The Dacron graft produced arterial blood shear rates (initial rate, ~265 s^{-1}) and accumulated thrombus composed predominantly of platelets, whereas the Teflon chamber exhibited a low shear rate (<30 s^{-1}), venous recirculation, and stasis that produced thrombus that was rich in fibrin and red cells.

thrombi; the proximal segment of vascular graft selectively accumulates platelets, and the distal expanded chamber of disturbed flow selectively accumulates fibrin (Fig. 5).

The thrombogenic surface incorporated into the proximal segment is composed of Dacron vascular graft. This thrombogenic segment was selected because it induces thrombus that is highly reproducible and resistant to aspirin and heparin. The thrombus formed on segments of vascular graft is thrombin-mediated and platelet-selective, whereas thrombus forming in the expanded chamber is thrombin-mediated and fibrin-selective.

The extent of acute thrombus formation on the graft and in the chamber was measured in real time by (1) scintillation camera imaging of deposited autologous indium 111-labeled platelets; and (2) determination of iodine 125–labeled fibrinogen accumulation in forming thrombus. In addition, the species specificity is less of a problem in the nonhuman primates compared with other species [93,94], and the blood tests of thrombosis for humans can be used to quantitate plasma levels of platelet factor 4, beta-thromboglobulin, and thrombin:antithrombin complex, and D-dimer levels [82].

References

[1] Bates SM, Weitz JI. New anticoagulants: beyond heparin, low-molecular-weight heparin and warfarin. Br J Pharmacol 2005;144(8):1017–28.
[2] Butenas S, van't Veer C, Mann KG. "Normal" thrombin generation. Blood 1999;94(7):2169–78.
[3] Di Cera E. Thrombin interactions. Chest 2003;124(3 Suppl):11S–7S.
[4] Krishnaswamy S. Exosite-driven substrate specificity and function in coagulation. J Thromb Haemost 2005;3(1):54–67.
[5] Lane DA, Philippou H, Huntington JA. Directing thrombin. Blood 2005;106(8):2605–12.
[6] Murano G, Williams L, Miller-Andersson M, et al. Some properties of antithrombin-III and its concentration in human plasma. Thromb Res 1980;18(1–2):259–62.
[7] Menache D, O'Malley JP, Schorr JB, et al. Evaluation of the safety, recovery, half-life, and clinical efficacy of antithrombin III (human) in patients with hereditary antithrombin III deficiency. Blood 1990;75(1):33–9.
[8] Rand MD, Lock JB, van't Veer C, et al. Blood clotting in minimally altered whole blood. Blood 1996;88(9):3432–45.
[9] Brummel KE, Paradis SG, Butenas S, et al. Thrombin functions during tissue factor-induced blood coagulation. Blood 2002;100(1):148–52.
[10] Huntington JA, Read RJ, Carrell RW. Structure of a serpin-protease complex shows inhibition by deformation. Nature 2000;407(6806):923–6.
[11] Langdown J, Johnson DJD, Baglin TP, et al. Allosteric activation of antithrombin critically depends upon hinge region extension. J Biol Chem 2004;279(45):47288–97.
[12] Ishiguro K, Kojima T, Kadomatsu K, et al. Complete antithrombin deficiency in mice results in embryonic lethality. J Clin Invest 2000;106(7):873–8.
[13] Hirsh J, Piovella F, Pini M. Congenital antithrombin III deficiency. Incidence and clinical features. Am J Med 1989;87(3B):34S–8S.
[14] Dietrich W, Spannagl M, Schramm W, et al. The influence of preoperative anticoagulation on heparin response during cardiopulmonary bypass. J Thorac Cardiovasc Surg 1991;102(4):505–14.
[15] Staples MH, Dunton RF, Karlson KJ, et al. Heparin resistance after preoperative heparin therapy or intraaortic balloon pumping. Ann Thorac Surg 1994;57(5):1211–6.

[16] Tanaka KA, Szlam F, Katori N, et al. The effects of argatroban on thrombin generation and hemostatic activation in vitro. Anesth Analg 2004;99(5):1283–9.

[17] Weitz JI, Hudoba M, Massel D, et al. Clot-bound thrombin is protected from inhibition by heparin-antithrombin III but is susceptible to inactivation by antithrombin III-independent inhibitors. J Clin Invest 1990;86(2):385–91.

[18] Berry CN, Girardot C, Lecoffre C, et al. Effects of the synthetic thrombin inhibitor argatroban on fibrin- or clot-incorporated thrombin: comparison with heparin and recombinant hirudin. Thromb Haemost 1994;72(3):381–6.

[19] Salzman EW, Rosenberg RD, Smith MH, et al. Effect of heparin and heparin fractions on platelet aggregation. J Clin Invest 1980;65(1):64–73.

[20] Matsuo T, Nakao K, Yamada T, et al. Effect of a new anticoagulant (MD 805) on platelet activation in the hemodialysis circuit. Thromb Res 1986;41(1):33–41.

[21] Xiao Z, Theroux P. Platelet activation with unfractionated heparin at therapeutic concentrations and comparisons with a low-molecular-weight heparin and with a direct thrombin inhibitor. Circulation 1998;97(3):251–6.

[22] Stafford-Smith M, Lefrak EA, Qazi AG, et al. Efficacy and safety of heparinase I versus protamine in patients undergoing coronary artery bypass grafting with and without cardiopulmonary bypass. Anesthesiology 2005;103(2):229–40.

[23] Edmunds T, Van Patten SM, Pollock J, et al. Transgenically produced human antithrombin: structural and functional comparison to human plasma-derived antithrombin. Blood 1998; 91(12):4561–71.

[24] Levy JH, Despotis GJ, Szlam F, et al. Recombinant human transgenic antithrombin in cardiac surgery: a dose-finding study. Anesthesiology 2002;96(5):1095–102.

[25] Avidan MS, Levy JH, van Aken H, et al. Recombinant human antithrombin III restores heparin responsiveness and decreases activation of coagulation in heparin-resistant patients during cardiopulmonary bypass. J Thorac Cardiovasc Surg 2005;130(1):107–13.

[26] O'Keeffe D, Olson ST, Gasiunas N, et al. The heparin binding properties of heparin cofactor II suggest an antithrombin-like activation mechanism. J Biol Chem 2004;279(48): 50267–73.

[27] Sheffield WP, Blajchman MA. Deletion mutagenesis of heparin cofactor II: defining the minimum size of a thrombin inhibiting serpin. FEBS Lett 1995;365(2–3):189–92.

[28] Hoffman M, Loh KL, Bond VK, et al. Localization of heparin cofactor II in injured human skin: a potential role in wound healing. Exp Mol Pathol 2003;75(2):109–18.

[29] Halvorsen B, Aas UK, Kulseth MA, et al. Proteoglycans in macrophages: characterization and possible role in the cellular uptake of lipoproteins. Biochem J 1998;331(3):743–52.

[30] Zimmermann R, Sartipy P, Winkler R, et al. Endogenously produced glycosaminoglycans affecting the release of lipoprotein lipase from macrophages and the interaction with lipoproteins. Biochim Biophys Acta Mol Cell Biol Lipids 2000;1484(2–3):316–24.

[31] Abildgaard U. Binding of thrombin to antithrombin III. Scand J Clin Lab Invest 1969;24(1): 23–7.

[32] Kurachi K, Fujikawa K, Schmer G, et al. Inhibition of bovine factor IXa and factor Xabeta by antithrombin III. Biochemistry 1976;15(2):373–7.

[33] Stead N, Kaplan AP, Rosenberg RD. Inhibition of activated factor XII by antithrombin-heparin cofactor. J Biol Chem 1976;251(21):6481–8.

[34] Kondo S, Kisiel W. Regulation of factor VIIa activity in plasma: evidence that antithrombin III is the sole plasma protease inhibitor of human factor VIIa. Thromb Res 1987;46(2): 325–35.

[35] Parker KA, Tollefsen DM. The protease specificity of heparin cofactor II. Inhibition of thrombin generated during coagulation. J Biol Chem 1985;260(6):3501–5.

[36] Church FC, Noyes CM, Griffith MJ. Inhibition of chymotrypsin by heparin cofactor II. Proc Natl Acad Sci U S A 1985;82(19):6431–4.

[37] Liaw PC, Mather T, Oganesyan N, et al. Identification of the protein C/activated protein C binding sites on the endothelial cell protein C receptor. Implications for a novel mode of

ligand recognition by a major histocompatibility complex class 1-type receptor. J Biol Chem 2001;276(11):8364–70.

[38] Vicente CP, He L, Pavao MS, et al. Antithrombotic activity of dermatan sulfate in heparin cofactor II-deficient mice. Blood 2004;104(13):3965–70.

[39] Bertina RM, van der Linden IK, Engesser L, et al. Hereditary heparin cofactor II deficiency and the risk of development of thrombosis. Thromb Haemost 1987;57(2):196–200.

[40] Kondo S, Tokunaga F, Kario K, et al. Molecular and cellular basis for type I heparin cofactor II deficiency (heparin cofactor II Awaji). Blood 1996;87(3):1006–12.

[41] He L, Vicente CP, Westrick RJ, et al. Heparin cofactor II inhibits arterial thrombosis after endothelial injury. J Clin Invest 2002;109(2):213–9.

[42] Takamori N, Azuma H, Kato M, et al. High plasma heparin cofactor II activity is associated with reduced incidence of in-stent restenosis after percutaneous coronary intervention. Circulation 2004;109(4):481–6.

[43] Tanaka KA, Szlam F, Vinten-Johansen J, et al. Effects of antithrombin and heparin cofactor II levels on anticoagulation with Intimatan. Thromb Haemost 2005;94(4):808–13.

[44] Buchanan MR, Brister SJ. Anticoagulant and antithrombin effects of Intimatan, a heparin cofactor II agonist. Thromb Res 2000;99(6):603–12.

[45] Andersson TR, Sie P, Pelzer H, et al. Elevated levels of thrombin-heparin cofactor II complex in plasma from patients with disseminated intravascular coagulation. Thromb Res 1992;66(5):591–8.

[46] Taliani MR, Agnelli G, Nenci GG, et al. Dermatan sulphate in patients with heparin-induced thrombocytopenia. Br J Haematol 1999;104(1):87–9.

[47] Conway EM, Van de Wouwer M, Pollefeyt S, et al. The lectin-like domain of thrombomodulin confers protection from neutrophil-mediated tissue damage by suppressing adhesion molecule expression via nuclear factor kappaB and mitogen-activated protein kinase pathways. J Exp Med 2002;196(5):565–77.

[48] Weiler H, Isermann BH. Thrombomodulin. J Thromb Haemost 2003;1(7):1515–24.

[49] Healy AM, Rayburn HB, Rosenberg RD, et al. Absence of the blood-clotting regulator thrombomodulin causes embryonic lethality in mice before development of a functional cardiovascular system. Proc Natl Acad Sci U S A 1995;92(3):850–4.

[50] Isermann B, Hendrickson SB, Zogg M, et al. Endothelium-specific loss of murine thrombomodulin disrupts the protein C anticoagulant pathway and causes juvenile-onset thrombosis. J Clin Invest 2001;108(4):537–46.

[51] Esmon CT. Inflammation and thrombosis. J Thromb Haemost 2003;1(7):1343–8.

[52] Campbell W, Okada N, Okada H. Carboxypeptidase R is an inactivator of complement-derived inflammatory peptides and an inhibitor of fibrinolysis. Immunol Rev 2001;180:162–7.

[53] Riewald M, Petrovan RJ, Donner A, et al. Activation of endothelial cell protease activated receptor 1 by the protein C pathway. Science 2002;296(5574):1880–2.

[54] Mosnier LO, Gale AJ, Yegneswaran S, et al. Activated protein C variants with normal cytoprotective but reduced anticoagulant activity. Blood 2004;104(6):1740–4.

[55] Guo H, Liu D, Gelbard H, et al. Activated protein C prevents neuronal apoptosis via protease activated receptors 1 and 3. Neuron 2004;41(4):563–72.

[56] Ludeman MJ, Kataoka H, Srinivasan Y, et al. PAR1 cleavage and signaling in response to activated protein C and thrombin. J Biol Chem 2005;280(13):13122–8.

[57] Riewald M, Ruf W. Protease-activated receptor-1 signaling by activated protein C in cytokine-perturbed endothelial cells is distinct from thrombin signaling. J Biol Chem 2005;280(20):19808–14.

[58] Esmon CT. The protein C pathway. Chest 2003;124(3 Suppl):26S–32S.

[59] Salomaa V, Matei C, Aleksic N, et al. Soluble thrombomodulin as a predictor of incident coronary heart disease and symptomless carotid artery atherosclerosis in the Atherosclerosis Risk in Communities (ARIC) Study: a case-cohort study. Lancet 1999;353(9166):1729–34.

[60] Boldt J, Zickmann B, Schindler E, et al. Influence of aprotinin on the thrombomodulin/protein C system in pediatric cardiac operations. J Thorac Cardiovasc Surg 1994;107(5): 1215–21.

[61] Liaw PCY, Esmon CT, Kahnamoui K, et al. Patients with severe sepsis vary markedly in their ability to generate activated protein C. Blood 2004;104(13):3958–64.

[62] Bernard GR, Vincent JL, Laterre PF, et al. Efficacy and safety of recombinant human activated protein C for severe sepsis. N Engl J Med 2001;344(10):699–709.

[63] Dhainaut JF, Yan SB, Margolis BD, et al. Drotrecogin alfa (activated) (recombinant human activated protein C) reduces host coagulopathy response in patients with severe sepsis. Thromb Haemost 2003;90(4):642–53.

[64] Asakura H, Ontachi Y, Mizutani T, et al. Decreased plasma activity of antithrombin or protein C is not due to consumption coagulopathy in septic patients with disseminated intravascular coagulation. Eur J Haematol 2001;67(3):170–5.

[65] Wada H, Sakakura M, Kushiya F, et al. Thrombomodulin accelerates activated protein C production and inhibits thrombin generation in the plasma of disseminated intravascular coagulation patients. Blood Coagul Fibrinolysis 2005;16(1):17–24.

[66] Maruyama I. Recombinant thrombomodulin and activated protein C in the treatment of disseminated intravascular coagulation. Thromb Haemost 1999;82(2):718–21.

[67] Moll S, Lindley C, Pescatore S, et al. Phase I study of a novel recombinant human soluble thrombomodulin, ART-123. J Thromb Haemost 2004;2(10):1745–51.

[68] Kearon C, Comp P, Douketis J, et al. Dose-response study of recombinant human soluble thrombomodulin (ART-123) in the prevention of venous thromboembolism after total hip replacement. J Thromb Haemost 2005;3(5):962–8.

[69] Tanaka KA, Fernandez JA, Marzec UM, et al. Soluble thrombomodulin is antithrombotic in the presence of neutralising antibodies to protein C and reduces circulating activated protein C levels in primates. Br J Haematol 2006;132:197–203.

[70] Aritomi M, Watanabe N, Ohishi R, et al. Recombinant human soluble thrombomodulin delivers bounded thrombin to antithrombin III: thrombomodulin associates with free thrombin and is recycled to activate protein C. Thromb Haemost 1993;70(3):418–22.

[71] Warren BL, Eid A, Singer P, et al. Caring for the critically ill patient. High-dose antithrombin III in severe sepsis: a randomized controlled trial. JAMA 2001;286(15):1869–78.

[72] Okamoto S, Hijikata A, Kikumoto R, et al. Potent inhibition of thrombin by the newly synthesized arginine derivative No. 805. The importance of stereo-structure of its hydrophobic carboxamide portion. Biochem Biophys Res Commun 1981;101(2):440–6.

[73] Okamoto S. Strategies for creating new medicines. Kobe Research Project on Thrombosis and Hemostasis; 2003.

[74] Kikumoto R, Tamao Y, Tezuka T, et al. Selective inhibition of thrombin by (2R, 4R)-4-methyl-1-[N^2-[(3-methyl-1,2,3,4-tetrahydro-8-quinolinyl)sulfonyl]-L-arginyl]]-2-piperidinecarboxylic acid. Biochemistry 1984;23(1):85–90.

[75] Hofsteenge J, Stone SR, Donella-Deana A, et al. The effect of substituting phosphotyrosine for sulphotyrosine on the activity of hirudin. Eur J Biochem 1990;188(1):55–9.

[76] Lefevre G, Duval M, Gauron S, et al. Effect of renal impairment on the pharmacokinetics and pharmacodynamics of desirudin. Clin Pharmacol Ther 1997;62(1):50–9.

[77] Parry MA, Maraganore JM, Stone SR. Kinetic mechanism for the interaction of hirulog with thrombin. Biochemistry 1994;33(49):14807–14.

[78] Kelly AB, Maraganore JM, Bourdon P, et al. Antithrombotic effects of synthetic peptides targeting various functional domains of thrombin. Proc Natl Acad Sci U S A 1992;89(13): 6040–4.

[79] Witting JI, Bourdon P, Brezniak DV, et al. Thrombin-specific inhibition by and slow cleavage of hirulog-1. Biochem J 1992;283(Pt 3):737–43.

[80] Warkentin TE, Greinacher A, Craven S, et al. Differences in the clinically effective molar concentrations of four direct thrombin inhibitors explain their variable prothrombin time prolongation. Thromb Haemost 2005;94:958–64.

[81] Noeske-Jungblut C, Haendler B, Donner P, et al. Triabin, a highly potent exosite inhibitor of thrombin. J Biol Chem 1995;270(48):28629–34.

[82] Hanson SR, Griffin JH, Harker LA, et al. Antithrombotic effects of thrombin-induced activation of endogenous protein C in primates. J Clin Invest 1993;92(4):2003–12.

[83] Cantwell AM, Di Cera E. Rational design of a potent anticoagulant thrombin. J Biol Chem 2000;275(51):39827–30.

[84] Pineda AO, Chen ZW, Caccia S, et al. The anticoagulant thrombin mutant W215A/E217A has a collapsed primary specificity pocket. J Biol Chem 2004;279(38):39824–8.

[85] Gruber A, Cantwell AM, Di Cera E, et al. The thrombin mutant W215A/E217A shows safe and potent anticoagulant and antithrombotic effects in vivo. J Biol Chem 2002;277(31):27581–4.

[86] Macias WL, Dhainaut JF, Yan SC, et al. Pharmacokinetic-pharmacodynamic analysis of drotrecogin alfa (activated) in patients with severe sepsis. Clin Pharmacol Ther 2002;72(4):391–402.

[87] Shim K, Zhu H, Westfield LA, et al. A recombinant murine meizothrombin precursor, prothrombin R157A/R268A, inhibits thrombosis in a model of acute carotid artery injury. Blood 2004;104(2):415–9.

[88] Hosokawa K, Ohnishi T, Shima M, et al. Preparation of anhydrothrombin and characterization of its interaction with natural thrombin substrates. Biochem J 2001;354(Pt 2):309–13.

[89] Sakurai Y, Shima M, Giddings J, et al. A critical role for thrombin in platelet aggregation under high shear stress. Thromb Res 2004;113(5):311–8.

[90] Krem MM, Cera ED. Evolution of enzyme cascades from embryonic development to blood coagulation. Trends Biochem Sci 2002;27(2):67–74.

[91] Coughlin SR, Camerer E. Participation in inflammation. J Clin Invest 2003;111(1):25–7.

[92] Hemker HC, Giesen P, Al Dieri R, et al. Calibrated automated thrombin generation measurement in clotting plasma. Pathophysiol Haemost Thromb 2003;33(1):4–15.

[93] Fernandez JA, Xu X, Liu D, et al. Recombinant murine-activated protein C is neuroprotective in a murine ischemic stroke model. Blood Cells Mol Dis 2003;30(3):271–6.

[94] Malm K, Dahlback B, Arnljots B. Prevention of thrombosis following deep arterial injury in rats by bovine activated protein C requiring co-administration of bovine protein S. Thromb Haemost 2003;90(2):227–34.

Hematol Oncol Clin N Am 21 (2007) 51–63

HEMATOLOGY/ONCOLOGY CLINICS
OF NORTH AMERICA

LSEVIER
AUNDERS

Platelet Inhibitors and Monitoring Platelet Function: Implications for Bleeding

Linda Shore-Lesserson, MD

Department of Anesthesiology, Cardiothoracic Anesthesiology,
Montefiore Medical Center, 111 East 210th Street, Bronx, NY 10467, USA

C ardiovascular disease is prevalent in our medical and surgical patient populations. Patients who have atherosclerotic heart disease suffer from endothelial disorders that predispose them to plaque and thrombus formation in diseased arteries. The propagation of thrombus occurs by means of deposition and activation of platelets and other cellular elements at the site of injury. The formation of a thrombus, with activation of thrombin, platelet degranulation, and subsequent platelet aggregation, is a self-perpetuating positive feedback loop that results ultimately in arterial occlusion. As our knowledge of platelet physiology improves, we can understand the contribution of platelet activation to arterial disease and we can specifically inhibit that activation with platelet-inhibitory drugs. The recent increase in the number of coronary interventional procedures performed has spawned the increasing use of antiplatelet medication as prophylaxis against thrombus formation in the instrumented artery.

Circulating platelets are anucleate discoid-shaped cells that are formed from megakaryocytes. A normal component of platelets includes a normal count $(150,000–450,000/\mu L)$ and normal function. It is important to appreciate the many different roles that platelets have in preserving circulation and hemostasis. Platelets form the primary phase of hemostasis, the platelet plug. This early adhesion of platelets to the injured endothelium is responsible for the physical "healing" of the wound and the biochemical signaling that occurs when other cells and coagulation factors are summoned to the site of injury. The platelet surface phospholipid is a critical surface on which the coagulation cascade proteases become activated and form a fibrin clot.

Cell-based theories of coagulation describe tissue factor release as being responsible for the initiation phase of coagulation. Cellular hemostasis is believed to occur in three stages: initiation, amplification, and propagation.

E-mail address: lshore@montefiore.org

0889-8588/07/$ – see front matter
doi:10.1016/j.hoc.2006.11.012

The initiation stage takes place on tissue-factor bearing cells, which come into contact with tissue factor when endothelial injury occurs. The initiation stage is characterized by presentation of tissue factor to its ligand factor VII and the subsequent activation of factors IX and X on the tissue-factor bearing cell [1]. The activation of factor X to Xa causes thrombin production and activation. Thrombin activation is then sufficient to activate factors VIII, V, and platelets. The amplification stage then occurs on the surface of the activated platelet, which exposes surface phospholipids that act as receptors for the activated factors VIIIa and IXa. The platelet surface allows for thrombin formation, therefore amplifying coagulation. The activation of thrombin causes further positive feedback mechanisms to occur that ensure formation of a stable clot. These include fibrinogen cleavage, release of factor XIII for fibrinogen cross-linkage, and the release of a fibrinolysis inhibitor.

PLATELET DYSFUNCTION

Thrombocytopenia exists, by definition, if the platelet count decreases to less than 150,000/μL. A minimum platelet count of 50,000/μL to 100,000/μL is recommended before elective surgery. Spontaneous bleeding can occur with platelet counts less than 30,000/μL. In the cancer chemotherapy patient, however, spontaneous bleeding may not be seen until the platelet count is well below 5000/μL. Bleeding may not be an issue until such low levels are reached if all other factors are normal. Most anesthesiologists and surgeons would prefer not to be at the absolute limit of normal coagulation, and the standard recommendations in texts are a minimum of 20,000/μL to 50,000/μL for elective surgery and 100,000/μL for cardiopulmonary bypass (CPB). Of course, if the platelet function is abnormal, a platelet count of even 150,000/μL or greater may be insufficient to ensure normal coagulation.

Platelet counts are readily available using automated devices with laser technology. These Coulter counters separate populations of particles based on size. Computer programming of the systems means that certain sized particles are deemed platelets, others white cells, and still others erythrocytes.

THE PLATELET AND CARDIOPULMONARY BYPASS

The hemostatic defect of CPB is largely attributable to platelet dysfunction. Aspects of CPB that are known to affect platelet function include hypothermia, drugs, fibrinolysis, materials-induced activation, and activation-related receptor alterations. The following briefly summarizes these adverse platelet effects. The remainder of the discussion introduces antiplatelet therapeutics and their synergistic platelet inhibiting effects with CPB. Methods of platelet analysis are also covered. Hypothermia causes reversible inhibition of platelet aggregation and slows the thrombin-induced platelet activation changes that occur at normothermia. In volunteers, Michelson and colleagues [2] have shown that hypothermia results in reduced platelet P-selectin expression and reduced GPIb down-regulation. These hypothermia-induced changes have been demonstrated in vivo and in vitro, in animals and in humans [3]. In a clinical study,

Boldt and colleagues [4] showed that hypothermic CPB caused reduced platelet aggregation in response to adenosine diphosphate (ADP), collagen, and epinephrine, which was accompanied by a higher volume of blood loss compared with normothermic CPB. Improvements in aggregation responses and in bleeding parameters were noted with the use of high-dose aprotinin during hypothermia but not during normothermia.

In an in vitro study, however, Faraday and Rosenfeld [5] demonstrated that agonist-induced platelet aggregation and fibrinogen binding are significantly *enhanced* during hypothermia (22°C). Flow cytometry results showed that activation-specific platelet receptors are upregulated during hypothermia. This might lead to the conclusion that either hypothermia is not likely to be responsible for CPB-induced platelet dysfunction or that the results of an in vitro investigation may not be applicable to the in vivo environment.

Heparin induces platelet dysfunction through various mechanisms. Heparin inactivates circulating thrombin and induces a fibrinolytic state, both of which make platelets dysfunctional [6]. At heparin concentrations of 1 U/mL to 70 U/mL, activation and degranulation of platelets does occur. Another study has shown that at heparin concentrations of 100 U/mL, degranulation is suppressed [7].

Protamine-induced platelet dysfunction has also been demonstrated as a defect in thrombin-induced platelet aggregation and a reduction in thrombin receptor agonist peptide (TRAP)-induced P-selectin expression [8]. Protamine administration to reverse heparin effect potentiates the antiplatelet effects of heparin [9]. These data suggest that protamine itself has independent properties that render platelets dysfunctional.

CPB is associated with several platelet receptor defects, namely decreases in the GPIIbIIIa and the GPIb receptor, which have been characterized by Rinder and colleagues [10] and others. Ferraris and colleagues [11], however, have characterized a thrombin receptor defect that may be responsible for post-CPB bleeding.

Fibrinolysis has adverse effects on platelet function, although its contribution to postoperative blood loss has been diminished through the widespread use of antifibrinolytic agents. Plasmin's effects on platelets are concentration- and temperature-dependent. At low concentrations, plasmin *inhibits* platelet activation induced by thrombin or collagen, except at 22°C, where low concentrations of plasmin fully activate platelets. At high plasmin concentrations, platelets are activated.

A reduced concentration of active GPIb on the platelet surface occurs during CPB. This is probably the result of platelet activation by plasmin and other substances, because platelet activation is known to cause internalization of this receptor. The use of aprotinin and the synthetic antifibrinolytic agents should yield platelet protective effects at least by an indirect mechanism, that of inhibition of plasmin.

Aprotinin also has platelet protective effects that are independent of its ability to inhibit plasmin. These effects include retention of GPIb and GPIIbIIIa receptors on the platelet surface after CPB [12]. Also, aprotinin prevents platelet activation of the protease activated receptor type I (PAR 1) by thrombin [13]. PAR 1 protection renders platelets more functional after CPB.

Materials-induced platelet activation is another component of CPB-induced platelet dysfunction that is seemingly preventable through attenuation of leukocyte-platelet interactions.

ANTI-PLATELET THERAPEUTICS
Glycoprotein IIb/IIIa Receptor Inhibitors
The GPIIb/IIIa receptor on the platelet surface is the base for the fibrin cross-linking responsible for platelet aggregation. Platelet antagonists directly block the fibrinogen receptor on platelets, thereby preventing ligand binding and preventing aggregation. Currently available GPIIb/IIIa antagonists include abciximab (ReoPro, Eli Lilly and Co., Indianapolis, IN), eptifibatide (Integrelin, Millennium Pharmaceuticals, Inc., Cambridge, MA) and tirofiban (Aggrastat, Merck & Co., Inc., Whitehouse Station, NJ).

Abciximab (ReoPro)
Abciximab is a human-murine chimeric monoclonal Fab antibody fragment that binds nonspecifically to the GPIIb/IIIa receptor (the fibrinogen receptor), preventing platelet aggregation. Abciximab is a large molecule. When it binds to the GPIIb/IIIa receptor, it sterically inhibits binding of other ligands to adjacent platelet receptors and thus causes even more profound platelet inhibitory effects. The effective half-life is approximately 12 hours, with approximately 50% inhibition of platelet function remaining 24 hours after stopping the infusion [14]. Once the infusion is stopped, the anticoagulant effects of abciximab *can* be reversed by transfusion of fresh platelets [15], though the already bound platelets remain inhibited during their lifespan.

Eptifibatide (Integrelin) and Tirofiban (Aggrastat)
Eptifibatide is a cyclic heptapeptide based on the KGD amino acid sequence that binds selectively to the GPIIb/IIIa receptor. The effective half-life is approximately 2 hours, with platelet function returning to more than 50% of normal within 4 hours after discontinuation. Despite the short half-life, the effects of eptifibatide are *not* reversible by transfusion of fresh platelets until several hours following discontinuation of the infusion. This is because of the high affinity of drug for the platelet receptor and the binding to transfused platelets if active drug is still circulating. Eptifibatide clearance depends on renal elimination.

Tirofiban is a non-peptide tyrosine derivative that binds selectively to the GPIIb/IIIa receptor and is cleared by way of renal and biliary elimination. Like eptifibatide, the effective half-life is approximately 2 hours and platelet function returns to more than 50% of normal within 4 hours after discontinuation.

The differential ability of platelet transfusion to reverse the effects of these agents stems from the stoichiometric ratios of drug:receptor in vivo. With abciximab, the ratio of drug to receptor is nearly 1:1, because unbound drug is degraded by plasma proteases. Because less than 4% of the administered dose remains unbound after 2 hours, the overall effects of this long-acting and "irreversible" agent can be "reversed" once the infusion is discontinued. In contrast, the short-acting competitive agents eptifibatide and tirofiban continually bind and dissociate from the GPIIb/IIIa receptor and the free drug to receptor ratio is greater than 1:1. Transfused platelets therefore are antagonized by these agents for a few hours following discontinuation of their infusion. Fortunately the short half-life of these two agents makes emergent platelet transfusion a rare and unnecessary action in real life situations; one can simply allow these agents to wear off.

Although some centers reserve the GPIIb/IIIa antagonists for those cases believed to be high risk (eg, acute coronary syndrome, diabetics, bifurcation lesions, re-stentings), some routinely use these potent platelet antagonists during every case, because their use during stenting has been associated with significant reductions in myocardial infarction and ischemic events [16].

Large-scale multicenter studies have shown that re-thrombosis and infarction rates after percutaneous angioplasty and after stent procedures have been reduced with the use of these drugs. Additionally, a decrease in the mortality rate for patients who have diabetes during interventional procedures was demonstrated for abciximab (2.5%) versus placebo (4.5%) [17].

Thienopyridine AntiPlatelet Agents

There are three described ADP receptors on the platelet surface (Fig. 1). Normal activation of one of the ADP receptors (the G protein-linked stimulatory receptor, P2Y1), is responsible for platelet shape change and initiation of aggregation. Maintaining the aggregatory state occurs by stimulating the G protein-linked ADP receptor the P2Y12 receptor. Stimulation of this receptor inhibits

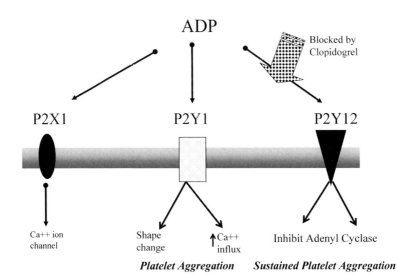

Fig. 1. The three ADP receptors on the platelet surface: P2X1, P2Y1, P2Y12.

adenyl cyclase and inhibits formation of cyclic adenosine monophosphate (cAMP). Inhibition of cAMP allows for platelet activation, increased expression of the GPIIb/IIIa receptor (fibrinogen receptor), and platelet aggregation [18]. The thienopyridines ticlopidine and clopidogrel irreversibly bind to the P2Y12 receptor and prevent platelet activation from being a sustained process. The alteration in the platelet P2Y12 receptor is permanent for the lifespan of the affected platelet.

The thienopyridine ticlopidine hydrochloride (Ticlid, Roche Pharmaceuticals; Nutley, NJ) is rarely used because of undesirable side effects (eg, aplastic anemia, neutropenia, and thrombotic thrombocytopenic purpura) and the need for three-times daily dosing. Its efficacy has been recently compared with equipotent doses of clopidogrel, a drug in the same thienopyridine class. Studies have documented superiority of clopidogrel with respect to prevention of ischemic outcomes. This in combination with a more favorable side effect profile have caused ticlopidine to be replaced with clopidogrel in almost all clinical situations [19].

Clopidogrel bisulfate (Plavix, Sanofi-Aventis, Paris, France) is a thienopyridine pro-drug metabolized by hepatic cytochrome P-450 to an active compound that (like ticlopidine) irreversibly binds the P2Y12 ADP receptor on the platelet's surface, partially blocking platelet activation by ADP [20].

The efficacy of clopidogrel was demonstrated in the CAPRIE trial [21]. The effective half-life of the active metabolite of clopidogrel is short, and daily dosing is required to preserve the overall antiplatelet effects of the agent as new platelets are produced [22]. Although it is believed the antiplatelet activity of clopidogrel lasts nearly 7 days (the lifespan of a platelet), as with aspirin, transfusion of fresh platelets can effectively reverse the antiplatelet effects of clopidogrel on overall hemostatic competence, though circulating platelets already bound with clopidogrel remain inhibited.

Following implantation of a bare metal stent (BMS), the incidence of death, emergent coronary artery bypass grafting (CABG), myocardial infarction (MI), and angiographic stent thrombosis has been demonstrated to be significantly decreased by administration of dual antiplatelet therapy with a thienopyridine plus aspirin, when compared with aspirin alone or aspirin plus Coumadin [23]. It has also been demonstrated that administration of clopidogrel and aspirin before stent placement decreases the overall incidence of MI, death, and the need for target vessel revascularization [24].

The duration of clopidogrel therapy depends not only on the stent (BMS versus drug-eluting stent [DES]), but on the preference of the cardiologist and local patterns of practice. Although manufacturers' recommendations suggest that clopidogrel should be maintained for at least 3 months following placement of a sirolimus-eluting stent, and for at least 6 months following a paclitaxel-eluting stent, different centers have their own maintenance regimens and some interventionalists are recommending that clopidogrel be continued indefinitely, because clopidogrel therapy alone has been shown to decrease the incidence of ischemic stroke, MI, and death in patients who have atherosclerotic disease. The 2005

ACC/AHA/SCAI guidelines recommend 12 months of clopidogrel therapy under ideal circumstances [25]. Rare case reports of in-stent thromboses have been documented more than 1 year after DES implantation when antiplatelet therapy was discontinued [26].

The effects of clopidogrel plus aspirin are not just additive, they are synergistic [27] and this may explain why cardiac surgical patients having received this combination of drugs have excessive postoperative bleeding [28,29]. Patients on these medications who then present for cardiac surgery are at increased risk for bleeding complications. It is in these situations that specific platelet function monitoring could guide platelet transfusion therapy. Alternatively, patients on these medications who do not present for surgery could simply be monitored by specific platelet function testing to best guide therapy for safety and efficacy.

PLATELET FUNCTION TESTING

The ideal platelet function test is one that is measurable at the point-of-care and one that specifically measures the platelet defect in question. Incorporating platelet function testing into blood transfusion algorithms in cardiac surgery has been demonstrated to reduce overall transfusion requirements [30]. Much of this reduction in transfusion arises from eliminating empiric transfusions of platelet concentrates in patients who have received antiplatelet agents. Without a measurable platelet defect, most cardiac surgical patients stop bleeding, if given a modest period of time.

Also, the measure of platelet function preoperatively has a multitude of benefits for general surgical patients. The absence of a defect or demonstration of a minimal defect may allow performing regional anesthetic techniques for patients in whom this is deemed the most suitable anesthetic. The temptation to transfuse these patients with platelet concentrates at the first sign of bleeding also might be avoided.

The bleeding time is a crude test of platelet plug formation that has been of historical and clinical interest. The bleeding time is prolonged in individuals who have received clopidogrel or aspirin; however, the literature so far has not demonstrated an association of the bleeding time with risk for abnormal hemorrhage during or after surgery [31–33]. The physiology of the platelet plug as an isolated event in hemostasis has little to no relationship to the risk for bleeding in the in vivo physiologic situation of surgery or regional anesthesia. The bleeding time is too crude and nonspecific to be used to determine the risk for bleeding in patients having recently been exposed to antiplatelet medication.

Platelet aggregometry can be performed to evaluate certain platelet function abnormalities. These tests use the patient's platelet-rich plasma to which a certain known concentration of the patient's own plasma has been added back to control platelet count. An aggregometer is a warmed chamber through which a light is shone and detected on the other side of the sample. The turbidity of the system and so the density of the platelets determines light transmission.

When a stimulating chemical is added to the system, the platelets begin to clump and precipitate, decreasing the turbidity of the sample. One can perform platelet aggregometry without any in vitro stimulus. Recently it has been shown that if patients have an abnormally fast spontaneous platelet aggregometry, then their risk for MI and unstable angina may be increased [34]. That means that spontaneous platelet aggregometry may be a test for increased platelet activity or "stickiness." Many other compounds can be added as stimuli for platelet aggregometry, including ADP, arachidonic acid, collagen, epinephrine, serotonin, ristocetin, platelet activating factor, fibrinogen, and thromboxane. Although abnormalities may be demonstrated in one or more of these artificially stimulated platelet aggregation tests, it is difficult to infer from any one test a certain increased risk for bleeding. If a specific platelet antagonist drug is being used, then the agonist whose effect on the platelet is inhibited by that drug should be used in the assay. This makes the test specific for measuring drug effects. ADP-stimulated aggregometry thus can be used to measure the platelet inhibitory effects of clopidogrel, and arachidonic acid-stimulated aggregometry for measuring the effects of aspirin. Because these require precise measurement of platelet concentration and resuspension of platelets in plasma, the technician time needed to perform these tests restricts them from being of usefulness during surgery.

THROMBOELASTOGRAPHY

The thromboelastograph (TEG) is a test of whole blood clot strength whose mechanism uses a warmed cup made of disposable plastic. Suspended inside the cup is a piston that does not touch the walls of the cup. The cup moves through an arc of 4.5° once every second, pauses for 1 second, and then moves back through the arc in the opposite direction. There is no connection between the cup and the piston until whole blood is placed in the cup and coagulation begins. A small amount of blood is needed to perform this test (0.36 mL). With the current disposables, an activator is needed because the onset to coagulation varies, probably because of defects in the plastic. Celite, kaolin, or tissue factor have all been used to activate the TEG.

The TEG measures clot strength over time by keeping the piston stable in an electromagnetic field. A paper tracing relates the power necessary to preserve that as the rotational motion of the cup is transferred to the piston. Standard parameters and a signature tracing are generated. The maximum amplitude (MA) measures the maximum clot strength. The TEG examines whole blood coagulation from the time of initiation through acceleration, control, and eventual lysis.

The physical strength of clot depends on the interaction of platelets and fibrin. Work has shown that platelets have approximately twice as much effect on the MA as does the fibrinogen concentration alone [35,36]. Recent work with glycoprotein-blocking agents has shown that the TEG MA relates closely to the dosage of blocking agent administered, whereas the TEG MA has little or no relationship to changes in ADP platelet aggregation [37]. TEG with tissue factor acceleration speeds the appearance of MA and is accurate for monitoring the platelet inhibition by large concentrations of GPIIb/IIIa receptor blockers. Comparison with the baseline MA yields a relative measure of the degree of platelet inhibition. TRAP-induced aggregation correlates strongly with the TEG values measured in this fashion [37].

In native activated form, the TEG is insensitive to the effects of aspirin and clopidogrel, because thrombin formation in the cup is enough to stimulate clot formation even in the presence of antiplatelet drug therapy. The TEG assay, however, can be modified to interrogate the specific pathway of platelet activation that is inhibited by drug therapy.

THROMBOELASTOGRAPHY MODIFICATIONS

The thienopyridine ADP-receptor blockers clopidogrel and ticlopidine are widely used in cardiovascular medicine. The ability to measure the platelet defect induced by these drugs is difficult unless sophisticated laboratory techniques such as ADP-aggregometry are used. Aggregometry yields accurate results; however, it is not readily available in the perioperative period as a point-of-care test. Native TEG analysis does not measure the thienopyridine-induced platelet defect, because forming thrombin in the assay has an overwhelming effect on developing the TEG MA. A modification of the TEG removes thrombin from the assay and studies a non-thrombin clot, strengthened by adding ADP. Fig. 2 depicts the different signature TEG tracings that are used to calculate the platelet contribution to MA when a platelet inhibitor is present. This assay was specifically created to measure the platelet inhibition by ADP antagonists such as clopidogrel. It is commercially referred to as the "Platelet Mapping Assay." The MA_{kh} is the maximal activation of platelets and fibrin and is the largest amplitude that can be achieved. The MA_f is the maximal amplitude that is obtained when a thrombin-depleted fibrin

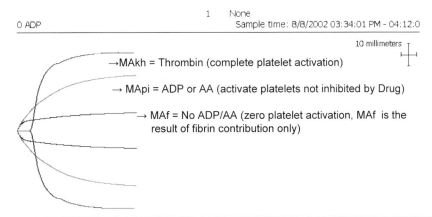

Fig. 2. The different signature TEG tracings that are used to calculate the platelet contribution to MA when a platelet inhibitor is present. (*Courtesy of* Haemoscope Co., Skokie (IL); with permission.)

clot is formed without a platelet contribution. The MA_{pi} is the MA_f contribution plus the platelet contribution. MA_{pi} is created by adding an activator such as ADP to the MA_f assay (for clopidogrel testing). Only platelets that can be activated by ADP contribute to the MA_{pi}. The following formula calculates the percent reduction in platelet activity using this assay.

$$100 - [(MA_{pi} - MA_f)/(MA_{kh} - MA_f)] \times 100$$

Clopidogrel, ticlopidine, and even aspirin inhibition can now be studied at the point-of-care using this modification [38,39]. (This class of drug inhibits platelet aggregation through inhibition of the P2Y12 ADP receptor) (see Fig. 1).

Ultegra (Accumetrics, San Diego, CA), is a point-of-care monitor that was designed specifically to measure the platelet response to a thrombin receptor agonist. This technology, using an adjunctive cartridge containing ADP, was recently approved by the US Food and Drug Administration (FDA) for use as a platelet function assay for measuring the platelet defect of clopidogrel. This activation process is specific for the P2Y12 receptor, which is the ADP receptor blocked by thienopyridine therapy. In whole blood, it measures activation-induced platelet agglutination of fibrinogen-coated beads using an optical detection system. Because of the importance of the GPIIb/IIIa receptor in mediating fibrinogen-platelet interactions, the Ultegra has been especially useful in accurately measuring receptor inhibition in the invasive cardiology patients receiving GPIIb/IIIa inhibiting drugs [14,40]. The platelet inhibition measured by Ultegra has been demonstrated to correlate inversely with adverse outcomes after percutaneous coronary intervention [24,41].

The Platelet Function Analyzer (PFA-100) (Dade Behring, Miami, FL) is a monitor of platelet adhesive capacity that is approved by the US FDA and is valuable in its diagnostic abilities to identify drug-induced platelet abnormalities, von Willebrand disease platelet dysfunction, and other acquired and congenital platelet defects [42,43]. The test is conducted as an adapted in vitro bleeding time. Whole blood is drawn through a chamber by vacuum and is perfused across an aperture in a collagen membrane coated with an agonist (epinephrine or ADP). Platelet adhesion and formation of aggregates seals the aperture, thus signaling the "closure time" measured by the PFA-100. Preliminary evidence with post-CPB sampling and with in vitro addition of glycoprotein IIb/IIIa inhibiting drugs, however, suggests that these closure times may exceed those measurable using standard testing with the PFA-100 [44].

"Platelet Works" Ichor (Array Medical, Somerville, NJ) is a test that uses the principle of the platelet count ratio to assess platelet reactivity. The instrument is a Coulter counter that measures the platelet count in a standard EDTA-containing tube. Platelet count is also measured in tubes containing the platelet agonists ristocetin, ADP, arachidonic acid, or collagen. Addition of blood to these agonist tubes causes platelets to activate, adhere to the tube, and to be effectively eliminated from the platelet count. The ratio of the activated platelet count to the nonactivated platelet count is a function of the reactivity of the platelets. Early investigation in cardiac surgical patients indicates that this assay is useful in providing a platelet count, and that it is capable of measuring the platelet dysfunction that accompanies CPB [45]. The ADP activator tube has been shown to measure the platelet defect in patients receiving clopidogrel therapy. There is also an arachidonic acid tube used to measure the effects of aspirin. Clinical data using the arachidonic acid tube are lacking, but anecdotal use favors the applicability of this test.

It is essential to understand the complex array of hemostatic insults that occur because of extracorporeal circulation before selecting a suitable platelet function monitor during cardiac surgery. Even in hemostatically normal individuals, CPB induces a heparin effect, platelet dysfunction, fibrinolysis, and coagulation factor defects for which there are many clinical laboratory tests available for accurate diagnoses. With the recent increase in prescription of antithrombotic platelet inhibitors, the hemostatic defect after CPB is even more pronounced. When microvascular bleeding does occur, rapid diagnosis and therapeutic intervention are made possible by point-of-care hemostasis testing, which can take place directly in the operating theater. If on-site testing is not available or does not provide sufficient timely information regarding the patient's coagulation defect, transfusion therapy for cardiac surgical patients remains indiscriminate and empiric, at best.

References

[1] Hoffman M. A cell-based model of coagulation and the role of factor VIIa. Blood Rev 2003;17:S1–5.
[2] Michelson AD, MacGregor H, Barnard MR, et al. Reversible inhibition of human platelet activation by hypothermia in vivo and in vitro. Thromb Haemost 1994;71:633–40.
[3] Valeri CR, Bougas JA, Talarico L, et al. Behavior of previously frozen erythrocytes used during open-heart surgery. Transfusion 1970;10:238–46.
[4] Boldt J, Zickmann B, Czeke A, et al. Blood conservation techniques and platelet function in cardiac surgery. Anesthesiology 1991;75:426–32.
[5] Faraday N, Rosenfeld BA. In vitro hypothermia enhances platelet GPIIb-IIIa activation and P-selectin expression. Anesthesiology 1998;88:1579–85.
[6] Upchurch GR, Valeri CR, Khuri SF, et al. Effect of heparin on fibrinolytic activity and platelet function in vivo. Am J Physiol 1996;271:H528–34.
[7] John LC, Rees GM, Kovacs IB. Inhibition of platelet function by heparin. An etiologic factor in postbypass hemorrhage. J Thorac Cardiovasc Surg 1993;105:816–22.
[8] Ammar T, Fisher CF. The effects of heparinase 1 and protamine on platelet reactivity. Anesthesiology 1997;86:1382–6.
[9] Carr ME Jr, Carr SL. At high heparin concentrations, protamine concentrations which reverse heparin anticoagulant effects are insufficient to reverse heparin anti-platelet effects. Thromb Res 1994;75:617–30.
[10] Rinder CS, Mathew JP, Rinder HM, et al. Modulation of platelet surface adhesion receptors during cardiopulmonary bypass. Anesthesiology 1991;75:563–70.
[11] Ferraris VA, Ferraris SP, Singh A, et al. The platelet thrombin receptor and postoperative bleeding. Ann Thorac Surg 1998;65:352–8.
[12] Landis RC, Asimakopoulos G, Poullis M, et al. The antithrombotic and antiinflammatory mechanisms of action of aprotinin. Ann Thorac Surg 2001;72:2169–75.

[13] Poullis M, Manning R, Laffan M, et al. The antithrombotic effect of aprotinin: actions mediated via the protease-activated receptor 1. J Thorac Cardiovasc Surg 2000;120:370–8.

[14] Coller BS, Folts JD, Scudder LE, et al. Antithrombotic effect of a monoclonal antibody to the platelet glycoprotein IIb/IIIa receptor in an experimental animal model. Blood 1986;68:783–6.

[15] Tcheng JE, Campbell ME. Platelet inhibition strategies in percutaneous coronary intervention: competition or coopetition? J Am Coll Cardiol 2003;42:1196–8.

[16] Chan AW, Moliterno DJ, Berger PB, et al. Triple antiplatelet therapy during percutaneous coronary intervention is associated with improved outcomes including one-year survival: results from the Do Tirofiban and ReoProGive Similar Efficacy Outcome Trial (TARGET). J Am Coll Cardiol 2003;42:1188–95.

[17] Bhatt DL, Marso SP, Lincoff AM, et al. Abciximab reduces mortality in diabetics following percutaneous coronary intervention. J Am Coll Cardiol 2000;35:922–8.

[18] Savi P, Herbert JM. Clopidogrel and ticlopidine: P2Y12 adenosine diphosphate-receptor antagonists for the prevention of atherothrombosis. Semin Thromb Hemost 2005;31:174–83.

[19] Bertrand ME, Rupprecht HJ, Urban P, et al. Double-blind study of the safety of clopidogrel with and without a loading dose in combination with aspirin compared with ticlopidine in combination with aspirin after coronary stenting: the Clopidogrel Aspirin Stent International Cooperative Study (CLASSICS). Circulation 2000;102:624–9.

[20] Savi P, Combalbert J, Gaich C, et al. The antiaggregating activity of clopidogrel is due to a metabolic activation by the hepatic cytochrome P450-1A. Thromb Haemost 1994;72:313–7.

[21] Hirsh J, Bhatt DL. Comparative benefits of clopidogrel and aspirin in high-risk patient populations: lessons from the CAPRIE and CURE studies. Arch Intern Med 2004;164:2106–10.

[22] Savi P, Pereillo JM, Uzabiaga MF, et al. Identification and biological activity of the active metabolite of clopidogrel. Thromb Haemost 2000;84:891–6.

[23] Mehta SR, Yusuf S, Peters RJ, et al. Effects of pretreatment with clopidogrel and aspirin followed by long-term therapy in patients undergoing percutaneous coronary intervention: the PCI-CURE study. Lancet 2001;358:527–33.

[24] Steinhubl SR, Berger PB, Mann JT 3rd, et al. Early and sustained dual oral antiplatelet therapy following percutaneous coronary intervention: a randomized controlled trial. JAMA 2002;288:2411–20.

[25] Smith SC, Feldman TE, Hirshfeld JW, et al. ACC/AHA/SCAI 2005 guideline update for percutaneous coronary intervention—summary article: a report of the American College of Cardiology/American Heart Association Task Force on Practice Guidelines. Circulation 2006;113:156–75.

[26] McFadden EP, Stabile E, Regar E, et al. Late thrombosis in drug-eluting coronary stents after discontinuation of antiplatelet therapy. Lancet 2004;364:1519–21.

[27] Herbert JM, Dol F, Bernat A, et al. The antiaggregating and antithrombotic activity of clopidogrel is potentiated by aspirin in several experimental models in the rabbit. Thromb Haemost 1998;80:512–8.

[28] Hongo RH, Ley J, Dick SE, et al. The effect of clopidogrel in combination with aspirin when given before coronary artery bypass grafting. J Am Coll Cardiol 2002;40:231–7.

[29] Purkayastha S, Athanasiou T, Malinovski V, et al. Does clopidogrel affect outcome after coronary artery bypass grafting? A meta-analysis. Heart 2006;92:531–2.

[30] Chen L, Bracey AW, Radovancevic R, et al. Clopidogrel and bleeding in patients undergoing elective coronary artery bypass grafting. J Thorac Cardiovasc Surg 2004;128:425–31.

[31] Rodgers RP, Levin J. Bleeding time revisited. Blood 1992;79:2495–7.

[32] Rodgers RP. Bleeding time tables. A tabular summary of pertinent literature. Semin Thromb Hemost 1990;16:21–138.

[33] Rodgers RP. Supplementary bleeding time bibliography. Semin Thromb Hemost 1990;16: 139–44.
[34] Elwood PC, Beswick AD, Sharp DS, et al. Whole blood impedance platelet aggregometry and ischemic heart disease. The Caerphilly Collaborative Heart Disease Study. Arteriosclerosis 1990;10:1032–6.
[35] Chandler WL. The thromboelastography and the thromboelastograph technique. Semin Thromb Hemost 1995;21(Suppl 4):1–6.
[36] Davis CL, Chandler WL. Thromboelastography for the prediction of bleeding after transplant renal biopsy. J Am Soc Nephrol 1995;6:1250–5.
[37] Khurana S, Mattson JC, Westley S, et al. Monitoring platelet glycoprotein IIb/IIIa-fibrin interaction with tissue factor-activated thromboelastography. J Lab Clin Med 1997;130: 401–11.
[38] Mobley JE, Bresee SJ, Wortham DC, et al. Frequency of nonresponse antiplatelet activity of clopidogrel during pretreatment for cardiac catheterization. Am J Cardiol 2004;93: 456–8.
[39] Shore-Lesserson L, Fischer G, Sanders J, et al. Clopidogrel induces a platelet aggregation defect that is partially mitigated by ex-vivo addition of aprotinin [abstract]. Anesthesiology 2004;101:A-268.
[40] Smith SM, Judge HM, Peters G, et al. Multiple antiplatelet effects of clopidogrel are not modulated by statin type in patients undergoing percutaneous coronary intervention. Platelets 2004;15:465–74.
[41] Steinhubl SR, Talley JD, Braden GA, et al. Point-of-care measured platelet inhibition correlates with a reduced risk of an adverse cardiac event after percutaneous coronary intervention: results of the GOLD (AU-Assessing Ultegra) multicenter study. Circulation 2001;103: 2572–8.
[42] Bock M, De Haan J, Beck KH, et al. Standardization of the PFA-100(R) platelet function test in 105 mmol/l buffered citrate: effect of gender, smoking, and oral contraceptives. Br J Haematol 1999;106:898–904.
[43] Escolar G, Cases A, Vinas M, et al. Evaluation of acquired platelet dysfunctions in uremic and cirrhotic patients using the platelet function analyzer (PFA-100): influence of hematocrit elevation. Haematologica 1999;84:614–9.
[44] Campbell CL, Berger PB, Nuttall GA, et al. Can N-acetylcysteine reverse the antiplatelet effects of clopidogrel? An in vivo and vitro study. Am Heart J 2005;150:796–9.
[45] Carville DG, Schleckser PA, Guyer KE, et al. Whole blood platelet function assay on the ICHOR point-of-care hematology analyzer. J Extra Corpor Technol 1998;30:171–7.

Hematol Oncol Clin N Am 21 (2007) 65–88

HEMATOLOGY/ONCOLOGY CLINICS
OF NORTH AMERICA

Heparin-induced Thrombocytopenia, a Prothrombotic Disease

Jerrold H. Levy, MD[a,b,*], Marcie J. Hursting, PhD[c]

[a]Department of Anesthesiology, Emory University School of Medicine, 1364 Clifton Road N.E., Atlanta, GA 30322, USA
[b]Cardiothoracic Anesthesiology and Critical Care, Emory Healthcare, 1364 Clifton Road N.E., Atlanta, GA 30322, USA
[c]Clinical Science Consulting, 3001 Loveland Cove, Austin, TX 78746, USA

Heparin-induced thrombocytopenia (HIT) is a serious, immune-mediated prothrombotic disease, frequently resulting in limb- or life-threatening thromboembolic complications. Because heparins are used so widely, with more than 12 million patients treated annually in the United States [1], and because HIT all too often manifests devastating thrombotic sequelae [2], this complication of heparin therapy ranks among the most important adverse drug reactions of today. Yearly in the United States, an estimated 600,000 new cases of HIT occur, with as many as 300,000 patients developing thrombotic complications, and 90,000 patients dying [3]. By comparison, approximately 216,000 new cases of invasive breast cancer occurred in the United States in 2004 [3]. HIT is also quite costly. In the United States, the annual total cost when HIT complicates cardiac surgery alone is estimated to be $100 to $300 million, and the potential financial loss is estimated to be $33 to $100 million [4]. To ensure the prompt recognition, diagnosis, and treatment of this prothrombotic condition, increased awareness and a high degree of suspicion are critical. This article discusses the pathogenesis, frequency, presentations, sequelae, diagnosis, and treatment of HIT.

Immune-mediated HIT sometimes has been called HIT type II to distinguish it from so-called HIT type I, a nonimmune-mediated, asymptomatic, transient drop in platelet count that occurs in some heparin-treated patients. Unfractionated heparin is a complex array of larger and smaller molecular weight fractions, of which the large fractions can bind and activate platelets. Now the term

---

Dr. Levy is on the speakers bureau for GlaxoSmithKline. Dr. Hursting has received consultancy fees from GlaxoSmithKline.

*Corresponding author. Department of Anesthesiology, Emory University School of Medicine, 1364 Clifton Road N.E., Atlanta, GA 30322. E-mail address: jerrold.levy@emoryhealthcare.org (J.H. Levy).

0889-8588/07/$ – see front matter
doi:10.1016/j.hoc.2006.11.003

HIT is preferably reserved for the immune-mediated condition [1], and this article adheres to that convention.

PATHOGENESIS AND HEPARIN-PLATELET FACTOR 4 ANTIBODIES

HIT is triggered by heparin usage and mediated by antibodies, typically IgG, to the complex of heparin and platelet factor 4 (PF4) (Fig. 1) [5]. PF4 is a basic protein stored in platelet alpha-granules that can be expressed on the surface of platelets and endothelial cells following platelet activation. Heparins are negatively charged, sulfated gylcosaminoglycans that have high affinity for PF4. When heparin and PF4 bind, a conformational change occurs in PF4, exposing antigenic neoepitopes that promote generation of antiheparin-PF4 antibodies [6].

Some heparin-PF4 antibodies (sometimes called HIT antibodies) are capable of activating platelets by means of their FcγIIa receptors. On the platelet surface, PF4 and unfractionated heparin form ultralarge, stable complexes that presumably enhance the ability of the antibodies to occupy and crosslink the FcγIIa receptors [7]. By contrast, ultralarge complexes form inefficiently with PF4 and low molecular weight heparins and not at all with the pentasaccharide fondaparinux, which may contribute to the relative differences in HIT frequency among these agents (further discussed subsequently). When activated, the platelets release prothrombotic platelet-derived microparticles, and excessive thrombin generation, platelet consumption, thrombocytopenia, and frequently thrombosis follow [8,9]. Processes that further promote

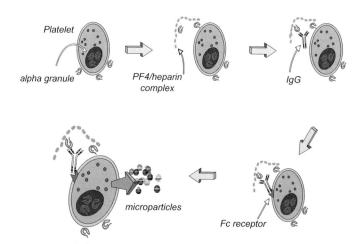

Fig. 1. Pathogenesis of heparin-induced thrombocytopenia. Heparin and platelet factor 4 (PF4) bind, exposing neoepitopes on PF4, which leads to antibody formation. Heparin-PF4 and IgG form immune complexes. The antibody in the immune complex binds to platelet Fc receptors, causing platelet activation. The activated platelet releases prothrombotic microparticles, leading to excessive thrombin generation and often thrombosis.

a prothrombotic state in HIT include tissue factor production, resulting from interactions between the immune complexes and monocytes [10], and antibody-mediated endothelial injury [11].

The prevalence of heparin-PF4 antibodies varies by patient population (cardiac surgery>orthopedic surgery>medical), type of heparin used (bovine unfractionated>porcine unfractionated>low molecular weight), and the assay used to detect the antibodies (antigen>platelet activation) [12–14]. Circulating heparin-PF4 antibodies are present in 2% to 13% of patients who have cardiovascular disease [15,16], 20% to 61% of cardiovascular surgery patients postoperatively [12,13,16–18], 0% to 12% of patients undergoing hemodialysis [19,20], and 7% of emergency department patients presenting with chest pain [21]. On admission to certain intensive care units, 2% of patients have the antibodies, increasing to 10% within a week [22]. Among patients presenting for cardiac catheterization, 3% are seropositive; this percentage increases to 10% within 5 days after catheterization [23].

Not all patients with heparin-PF4 antibodies progress to HIT; in fact, most do not. Antibody features favoring progression to HIT include a high titer and IgG isotype. The antibody's titer (by antigen assay) correlates with its ability to activate platelets [12] and also the extent of in vivo activation of the coagulation and fibrinolytic systems (as measured by prothrombin fragment 1.2, thrombin–antithrombin complex, and D-dimer) [24]. It is controversial if IgA or IgM antibodies mediate HIT in the absence of IgG antibodies [25–27]. PF4 polymorphism does not explain differences in susceptibility to HIT [28]. Limited data suggest that HIT is more likely to occur in women than in men, perhaps owing to increased immune response [25].

Even without inducing thrombocytopenia, heparin-PF4 antibodies are clinically important, increasing morbidity or mortality in various patient populations (Table 1). Rates of myocardial infarction at 30 days [29] and thrombotic outcomes at 1 year [30] are increased significantly in seropositive patients who have acute coronary syndromes without thrombocytopenia. Also among patients with, versus without, heparin-PF4 antibodies, irrespective of platelet count, there are significant increases in the length of hospitalization and in-hospital mortality after cardiac surgery [31], thrombosis in acutely ill pediatric patients [32], and thrombotic events perioperatively in vascular reconstruction patients [33] and postoperatively in orthopedic surgery patients [34]. Associations of seropositivity with thrombotic morbidity [20,35–37] and 2-year mortality [38] have been reported in hemodialysis patients, but they have not been observed consistently in this population [19,39]. Although the pathophysiologic basis of these untoward effects remains to be well characterized, early data suggest that antibody-associated endothelial cell activation plays a role, at least in patients with acute coronary syndromes [40].

Despite their association with long-term adverse effects, circulating heparin-PF4 antibodies are transient, detectable for a median 50 or 85 days by platelet activation or antigen assays, respectively [41].

Table 1
Adverse effects of heparin-PF4 antibodies, in the absence of thrombocytopenia

Patient population	Outcome	Antibody effect (irrespective of presence of thrombocytopenia)	Reference
Acute coronary syndrome	30-day death or MI	OR, 4.0 (95% CI, 1.4–11.3; P = .009)	[29]
	30-day MI	OR, 4.6 (95% CI, 1.4–15.0; P = .011)	[29]
	1-year thrombotic outcome[a]	66% versus 44% (P < .01)	[30]
Cardiovascular surgery	Death or postoperative hospitalization >10 days	OR, 1.98 (95% CI, 1.06–3.62; P = .03)	[31]
	Perioperative thrombotic events	2.6 fold increase	[33]
Orthopedic surgery	Symptomatic thrombosis after postoperative day 4	OR, 15.3 (95% CI, 2.9–25.2; P = .005)	[34]
Pediatrics	Thrombotic event	OR, 34 (95% CI, 4.4–262)	[32]
Hemodialysis	2-year[b] all-cause mortality	HR[b], 2.47 (P = .03)	[38]
	Cardiovascular death	HR[b], 4.14 (P = .02)	[38]
	Thrombotic death	28.6% versus 4.4% (P < .05)	[37]
	Thrombosis or bleeding	60% versus 8.7% (P < .05)	[37]
	Arteriovenous fistula failure	Positive correlation with titer (P < .001)	[36]
	Vascular access thrombosis	Positive correlation with titer (P > .05)	[20]
	Vascular access obstruction	0.49 versus 0.13 events/ year (P = .03)	[35]

Abbreviations: HIT, heparin-induced thrombocytopenia; HR, hazard ratio; MI, myocardial infarction; OR, odds ratio.
[a]Death, MI, recurrent angina, urgent revascularization, or stroke.
[b]Highest tertile of antibody content versus lower tertiles; follow-up for median of 798 days.

FREQUENCY

Patients of any age receiving any type of heparin at any dose by any route of administration are at risk of developing HIT [42]. HIT has been described in association with heparin exposure from a heparin-coated stent [43], a single 5000-unit injection [44], and flushes only [45], from subcutaneous [46] and intravenous [12] administration, and in pediatric [47–49] and elderly [50] patients.

In general though, approximately 0.5% to 5% of heparin-treated patients develop HIT, with the frequency particularly dependent on the patient population and heparin type used (Table 2) [12,14]. Some surgical populations, such as cardiac transplant or neurosurgery patients [51,52], and perhaps certain ethnic groups [53], have a somewhat higher risk. Interestingly, orthopedic surgery patients, compared with cardiac surgery patients, who are receiving unfractionated heparin postoperatively, are less likely to develop heparin-PF4

Table 2
Frequency of heparin-induced thrombocytopenia by patient population and type of heparin

Patient population	Frequency
Cardiac surgery	
Adults (unfractionated heparin postoperatively)	1.0%–2.4%
Pediatrics	1.3%
Orthopedic surgery	
Unfractionated heparin postoperatively	4.8%
Low molecular weight heparin postoperatively	0.6%
Medical	
Cardiovascular or cerebrovascular disease	0.3%–2.5%
Critical care	0.4%
Subcutaneous unfractionated heparin therapy	0.8%
Newly treated with hemodialysis	3.2%
Obstetrics	Rare
Higher risk	
Cardiac transplant	11%
Neurosurgery	15%
Indians	8%
Overall	
In-hospital (surveillance studies)	1.0%–1.2%
Unfractionated heparin (meta-analysis)	2.6%
Low molecular weight heparin (meta-analysis)	0.2%

Adapted from Jang IK, Hursting MJ. When heparins promote thrombosis: a review of heparin-induced thrombocytopenia. Circulation 2005;111:2671–83.

antibodies (14% versus 50% by antigen assay) yet more likely to develop HIT (4.9% versus 1.0%) [12]. Approximately 0.3% to 3% of medical patients receiving heparin therapy develop HIT [15,54–57]. HIT is rare, but has been reported, in obstetric patients [58,59]. Overall, a meta-analysis of studies of heparin thromboprophylaxis demonstrated that the absolute risk of HIT is 2.6% with heparin use and is substantially less, 0.2%, with low-molecular-weight heparins [60]. According to two hospital surveillance studies, each approximately 3 years in duration, 1.0% of all inpatients receiving heparin [61], and 1.2% of patients administered heparin at least 4 days [42], experience HIT.

Owing to the significantly lower frequency of HIT with low molecular weight heparins than unfractionated heparin both overall [60] and in orthopedic surgical patients [12,34], HIT is considered a largely preventable disease, at least for orthopedic patients.

PRESENTATIONS AND SEQUELAE

The clinical manifestations of HIT (ie, thrombocytopenia with or without an accompanying thrombotic event) typically develop 5 to 14 days after initiation of heparin therapy [14,41]. The thrombocytopenia may be relative (a platelet count drop of at least 50% from the preheparin level) or absolute (a count <150 × 10^9/L), and it is typically moderate in severity. In clinical studies in HIT, median platelet counts of approximately 50 to 80 × 10^9/L are reported [48,62,63]. Another temporal presentation of HIT, known as rapid-onset HIT, occurs in the first hours or days after heparin exposure and presumably is caused by enduring heparin-PF4 antibodies (particularly platelet-activating ones) from a previous heparin exposure [41,64]. Rapid-onset HIT, which most often is related to heparin exposure within the previous 3 months, also has been described after a 5.5-month heparin-free interval [65]. Delayed-onset HIT, associated with the presence of highly reactive heparin-PF4 antibodies, occurs days or up to 3 weeks after heparin cessation and often after the patient has been discharged from the hospital [44,66,67]. The patient subsequently re-presents, perhaps to the emergency department [68,69], with symptoms of thrombosis. Thrombocytopenia often, but not always, is present, and heparin re-exposure typically precipitates a rapid decline in the platelet count.

Heparin-induced Thrombocytopenia As a Prothrombotic Disease

HIT is among the more prothrombotic states known, with an odds ratio for thrombosis of 37 (95% confidence interval [CI], 5 to 1638) [70]. For perspective relative to other prothrombotic conditions, the likelihood of thrombosis increases 24 fold with congenital antithrombin deficiency, 14 fold with congenital protein C deficiency, 11 fold with dysfibrinogenemia, sevenfold with factor V Leiden, and fivefold with lupus anticoagulant [71]. No correlation has been detected between the risk of thrombosis in HIT and the presence of either platelet glycoprotein polymorphisms or clotting factor polymorphisms, including factor V Leiden, prothrombin G20210A, and methyltetrahydrofolate reductase C677T [72,73]. It is postulated that the excessive thrombin generated during HIT is so prothrombotic that less pronounced risk factors such as polymorphisms are overshadowed [73].

The thrombotic risk of HIT persists even after platelet counts have returned to normal, which typically occurs within a week of heparin cessation [74,75]. In HIT, there is an approximate 5% to 10% per day risk of a thromboembolic complication in the days immediately following heparin discontinuation [76], reaching a total risk of 38% to 76% at approximately a month [2]. Even for patients with isolated HIT (ie, thrombocytopenia only), the risk of thrombosis in the days to weeks following heparin cessation is 19% to 52% [2,74,77,78]. Patient groups at particular risk of suffering thromboembolic complications include females [73,79,80], orthopedic surgery patients [81,82], and individuals with higher-titer heparin-PF4 antibodies [81,83], more severe thrombocytopenia [80–82], or malignancy [84].

The site of HIT-related thrombotic events appears to be influenced by clinical factors including localized vascular injury. Venous and/or arterial thromboembolic complications occur in HIT, with venous events predominating in surgical patients [78] and arterial events predominating in patients with cardiovascular

disease [85]. Deep venous thrombosis, pulmonary embolism, myocardial infarction, thrombotic stroke, limb artery occlusion requiring amputation, and disseminated intravascular coagulation have been reported [62,63,74,86–88].
In patients who have HIT, a central venous catheter increases the risk of upper
extremity deep venous thrombosis [89], and there is a significantly increased risk
of saphenous vein graft occlusion, but not arterial conduit occlusion, after coronary artery bypass grafting [90].

Other HIT sequelae, each associated with the presence of platelet-activating
heparin-PF4 IgG antibodies, include heparin-induced erythematous or necrotic
skin lesions at a heparin injection site, acute systemic anaphylactoid reactions
following an intravenous heparin bolus, and warfarin-associated venous limb
ischemia [91]. Bleeding is rare in this prothrombotic condition, even if thrombocytopenia is severe. Hemorrhage following infarction and necrosis of the
adrenal glands has been described, however [92]. The thromboembolic complications of HIT contribute to high morbidity and mortality in affected patients.
Approximately 9% to 11% of patients who have HIT and thrombosis lose
a limb, and approximately 17% to 30% die [2,63,74,76].

DIAGNOSIS

The clinical diagnosis of HIT is based on the occurrence of absolute or relative
thrombocytopenia in a patient treated with a heparin product at least 5 days (or
less if there was recent heparin exposure), or acute thrombosis associated with
thrombocytopenia and a similar history, and other causes of thrombocytopenia
excluded. To ensure prompt diagnosis of HIT, routine platelet count monitoring, ideally including a preheparin baseline count, is recommended for patients
with at least a 0.1% risk of HIT, which means most patients receiving heparin
therapy [14,93].

Heparin use and thrombocytopenia are both common in hospitalized patients, and hence their combination does not necessarily indicate HIT. Other
explanations for thrombocytopenia, such as sepsis, perioperative hemodilution,
another drug-induced thrombocytopenia, or nonimmune heparin-associated
thrombocytopenia, should be excluded [91]. Clinical scoring systems have
been proposed to help differentiate patients with HIT from patients with
thrombocytopenia due to other causes. One such system, known as the 4 Ts
[94], awards points based on the degree of thrombocytopenia, timing of the
platelet count fall, presence of thrombosis or other sequelae, and whether other
causes for thrombocytopenia are excluded. A prospective evaluation of this system demonstrated that a low score is generally suitable for excluding HIT,
although the clinical implications of intermediate or high scores differ between
hospitals [95].

HIT also should be considered if a recently hospitalized patient returns
with thromboembolism [66–69]. Because of the pervasive use of heparins,
a fair assumption is that the patient received heparin during the previous
hospitalization [1]. Approximately 10% of patients who present to the emergency department with chest pain and have a history of recent hospitalization

also have heparin-PF4 antibodies [21]. A recent systematic literature review found that 13% of unfractionated heparin-treated patients who developed new or recurrent venous thromboembolism during short-term follow-up (typically in hospital and up to 90 days maximally) had laboratory-confirmed HIT [96].

Laboratory tests are available to confirm HIT, yet results may not be known rapidly. Because of the high risk of thrombosis early in the course of HIT [76] and the increased economic burden associated with delayed treatment [97], initiation of appropriate therapy for suspected HIT should not wait for laboratory confirmation. The College of American Pathologists recommends heparin-PF4 antibody testing for patients suspected of having HIT based on temporal features of the thrombocytopenia or the occurrence of new thrombosis during, or soon after heparin treatment [93]. Antigenic assays, including the ELISA, measure antibodies that are reactive to PF4 complexed with heparin or other polyanions. The ELISA, while having high sensitivity (>90%), also detects antibodies that do not induce HIT (false positives). A more rapid antigenic assay is the particle gel immunoassay, for which heparin-PF4 titers have been shown to correlate with clinical likelihood scores in patients with suspected HIT [98]. Functional tests, including the ^{14}C-serotonin release assay and platelet aggregometry, measure the platelet-activating ability of patient sera in the presence of heparin. The serotonin release assay, which is sensitive and specific (>95%), is rather technically demanding and time-consuming and often used as a confirmatory test only.

TREATMENT

When HIT is strongly suspected (or confirmed), whether or not complicated by thrombosis, all heparins should be stopped, and fast-acting, nonheparin alternative anticoagulation should be initiated immediately [14]. Importantly, heparin cessation alone is not sufficient therapy for this prothrombotic disease, even if a patient is diagnosed with isolated HIT [2,63,74,77,78,86,87]. Rather, prompt alternative anticoagulation is also critical for all presentations of HIT. The dual strategy of stopping heparin plus starting appropriate alternative anticoagulation significantly reduces the untoward outcomes of this prothrombotic disease [63,74,76,80,86,87] and its associated economic burdens [99]. When prompt, appropriate therapy is used for treating HIT patients with thrombosis, the estimated health care cost savings in the United States is approximately $400 million [99].

Low molecular weight heparins, which are less likely than unfractionated heparin to induce heparin-PF4 antibodies but typically cross-react with existing antibodies, should not be used to treat HIT [14]. Warfarin, which paradoxically can worsen the thrombosis and cause venous limb gangrene and skin necrosis, is also not appropriate therapy for acute HIT [14,100,101]. Rather, administration of vitamin K is recommended for patients receiving warfarin when HIT is suspected [14]. Appropriate alternative anticoagulant options, such as approved direct thrombin inhibitors, are discussed subsequently.

Heparins should continue to be avoided after an episode of HIT, at least for as long as heparin-PF4 antibodies are detectable by a sensitive assay [14,41], and many experts prefer longer heparin-free periods [65,102–104]. Patients who have a history of HIT do not invariably, but may, experience recurrent HIT if re-exposed to heparin [41,65]. Indeed, some patients who lack lingering heparin-PF4 antibodies have tolerated brief heparin exposures during cardiac surgery [105]. Until the risks involved with heparin re-exposure in patients who have a history of HIT are understood better, however, many physicians favor alternative, nonheparin anticoagulation when possible, even if the history is remote [65,102–104].

Avoiding heparin is generally possible in most patients, except perhaps in a few clinical situations (eg, cardiac surgery). If heparin exposure is unavoidable or planned, strategies to minimize exposure are recommended, such as using alternative anticoagulation before and after cardiac surgery conducted with heparin [14,106]. In the future, alternative anticoagulation may even be a reasonable option during cardiac surgery, based on the growing experience with bivalirudin in that setting for patients with [107] or without [108] HIT and patients either on or off cardiopulmonary bypass.

For longer term anticoagulation, warfarin can be introduced carefully after adequate alternative parenteral anticoagulation has been provided and after platelet counts have recovered substantially (ie, to 150×10^9/L) [14]. For patients who have isolated HIT, anticoagulation for at least a month is justified on the basis of the increased risk of thrombosis during that period [2]. Warfarin therapy for a minimum of 3 to 6 months is suggested for patients who experience HIT-associated thrombosis [109].

Direct Thrombin Inhibitors

The direct thrombin inhibitors argatroban (Argatroban), lepirudin (Refludan), and bivalirudin (Angiomax) are nonheparin anticoagulants that inhibit thrombin without need of a cofactor and that do not generate or interact with heparin-PF4 antibodies (Table 3) [110]. Argatroban is a hepatically metabolized, synthetic molecule derived from L-arginine. Lepirudin is a renally cleared, recombinant protein derived from leech hirudin, and bivalirudin is a 20-amino acid polypeptide with sequence homology to hirudin that is cleared renally and also undergoes proteolysis. These parenteral agents are monitored routinely using the activated partial thromboplastin time (aPTT), or at higher levels of anticoagulation, the activated clotting time (ACT) for argatroban or bivalirudin, or the ecarin clotting time for lepirudin.

In prospective, historical controlled studies, argatroban [63,74] and lepirudin [86,87,111] significantly improved outcomes in HIT, particularly reducing new thrombosis. Because no approved agent was available for use as a comparator when the studies were conducted, and because placebo control was unethical, historical control groups were used for comparisons. Fig. 2 presents the frequency of new thrombosis (35- to 37-day follow-up) in the control and treatment groups for the pivotal studies of direct thrombin inhibition in HIT.

Table 3
Direct thrombin inhibitors in heparin-induced thrombocytopenia

Property	Argatroban	Lepirudin	Bivalirudin
Molecular weight (Da)	526	6979	2180
Description	Synthetic molecule based on L-arginine	Recombinant hirudin	Polypeptide with sequence homology to hirudin
Primary route of elimination	Hepatic	Renal	Renal and proteolytic
Elimination half-life	39–51 min	1.7 h	36 min
Monitoring	aPTT or ACT	aPTT or ECT	aPTT or ACT
Approved uses in HIT[a]	Prophylaxis or treatment of thrombosis in patients with HIT Patients with or at risk for HIT undergoing PCI	Patients with HIT and associated TEC to prevent further TEC (Not approved for interventional use)	(Not approved for noninterventional use) Patients with or at risk for HIT undergoing PCI
Recommended infusion dosage	2 µg/kg/min, adjusted to achieve aPTTs 1.5 to 3 times the baseline value For PCI: 25 µg/kg/min (350-µg/kg initial bolus), adjusted to achieve ACTs of 300–450 s	0.15 mg/kg/h (0.4-mg/kg initial bolus), adjusted to achieve aPTT ratios of 1.5 to 2.5 —	For PCI: 1.75 mg/kg/h (0.75 mg/kg initial bolus)
Dose reduction recommended	Hepatic impairment	Renal impairment	Renal impairment
Induces antibodies to itself	No	Yes	Unclear
Effect on INR	Yes (sometimes pronounced)	Yes	Yes
Specific antidote	None	None	None

Abbreviations: ACT, activated clotting time; aPTT, activated partial thromboplastin time; ECT, ecarin clotting time; HIT, heparin-induced thrombocytopenia; INR, international normalized ratio; PCI, percutaneous coronary intervention; TEC, thromboembolic complications.
[a] In United States.

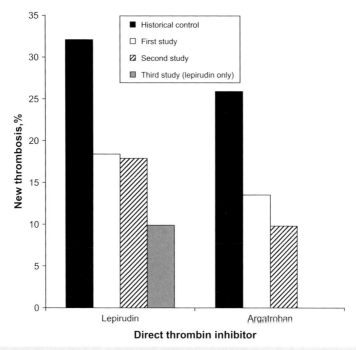

Fig. 2. Reduction of new thrombosis by lepirudin or argatroban therapy in historical controlled studies in HIT. Outcomes were assessed at 35 days (lepirudin studies) or 37 days (argatroban studies). Data sources for the lepirudin studies are as follows: first study (known as HAT-1, n = 71) and historical control (n = 120) [86]; second study (known as HAT-2, n = 95) [87]; third study (known as HAT-3, n = 191) [111]. Data sources for the argatroban studies are as follows: first study (known as Argatroban-911, n = 304) [63], and the second study (known as Argatroban-915, n = 418) and historical control (n = 183) [74].

These studies included 722 argatroban-treated patients (193 controls) and 357 lepirudin-treated patients (120 controls), respectively. In a combined analysis of the argatroban studies [80], the percentage of argatroban-treated patients who remained event-free of a 37-day composite endpoint of death caused by thrombosis, amputation caused by ischemic complications of HIT, or new thrombosis was 91% for individuals who had isolated HIT at enrollment (73% in control, $P < .001$) and 72% for patients who had HIT-associated thrombosis at enrollment (50% in control, $P < .001$). In a meta-analysis of two lepirudin studies in HIT [76], a 35-day composite endpoint of death, amputation, and new thromboembolic complications occurred in 21% of lepirudin-treated patients, compared with 48% of controls ($P = .004$). Major bleeding rates assessed by similar criteria were 6% to 7% with argatroban (7% in control) [63,74] and 13% to 19% with lepirudin (control not reported) [86,87,111].

Argatroban and lepirudin also have been evaluated prospectively in patients who had a history of HIT. In a prospective study of 36 patients who had history of HIT, intravenous argatroban provided adequate acute anticoagulation for venous or arterial thrombosis, without major bleeding or thrombotic complications [103]. In a prospective study of 19 patients who had current or previous HIT, subcutaneous lepirudin supported, without thrombotic or bleeding complications, long-term thromboprophylaxis after passivation of acute thromboembolism [112].

Although there has been no prospective, controlled study of bivalirudin in patients who have HIT, retrospective data describing its use in the noninterventional setting [113,114] and a prospective, open-label study in 52 patients with or at risk of HIT undergoing percutaneous coronary intervention (PCI) [115] have been published. The safety and efficacy of argatroban in patients with or at risk of HIT undergoing PCI were established in three similarly designed, multicenter, open-label prospective studies for which the combined study data of 91 patients were reported [116].

In the United States and other countries, argatroban and lepirudin are approved for use in patients who have HIT (argatroban) or HIT with thrombosis (argatroban and lepirudin). The recommended dosage for lepirudin in HIT with thrombosis is a 0.4 mg/kg initial bolus followed by a 0.15 mg/kg/h infusion (reduced or avoided in patients with renal impairment), adjusted to aPTT ratios of 1.5 to 2.5. Recent data suggest that a reduced initial dose may be safer for minimizing supratherapeutic aPTTs and bleeding risk, without compromising antithrombotic efficacy [117,118]. Lepirudin 0.1 mg/kg/h (without a bolus), adjusted to aPTTs of 1.5 to 2.5 times baseline, has been evaluated in patients who have isolated HIT [119], but it is not approved for use in those patients. Lepirudin was one of the first agents to be approved for HIT, but increased bleeding compared with other agents, refractory bleeding [117,120], and anaphylaxis on re-exposure [121] are complications.

The recommended initial dosage of argatroban for the prophylaxis or treatment of thrombosis in HIT is 2 µg/kg/min (0.5 µg/kg/min in patients who have hepatic impairment), adjusted to achieve aPTTs 1.5 to 3 times the baseline value. Emerging data indicate that a conservative initial dose, such as that recommended in hepatic impairment, may be prudent for patients with heart failure or multiple organ system failure, that is, conditions that may contribute to hepatic congestion and possible reduced argatroban clearance [122,123].

In the United States, argatroban and bivalirudin are approved for use in patients with or at risk of HIT undergoing PCI. The recommended dosage for argatroban during PCI is 25 µg/kg/min (350 µg/kg initial bolus), adjusted to achieve ACTs of 300 to 450 seconds. Lower doses may be adequate if glycoprotein IIb/IIIa receptor inhibitors are coadministered [124]. The recommended dosage for bivalirudin during PCI is an initial 0.75 mg/kg initial bolus followed by a 1.75 mg/kg/h infusion (reduced in patients with renal impairment).

Antithrombin-dependent Alternative Anticoagulants

Danaparoid (Orgaran), a heparinoid, was the first alternative agent approved for use in patients with HIT or a history of HIT in several countries, but it has been unavailable in the United States since 2002. This agent predominantly inhibits factor Xa by means of an antithrombin-dependent mechanism. In vitro cross-reactivity of danaparoid with HIT sera is approximately 10% to 50%, depending on the assay [125], however, for patients with strongly suspected (or confirmed) HIT, whether or not complicated by thrombosis, danaparoid has a Grade 1B recommendation based on ACCP Guidelines [14]. Clinical experience with danaparoid in HIT includes a compassionate use program [125,126], the only randomized clinical trial using dextran 70 as comparator [75], and a retrospective comparative trial with lepirudin [127]. From a summary analysis of 1478 clinical experiences with danaparoid for suspected or confirmed HIT between 1982 and 2004, 83.8% of the patients survived the treatment period; new thromboses developed during 9.7% of treatment episodes, and major bleeding occurred during 8.1% of the treatments [128]. Clinical outcomes of these case reports appear to be comparable with direct thrombin inhibitor therapy, especially when a sufficient danaparoid dosing intensity was used in patients with isolated HIT [128].

Fondaparinux (Arixtra), a synthetic pentasaccharide, is an antithrombin-dependent, selective, factor Xa inhibitor. In vitro cross-reactivity with HIT sera is negligible [129,130]. Fondaparinux induces formation of antibodies reactive with heparin-PF4 at a comparable, low frequency as do low molecular weight heparins. In contrast with low molecular weight heparin-induced antibodies, however, fondaparinux-induced antibodies do not promote HIT. There have been no episodes of HIT associated with fondaparinux use in greater than 1400 prospectively studied, orthopedic patients [131] and greater than 500,000 patients treated worldwide (data on file, GlaxoSmithKline, 2006). These findings suggest that fondaparinux, which is administered as a once-daily subcutaneous injection, may be useful as an alternative anticoagulant in patients who have HIT or a history of HIT, particularly for longer-term, outpatient needs. No prospective, controlled studies have been performed; therefore current data on the use of fondaparinux in HIT are limited yet encouraging [132–134].

Choosing an Alternative Anticoagulant

Key factors affecting the choice of alternative anticoagulant in HIT include its efficacy and safety in the intended use, availability of the drug and methods for its monitoring, and the patient's clinical status, including renal and hepatic function. Although retrospective comparisons of danaparoid and lepirudin [127], of argatroban and lepirudin [135,136], and of argatroban, lepirudin, and bivalirudin [114] have been published, only one prospective study compared danaparoid to dextran 70 [75].

Argatroban is primarily hepatically metabolized, and lepirudin and bivalirudin are primarily renally cleared. Patients who had hepatic impairment have been reported to be treated successfully with reduced doses of argatroban [123], and patients who had renal impairment have been reported to be treated successfully with reduced doses of lepirudin [137] or bivalirudin [113]. Such treatments, however, require careful monitoring and dose adjustments to minimize bleeding risk associated with potential drug accumulation from reduced elimination.

Approximately 50% of lepirudin-treated patients form antilepirudin antibodies that can increase plasma concentrations of lepirudin, and affected patients require careful monitoring and dose adjustments to avoid bleeding complications [138,139]. An estimated 0.2% of patients re-exposed to lepirudin experience anaphylactoid reactions, including possible death; omission of the bolus during lepirudin administration lessens the severity of the adverse reaction [121]. Argatroban, which does not induce antibodies to itself [140], has been used in patients with a history of HIT and anti-lepirudin antibodies [141]. Bivalirudin crossreacts in vitro with approximately 51% of antilepirudin antibodies [142].

Direct thrombin inhibitors as a class prolong the international normalized ratio (INR), and previously established relationships regarding bleeding risk and INRs during warfarin therapy do not apply during direct thrombin inhibition. This effect is particularly pronounced with argatroban [143], wherein INRs greater than 5 commonly occur during argatroban therapy and argatroban-warfarin cotherapy in HIT, without bleeding complications [144]. Methods for monitoring the transition from lepirudin or argatroban to coumarins, including warfarin, using the INR [86,87,145,146] or chromogenic factor Xa assay [147] have been published.

Prospective data on the use of bivalirudin and fondaparinux in HIT are limited, and neither is approved for use in HIT in the noninterventional setting. Bivalirudin has been studied extensively in non-HIT patients with unstable angina undergoing PCI [148], and it is approved in the United States in that setting, as well as in patients with or at risk of HIT undergoing PCI. Danaparoid is unavailable in the United States. Although cross-reactivity with heparin-PF4 antibodies have been reported [125,149], danaparoid use has been reported extensively in this patient population [14,128].

Direct thrombin inhibitors and fondaparinux lack a specific antidote, and danaparoid is neutralized only negligibly by protamine sulfate. If excessive levels of anticoagulation occur, with or without bleeding, the alternative anticoagulant should be stopped or its dose decreased. With argatroban (half-life, 39 to 51 minutes), lepirudin (half-life, 1.7 hours), and bivalirudin (half-life, 36 minutes), anticoagulant effects decrease to baseline typically within hours. This is not the case with danaparoid (half-life, 7 hours) or fondaparinux (half-life, 15 hours). Hemodialysis or hemofiltration sometimes reduces levels of lepirudin or bivalirudin [150]; high-flux, dialytic clearance of argatroban is clinically insignificant [151]. Recombinant factor VIIa has been used to treat severe bleeding in HIT patients who received direct thrombin inhibition [47,152] and also to reverse the effects of fondaparinux in healthy volunteers [153]. Fresh-frozen plasma also has been reported to be a nonspecific antidote following accidental overdose [154].

Prospective evaluation of the safety and efficacy of alternative anticoagulants in pediatric patients with HIT has not been reported, although a retrospective analysis [48] indicates that their use indeed reduces adverse outcomes in these patients. Single-center experiences [47], literature analyses [48,49], and case studies [155,156] provide limited guidance for alternative anticoagulant dosing in the pediatric HIT patient.

FUTURE DIRECTIONS

There is a growing body of literature indicating that heparin-platelet factor 4 antibodies are pathologic, irrespective of their ability to induce HIT. Studies are warranted to better characterize these adverse effects and their pathophysiologic basis and also to investigate the benefits and risks of antithrombotic therapy in seropositive patients without HIT.

Despite the availability of safe, effective treatment options for the patient who has HIT, the morbidity and mortality associated with this prothrombotic disease have not been eliminated. Continued research to identify additional therapies based on refined understandings of the pathophysiology of HIT is warranted [5,157]. Consideration should be given not only to treatment options but also to prevention approaches. Additional strategies to minimize heparin exposure, such as reconsidering routine use of heparin flush [45], and to minimize risk when heparins are administered, such as using porcine heparin rather than bovine heparin [13], and low-molecular-weight heparins rather than unfractionated heparin [34], are needed. Increasingly, unfractionated heparin is being replaced in various clinical settings by agents that are less likely or incapable of inducing heparin-PF4 antibodies or HIT (eg, low-molecular-weight heparins, direct thrombin inhibitors, and selective factor X inhibitors). Hopefully, as fewer patients are placed at risk, the burdens of HIT will be lessened further. This remains to be evaluated prospectively.

SUMMARY

Heparin-induced thrombocytopenia is a serious, yet treatable prothrombotic disease that dramatically increases a patient's risk of thrombosis (odds ratio, 37). This immune-mediated complication of heparin exposure occurs in approximately 0.5% to 5% of heparin-treated patients, and if left untreated, 38% to 76% of affected patients suffer thromboembolic complications within a month. The antibodies that mediate HIT (ie, heparin-PF4 antibodies) occur even more frequently than the overt disease itself, yet even in the absence of thrombocytopenia, they are associated with increased thrombotic morbidity and mortality.

Vigilance in monitoring the platelet count in heparin-treated patients is important for the prompt recognition of HIT. HIT should be suspected whenever the platelet count drops more than 50% from baseline (or to <150 × 10^9/L) beginning 5 to 14 days after starting heparin (or sooner if there was recent heparin exposure) and/or new thrombosis occurs during, or soon after heparin treatment, with other causes excluded. Laboratory tests for the presence (antigen) or platelet-activating ability (function) of heparin-PF4 antibodies are available for confirming HIT, but initiation of treatment should not be delayed pending the results. Rather, when HIT is strongly suspected, with or without complicating thrombosis, heparins should be discontinued immediately, and a fast-acting, nonheparin alternative anticoagulant should be initiated.

The choice of alternative anticoagulant should consider its efficacy and safety in the intended use, its availability, and the patient's clinical status including renal and hepatic function. In North America, the direct thrombin inhibitors argatroban and lepirudin are approved for use in HIT, and in the United States, argatroban and the direct thrombin inhibitor bivalirudin are approved for use in patients with or at risk for HIT undergoing PCI. Danaparoid, an antithrombin-dependent heparinoid, is approved for use in HIT in several countries (unavailable in the United States). Experience in treating HIT patients with fondaparinux is limited yet appears promising and needs further evaluation.

With prompt diagnosis of HIT and initiation of appropriate treatment, the adverse outcomes and economic burdens of this prothrombotic disease are reduced significantly. Future studies to identify means to further reduce or prevent these burdens and also to better characterize the pathologic nature of heparin-PF4 antibodies are warranted.

References

[1] Rice L. Heparin-induced thrombocytopenia. Myths and misconceptions (that will cause trouble for you and your patient). Arch Intern Med 2004;164:1961–4.

[2] Hirsh J, Heddle N, Kelton JG. Treatment of heparin-induced thrombocytopenia: a critical review. Arch Intern Med 2004;164:361–9.

[3] Levine RL. Finding haystacks full of needles. From Opus to Osler [editorial]. Chest 2005; 127:1488–90.

[4] Frame JN. The heparin-induced thrombocytopenia task force model: implementing quality improvement and economic outcome initiatives. Semin Hematol 2005;42:S28–35.

[5] Kelton JG. The pathophysiology of heparin-induced thrombocytopenia. Biological basis for treatment. Chest 2005;127:9S–20S.

[6] Horsewood P, Warkentin TE, Hayward CPM, et al. The epitope specificity of heparin-induced thrombocytopenia. Br J Haematol 1996;95:161–7.

[7] Rauova L, Poncz M, McKenzie SE, et al. Ultralarge complexes of PF4 and heparin are central to the pathogenesis of heparin-induced thrombocytopenia. Blood 2005;105:131–8.

[8] Chong BH, Fawaz I, Chesterman CN, et al. Heparin-induced thrombocytopenia: mechanism of interaction of the heparin-dependent antibody with platelets. Br J Haematol 1989;73:235–40.

[9] Warkentin TE, Hayward CPM, Boshkov LK, et al. Sera from patients with heparin-induced thrombocytopenia generate platelet-derived microparticles with procoagulant activity: an explanation for the thrombotic complications of heparin-induced thrombocytopenia. Blood 1994;84:3691–9.

[10] Arepally GM, Mayer IM. Antibodies from patients with heparin-induced thrombocytopenia stimulate monocytic cells to express tissue factor and secrete interleukin 8. Blood 2001;98:1252–4.

[11] Cines DB, Tomaski A, Tannenbaum S. Immune endothelial cell injury in heparin-associated thrombocytopenia. N Engl J Med 1987;316:581–9.

[12] Warkentin TE, Sheppard JI, Horsewood P, et al. Impact of the patient population on the risk for heparin-induced thrombocytopenia. Blood 2000;96:1703–8.

[13] Francis JL, Palmer GJ, Moroose R, et al. Comparison of bovine and porcine heparin in heparin antibody formation after cardiac surgery. Ann Thorac Surg 2003;75:17–22.

[14] Warkentin TE, Greinacher A. Heparin-induced thrombocytopenia: recognition, treatment, and prevention. Chest 2004;126:311S–37S.

[15] Kappers-Klunne MC, Boon DM, Hop WC, et al. Heparin-induced thrombocytopenia and thrombosis: a prospective analysis of the incidence in patients with heart and cerebrovascular diseases. Br J Haematol 1997;96:442–6.

[16] Everett BM, Foo SY, Criss D, et al. The prevalence of heparin/platelet factor 4 antibody is high in patients presenting for cardiac surgery and more than doubles after surgery [abstract]. Presented at the 77th Annual Scientific Sessions of the American Heart Association. New Orleans, LA, November 7, 2004.

[17] Visentin GP, Malik M, Cyganiak KA, et al. Patients treated with unfractionated heparin during open heart surgery are at high risk to form antibodies reactive with heparin:platelet factor 4 complexes. J Lab Clin Med 1996;128:376–83.

[18] Lindhoff-Last E, Eichler P, Stein M, et al. A prospective study on the incidence and clinical relevance of heparin-induced antibodies in patients after vascular surgery. Thromb Res 2000;97:387–93.

[19] O'Shea SI, Sands JJ, Nudo SA, et al. Frequency of antiheparin-platelet factor 4 antibodies in hemodialysis patients and correlation with recurrent vascular access thrombosis. Am J Hematol 2002;69:72–3.

[20] Yu A, Jacobson SH, Bygden A, et al. The presence of heparin-platelet factor 4 antibodies as a marker of hypercoagulability during hemodialysis. Clin Chem Lab Med 2002;40: 21–6.

[21] Francis JL, Drexler A, Walker JM, et al. Frequency of heparin–platelet factor 4 antibodies in patients with acute coronary syndromes presenting to the emergency department [abstract]. Blood 2004;104(Pt 1):569a.

[22] Hergenroeder GW, Francis JL, Miller CC, et al. Prevalence of heparin antibodies in intensive care unit patients (The HAICU study) [abstract]. Blood 2005;106(Pt 2):82b.

[23] Foo SY, Everett BM, Yeh R, et al. Prevalence of heparin-induced thrombocytopenia in patients undergoing cardiac catheterization. Am Heart J 2006;152:e1–7.

[24] Chilver-Stainer L, Lammle B, Alberio L. Titre of anti-heparin/PF4 antibodies and extent of in vivo activation of the coagulation and fibrinolytic systems. Thromb Haemost 2004;91: 276–82.

[25] Warkentin TE. Heparin-induced thrombocytopenia: pathogenesis and management. Br J Haematol 2003;121:535–55.

[26] Juhl D, Eichler P, Lubenow N, et al. Incidence and clinical significance of anti-PF4/heparin antibodies of the IgG, IgG, and IgA class in 755 consecutive patient samples referred for diagnostic testing for heparin-induced thrombocytopenia. Eur J Haematol 2006;76: 420–6.

[27] Amiral J, Wolf M, Fischer A, et al. Pathogenicity of IgA and/or IgM antibodies to heparin-PF4 complexes in patients with heparin-induced thrombocytopenia. Br J Haematol 1996; 92:954–9.

[28] Horsewood P, Kelton JG. Investigation of a platelet factor 4 polymorphism on the immune response in patients with heparin-induced thrombocytopenia. Platelets 2000;11:23–7.

[29] Williams RT, Damaraju LV, Mascelli MA, et al. Anti-platelet factor 4/heparin antibodies: an independent predictor of 30-day myocardial infarction after acute coronary ischemic syndromes. Circulation 2003;107:2307–12.

[30] Mattioli AV, Bonetti L, Sternieri S, et al. Heparin-induced thrombocytopenia in patients treated with unfractionated heparin: prevalence of thrombosis in a 1 year follow-up. Ital Heart J 2000;1:39–42.

[31] Bennett-Guerrero E, Slaughter TF, White WD, et al. Preoperative anti-PF4/heparin antibody level predicts adverse outcome after cardiac surgery. J Thorac Cardiovasc Surg 2005;130:1567–72.

[32] Risch L, Fischer JE, Schmugge M, et al. Association of anti-heparin platelet factor 4 antibody levels and thrombosis in pediatric intensive care patients without thrombocytopenia. Blood Coagul Fibrinolysis 2003;14:113–6.

[33] Calaitges JG, Liem TK, Spadone D, et al. The role of heparin-associated antiplatelet antibodies in the outcome of arterial reconstruction. J Vasc Surg 1999;29:779–85.

[34] Greinacher A, Eichler P, Lietz T, et al. Replacement of unfractionated heparin by low molecular weight heparin for postorthopedic surgery antithrombotic prophylaxis lowers the overall risk of symptomatic thrombosis because of a lower frequency of heparin-induced thrombocytopenia [letter]. Blood 2005;106:2921–2.

[35] Lee EY, Hwang KY, Yang JO, et al. Antiheparin platelet factor 4 antibody is a risk factor for vascular access obstruction in patients undergoing hemodialysis. J Korean Med Sci 2003;18:69–72.

[36] Nakamoto H, Shimada Y, Kanno T, et al. Role of platelet factor 4-heparin complex antibody (HIT antibody) in the pathogenesis of thrombotic episodes in patients on hemodialysis. Hemodial Int 2005;9(Suppl 1):S2–7.

[37] Mureebe L, Coats RD, Silliman WR, et al. Heparin-associated antiplatelet antibodies increase morbidity and mortality in hemodialysis patients. Surgery 2004;136:848–53.

[38] Pena de la Vega L, Miller RS, Benda MM, et al. Association of heparin-dependent antibodies and adverse outcomes in hemodialysis patients: a population-based study. Mayo Clin Proc 2005;80:995–1000.

[39] Skouri H, Gandouz R, Abroug S, et al. A prospective study of the prevalence of heparin-induced antibodies and other associated thromboembolic risk factors in pediatric patients undergoing hemodialysis. Am J Hematol 2006;81:328–34.

[40] Mascelli MA, Deliargyris EN, Damaraju LV, et al. Antibodies to platelet factor 4-heparin are associated with elevated endothelial cell activation markers in patients with acute coronary ischemic syndromes. J Thromb Thrombolysis 2004;18:171–5.

[41] Warkentin TE, Kelton JG. Temporal aspects of heparin-induced thrombocytopenia. N Engl J Med 2001;344·1286–92.

[42] Shuster TA, Silliman WR, Coats RD, et al. Heparin-induced thrombocytopenia: twenty-nine years later. J Vasc Surg 2003;38:1316–22.

[43] Cruz D, Karlsberg R, Takano Y, et al. Subacute stent thrombosis associated with heparin-coated stent and heparin-induced thrombocytopenia. Catheter Cardiovasc Interv 2003;58:80–3.

[44] Warkentin TE, Bernstein RA. Delayed-onset heparin-induced thrombocytopenia and cerebral thrombosis after a single administration of unfractionated heparin. N Engl J Med 2003;348:1067–8.

[45] McNutly I, Katz E, Kim KY. Thrombocytopenia following heparin flush. Prog Cardiovasc Nurs 2005;20:143–7.

[46] Hruskesky WJ. Subcutaneous heparin-induced thrombocytopenia. Arch Intern Med 1978;138:1489–91.

[47] Alsoufi B, Boshkov LK, Kirby A, et al. Heparin-induced thrombocytopenia (HIT) in pediatric cardiac surgery: an emerging cause of morbidity and mortality. Semin Thorac Cardiovasc Surg Pediatr Card Surg Annu 2004;7:155–71.

[48] Risch L, Fischer JE, Herklotz R, et al. Heparin-induced thrombocytopenia in paediatrics: clinical characteristics, therapy and outcomes. Intensive Care Med 2004;30:1615–24.

[49] Hursting MJ, Dubb J, Verme-Gibboney CN. Argatroban anticoagulation in pediatric patients: a literature analysis. J Pediatr Hematol Oncol 2006;28:4–10.

[50] Tardy-Poncet B, Tardy B. Heparin-induced thrombocytopenia. Minimizing the risks in the elderly patient. Drugs Aging 2000;16:351–64.

[51] Hourigan LA, Walters DL, Keck SA, et al. Heparin-induced thrombocytopenia: a common complication in cardiac transplant recipients. J Heart Lung Transplant 2002;21:1283–9.

[52] Hoh BL, Aghi M, Pryor JC, et al. Heparin-induced thrombocytopenia type II in subarachnoid hemorrhage patients: incidence and complications. Neurosurgery 2005;57:243–8.

[53] Saxena R, Batra VV, Ahmed RPH. Heparin-induced thrombocytopenia: prevalence in India [letter]. Am J Hematol 2001;68:215–7.

[54] Verma AK, Levine M, Shalansky SJ, et al. Frequency of heparin-induced thrombocytopenia in critical care patients. Pharmacotherapy 2003;23:745–53.

[55] Girolami B, Prandoni P, Stefani PM, et al. The incidence of heparin-induced thrombocytopenia in hospitalized medical patients treated with subcutaneous unfractionated heparin: a prospective cohort study. Blood 2003;101:2955–9.

[56] Yamamoto S, Koide M, Matsuo M, et al. Heparin-induced thrombocytopenia in hemodialysis patients. Am J Kidney Dis 1996;28:82–5.

[57] Harbrecht U, Bastians B, Kredteck A, et al. Heparin-induced thrombocytopenia in neurologic disease treated with unfractionated heparin. Neurology 2004;62:657–9.

[58] Gill J, Kovacs MJ. Successful use of danaparoid in treatment of heparin-induced thrombocytopenia during twin pregnancy. Obstet Gynecol 1997;90:648–50.

[59] Fausett MB, Vogtlander M, Lee RM, et al. Heparin-induced thrombocytopenia is rare in pregnancy. Am J Obstet Gynecol 2001;185:148–52.

[60] Martel N, Lee J, Wells PS. Risk for heparin-induced thrombocytopenia with unfractionated and low molecular weight heparin thromboprophylaxis: a meta-analysis. Blood 2005; 106:2710–5.

[61] Andreescu AC, Possidente C, Hsieh M, et al. Evaluation of a pharmacy-based surveillance program for heparin-induced thrombocytopenia. Pharmacotherapy 2002;20:974–80.

[62] Warkentin TE. Heparin-induced thrombocytopenia: a clinicopathologic syndrome. Thromb Haemost 1999;82:439–47.

[63] Lewis BE, Wallis DE, Berkowitz SD, et al. Argatroban anticoagulant therapy in patients with heparin-induced thrombocytopenia. Circulation 2001;103:1838 43.

[64] Lubenow N, Kempf R, Fichner A, et al. Heparin-induced thrombocytopenia: temporal pattern of thrombocytopenia in relation to initial use or re-exposure to heparin. Chest 2002;122:37–42.

[65] DeEugenio DL, Ruggiero N, Thomson LJ, et al. Early-onset heparin-induced thrombocytopenia after a 165-day heparin-free interval: case report and review of the literature. Pharmacotherapy 2005;25:615–9.

[66] Warkentin TE, Kelton JG. Delayed-onset heparin-induced thrombocytopenia and thrombosis. Ann Intern Med 2001;135:502–6.

[67] Rice L, Attisha WK, Drexler A, et al. Delayed-onset heparin-induced thrombocytopenia. Ann Intern Med 2002;136:210–5.

[68] Smythe MA, Stephens JL, Mattson JC. Delayed-onset heparin-induced thrombocytopenia. Ann Emerg Med 2005;45:417–9.

[69] Levine RL, Hursting MJ, Drexler A, et al. Heparin-induced thrombocytopenia in the emergency department. Ann Emerg Med 2004;44:511–5.

[70] Warkentin TE, Levine MN, Hirsh J, et al. Heparin-induced thrombocytopenia in patients treated with low molecular weight heparin or unfractionated heparin. N Engl J Med 1995;332:1330–5.

[71] Warkentin TE. Clinical picture of HIT. In: Warkentin TE, Greinacher A, editors. Heparin-induced thrombocytopenia. 3rd edition. New York: Marcel Dekker; 2004. p. 53–106.

[72] Lee DH, Warkentin TE, Denomme GA, et al. Factor V Leiden and thrombotic complications in heparin-induced thrombocytopenia. Thromb Haemost 1998;79:50–3.

[73] Carlsson LE, Lubenow N, Blumentritt C, et al. Platelet receptor and clotting factor polymorphisms as genetic risk factors for thromboembolic complications in heparin-induced thrombocytopenia. Pharmacogenetics 2003;13:253–8.

[74] Lewis BE, Wallis DE, Leya F, et al. Argatroban anticoagulation in patients with heparin-induced thrombocytopenia. Arch Intern Med 2003;163:1849–56.

[75] Chong BH, Gallus AS, Cade JF, et al. Prospective randomized open-label comparison of danaparoid with dextran 70 in the treatment of heparin-induced thrombocytopenia with thrombosis. Thromb Haemost 2001;86:1170–5.

[76] Greinacher A, Eichler P, Lubenow N, et al. Heparin-induced thrombocytopenia with thromboembolic complications: meta-analysis of 2 prospective trials to assess the value of parenteral treatment with lepirudin and its therapeutic aPTT range. Blood 2000;96: 846–51.

[77] Wallis DE, Workman DL, Lewis BE, et al. Failure of early heparin cessation as treatment for heparin-induced thrombocytopenia. Am J Med 1999;106:629–35.

[78] Warkentin TE, Kelton JG. A 14-year study of heparin-induced thrombocytopenia. Am J Med 1996;101:502–7.

[79] LaMonte MP, Brown PM, Hursting MJ. Stroke in patients with heparin-induced thrombocytopenia and the effect of argatroban therapy. Crit Care Med 2004;32:976–80.

[80] Lewis BE, Wallis DE, Hursting MJ, et al. Effects of argatroban therapy, demographic variables, and platelet count on thrombotic risks in heparin-induced thrombocytopenia. Chest 2006;129:1407–16.

[81] Fabris F, Luzzatto G, Soini B, et al. Risk factors for thrombosis in patients with immune-mediated heparin-induced thrombocytopenia. J Intern Med 2002;252:149–54.

[82] Greinacher A, Farner B, Kroll H, et al. Clinical features of heparin-induced thrombocytopenia including risk factors for thrombosis. Thromb Haemost 2005;94:132–5.

[83] Zwicker JI, Uhl L, Huang WY, et al. Thrombosis and ELISA optical density values in hospitalized patients with heparin-induced thrombocytopenia. J Thromb Haemost 2004;2: 2133–7.

[84] Opatrny L, Warner MN. Risk of thrombosis in patients with malignancy and heparin-induced thrombocytopenia. Am J Hematol 2004;76:240–4.

[85] Boskhov LK, Warkentin TE, Hayward CPM, et al. Heparin-induced thrombocytopenia and thrombosis: clinical and laboratory studies. Br J Haematol 1993;84:322–8.

[86] Greinacher A, Volpel H, Janssens U, et al. Recombinant hirudin (lepirudin) provides safe and effective anticoagulation in patients with heparin-induced thrombocytopenia: a prospective study. Circulation 1999;99:73–80.

[87] Greinacher A, Janssens U, Berg G, et al. Lepirudin (recombinant hirudin) for parenteral anticoagulation in patients with heparin-induced thrombocytopenia. Circulation 1999;100: 587–93.

[88] Mukundan S, Zeigler ZR. Direct antithrombin agents ameliorate disseminated intravascular coagulation in suspected heparin-induced thrombocytopenia thrombosis syndrome. Clin Appl Thromb Hemost 2002;8:287–9.

[89] Hong AP, Cook DJ, Sigouin CS, et al. Central venous catheters and upper-extremity deep-vein thrombosis complicating immune heparin-induced thrombocytopenia. Blood 2003; 101:3049–51.

[90] Liu JC, Lewis BE, Steen LH, et al. Patency of coronary artery bypass grafts in patients with heparin-induced thrombocytopenia. Am J Cardiol 2002;89:979–81.

[91] Warkentin TE. New approaches to the diagnosis of heparin-induced thrombocytopenia. Chest 2005;127(2 Suppl):35S–45S.

[92] Warkentin TE, Sikov WM, Lillicrap DP. Multicentric warfarin-induced skin necrosis complicating heparin-induced thrombocytopenia. Am J Hematol 1999;62:44–8.

[93] Warkentin TE. Platelet count monitoring and laboratory testing for heparin-induced thrombocytopenia: recommendations of the College of American Pathologists. Arch Pathol Lab Med 2002;126:1415–23.

[94] Warkentin TE, Aird WC, Rand JH. Platelet-endothelial interactions: sepsis, HIT, and antiphospholipid syndrome. Hematology Am Soc Hematol Educ Program 2003:497–519.

[95] Lo GK, Juhl D, Warkentin TE, et al. Evaluation of pretest clinical score (4 Ts) for the diagnosis of heparin-induced thrombocytopenia in two clinical settings. J Thromb Haemost 2006;4:759–65.

[96] Levine RL, McCollum D, Hursting MJ. How frequently is venous thromboembolism in heparin-treated patients associated with heparin-induced thrombocytopenia? Chest 2006;130:681–7.

[97] Arnold RJ, Kim R, Tang B. The cost-effectiveness of argatroban treatment in heparin-induced thrombocytopenia: the effect of early versus delayed treatment. Cardiol Rev 2006;14: 7–13.

[98] Alberio L, Kimmerle S, Baumann A, et al. Rapid determination of antiheparin/platelet factor 4 antibody titers in the diagnosis of heparin-induced thrombocytopenia. Am J Med 2003;114:528–36.

[99] Arnold R, Kim R, Zhou Y, et al. Budgetary impact of heparin-induced thrombocytopenia with thrombosis and treatment with the direct thrombin inhibitor argatroban [abstract]. Presented at the 39th Annual Meeting of the American Society of Health-System Pharmacists Midyear Clinical Meeting. Orlando, FL, December 8, 2004. P401E.

[100] Warkentin TE, Elavathil LJ, Hayward CPM, et al. The pathogenesis of venous limb gangrene associated with heparin-induced thrombocytopenia. Ann Intern Med 1997;127: 804–12.

[101] Srinivasan AF, Rice L, Bartholomew JR, et al. Warfarin-induced skin necrosis and venous limb gangrene in the setting of heparin-induced thrombocytopenia. Arch Intern Med 2004;164:66–70.

[102] Alving BM. How I treat heparin-induced thrombocytopenia and thrombosis. Blood 2003;101:21–37.

[103] Matthai WH, Lewis BE, Hursting MJ, et al. Argatroban anticoagulation in patients with a history of heparin-induced thrombocytopenia. Thromb Res 2005;116:121–6.

[104] Hassell K. The management of patients with heparin-induced thrombocytopenia who require anticoagulant therapy. Chest 2005;127:1S–8S.

[105] Potzsch B, Klovekorn WP, Madlener K. Use of heparin during cardiopulmonary bypass in patients with a history of heparin-induced thrombocytopenia [letter]. N Engl J Med 2000;343:515.

[106] Warkentin TE, Greinacher A. Heparin-induced thrombocytopenia and cardiac surgery. Ann Thorac Surg 2003;76:638–48.

[107] Dyke CM, Koster A, Veale JJ, et al. Preemptive use of bivalirudin for urgent on-pump coronary artery bypass grafting in patients with potential heparin-induced thrombocytopenia. Ann Thorac Surg 2005;80:299–303.

[108] Dyke CM, Smedira NG, Koster A, et al. A comparison of bivalirudin to heparin with protamine reversal in patients undergoing cardiac surgery with cardiopulmonary bypass: the EVOLUTION-ON study. J Thorac Cardiovasc Surg 2006;131:533–9.

[109] Greinacher A, Warkentin TE. Treatment of heparin-induced thrombocytopenia: an overview. In: Warkentin TE, Greinacher A, editors. Heparin-induced thrombocytopenia. 3rd edition. New York: Marcel Dekker; 2004. p. 335–70.

[110] Walenga JM, Kozu MJ, Lewis BE, et al. Relative heparin-induced thrombocytopenic potential of low molecular weight heparins and new antithrombotic agents. Clin Appl Thromb Hemost 1996;2(Suppl 1):S21–7.

[111] Greinacher A. Lepirudin for the treatment of heparin-induced thrombocytopenia. In: Warkentin TE, Greinacher A, editors. Heparin-induced thrombocytopenia. 3rd edition. New York: Marcel Dekker; 2004. p. 397–436.

[112] Huhle G, Hoffman U, Hoffman I, et al. A new therapeutic option by subcutaneous recombinant hirudin in patients with heparin-induced thrombocytopenia type II: a pilot study. Thromb Res 2000;99:325–34.

[113] Kiser TH, Fish DN. Evaluation of bivalirudin treatment for heparin-induced thrombocytopenia in critically ill patients with hepatic and/or renal dysfunction. Pharmacotherapy 2006;26:452–60.

[114] Dang CH, Durkalski VL, Nappi JM. Evaluation of treatment with direct thrombin inhibitors in patients with heparin-induced thrombocytopenia. Pharmacotherapy 2006;26: 461–8.

[115] Mahaffey KW, Lewis BE, Wildermann NM, et al. The anticoagulant therapy with bivalirudin to assist in the performance of percutaneous coronary intervention in patients with

heparin-induced thrombocytopenia (ATBAT) study: main results. J Invasive Cardiol 2003;
15:611–6.

[116] Lewis BE, Matthai WH, Cohen M, et al. Argatroban anticoagulation during percutaneous coronary intervention in patients with heparin-induced thrombocytopenia. Catheter Cardiovasc Interv 2002;57:177–84.

[117] Tardy B, Lecompte T, Boelhen F. Predictive factors for thrombosis and major bleeding in an observational study in 181 patients with heparin-induced thrombocytopenia treated with lepirudin. Blood 2006;108:1492–6.

[118] Lubenow N, Eichler P, Lietz T, et al. Lepirudin in patients with heparin-induced thrombocytopenia—results of the third prospective study (HAT-3) and a combined analysis of HAT-1, HAT-2, and HAT-3. J Thromb Haemost 2005;3:2428–36.

[119] Lubenow N, Eichler P, Lietz T, et al. Lepirudin for prophylaxis of thrombosis in patients with acute isolated heparin-induced thrombocytopenia: an analysis of three prospective studies. Blood 2004;104:3072–7.

[120] Oh JJ, Akers WS, Lewis D, et al. Recombinant factor VIIa for refractory bleeding after cardiac surgery secondary to anticoagulation with the direct thrombin inhibitor lepirudin. Pharmacotherapy 2006;26:569–77.

[121] Greinacher A, Lubenow N, Eichler P. Anaphylactic and anaphylactoid reactions associated with lepirudin in patients with heparin-induced thrombocytopenia. Circulation 2003;108:2062–5.

[122] Baghdasarian S, Singh I, Militello M, et al. Argatroban dosage in critically ill patients with HIT [abstract]. Blood 2004;104:493a.

[123] Levine RL, Hursting MJ, McCollum D. Argatroban therapy in heparin-induced thrombocytopenia with hepatic dysfunction. Chest 2006;129:1167–75.

[124] Jang IK, Lewis BE, Matthai WH, et al. Argatroban anticoagulation in conjunction with glycoprotein IIb/IIIa inhibition in patients undergoing percutaneous coronary intervention: an open-label, nonrandomized pilot study. J Thromb Thrombolysis 2004;18:31–7.

[125] Chong BH, Magnani HN. Danaparoid for the treatment of heparin-induced thrombocytopenia: an overview. In: Warkentin TE, Greinacher A, editors. Heparin-induced thrombocytopenia. 3rd edition. New York: Marcel Dekker; 2004. p. 371–96.

[126] Magnani HN. Heparin-induced thrombocytopenia (HIT): an overview of 230 patients treated with Orgaron (Org 10172). Thromb Haemost 1993;70:554–61.

[127] Farner B, Eichler P, Kroll H, et al. A comparison of danaparoid and lepirudin in heparin-induced thrombocytopenia. Thromb Haemost 2001;85:950–7.

[128] Magnani HN, Gallus A. Heparin-induced thrombocytopenia (HIT). A report of 1478 clinical outcomes of patients treated with danaparoid (Orgaran) from 1982 to mid-2004. Thromb Haemost 2006;95:967–81.

[129] Amiral J, Lormeua JC, Marfaing-Koka A, et al. Absence of cross-reactivity of SR90107A/ORG31540 pentasaccharide with antibodies to heparin-PF4 complexes developed in heparin-induced thrombocytopenia. Blood Coagul Fibrinolysis 1997;8:114–7.

[130] Savi P, Chong BH, Greinacher A, et al. Effect of fondaparinux on platelet activation in the presence of heparin-dependent antibodies. A blinded comparative multicenter study with unfractionated heparin. Blood 2005;105:139–44.

[131] Warkentin TE, Cook RJ, Marder VJ, et al. Antiplatelet factor 4-heparin antibodies in orthopedic surgery patients receiving antithrombotic prophylaxis with fondaparinux or enoxaparin. Blood 2005;106:3791–6.

[132] Harenberg J, Jorg I, Fenyvesi T. Treatment of heparin-induced thrombocytopenia with fondaparinux. Haematologica 2004;89:1017–8.

[133] Bradner J, Hallisey RK, Kuter DJ. Fondaparinux in the treatment of heparin-induced thrombocytopenia [abstract]. Blood 2004;104:492a.

[134] Kovacs MJ. Successful treatment of heparin-induced thrombocytopenia (HIT) with fondaparinux. Thromb Haemost 2005;93:999–1000.

[135] Warkentin TE. Management of heparin-induced thrombocytopenia: a critical comparison of lepirudin and argatroban. Thromb Res 2003;110:73–82.
[136] Smythe MA, Stephens JL, Koeber JM, et al. A comparison of lepirudin and argatroban outcomes. Clin Appl Thromb Hemost 2005;11:371–4.
[137] Dager WE, White RH. Use of lepirudin in patients with heparin-induced thrombocytopenia and renal failure requiring hemodialysis. Ann Pharmacother 2001;35:885–90.
[138] Song X, Huhle G, Wang L, et al. Generation of antihirudin antibodies in heparin-induced thrombocytopenic patients treated with r-hirudin. Circulation 1999;100:1528–32.
[139] Eichler P, Friesen HJ, Lubenow N, et al. Antihirudin antibodies in patients with heparin-induced thrombocytopenia treated with lepirudin: incidence, effects on aPTT and clinical relevance. Blood 2000;96:2373–8.
[140] Walenga JM, Ahmad S, Hoppensteadt DA, et al. Argatroban therapy does not generate antibodies that alter its anticoagulant activity in patients with heparin-induced thrombocytopenia. Thromb Res 2002;105:401–5.
[141] Harenberg J, Jorg I, Fenyvesi T, et al. Treatment of patients with a history of heparin-induced thrombocytopenia and antilepirudin antibodies with argatroban. J Thromb Thrombolysis 2005;19:65–9.
[142] Eichler P, Lubenow N, Strobel U, et al. Antibodies against lepirudin are polyspecific and recognize epitopes on bivalirudin. Blood 2004;103:613–6.
[143] Gosselin RC, Dager WE, King JH, et al. Effect of direct thrombin inhibitors, bivalirudin, lepirudin, and argatroban, on prothrombin time and INR values. Am J Clin Pathol 2004;121:593–9.
[144] Hursting MJ, Lewis BE, Macfarlane DE. Transitioning from argatroban to warfarin therapy in patients with heparin induced thrombocytopenia. Clin Appl Thromb Hemost 2005;11:279–87.
[145] Sheth SB, DiCicco RA, Hursting MJ, et al. Interpreting the International Normalized Ratio (INR) in individuals receiving argatroban and warfarin. Thromb Haemost 2001;85:435–40.
[146] Harder S, Graff J, Klinkhardt U, et al. Transition from argatroban to oral anticoagulation with phenprocoumon or acenocoumarol: effects on prothrombin time, activated partial thromboplastin time, and ecarin clotting time. Thromb Haemost 2004;91:1137–45.
[147] Arpino PA, Demirjian Z, Van Cott EM. Use of the chromogenic factor X assay to predict the International Normalized Ratio in patients transitioning from argatroban to warfarin. Pharmacotherapy 2005;25:157–64.
[148] Bittl JA, Chaitman BR, Feit F, et al. Bivalirudin versus heparin during coronary angioplasty for unstable or postinfarction angina: final report reanalysis of the Bivalirudin Angioplasty Study. Am Heart J 2001;142:952–9.
[149] Kodityal S, Manhas AH, Udden M, et al. Danaparoid for heparin-induced thrombocytopenia: an analysis of treatment failures. Eur J Haematol 2003;71:109–13.
[150] Fischer KG. Hirudin in renal insufficiency. Semin Thromb Hemost 2002;28:467–82.
[151] Murray PM, Reddy BV, Grossman EJ, et al. A prospective comparison of three argatroban treatment regimens during end-stage renal disease. Kidney Int 2004;66:2446–53.
[152] Stratmann G, diSilva AM, Tseng EE, et al. Reversal of direct thrombin inhibition after cardiopulmonary bypass in a patient with heparin-induced thrombocytopenia. Anesth Analg 2004;98:1635–9.
[153] Bijsterveld NR, Moons AH, Boekholdt SM, et al. Ability of recombinant factor VIIa to reverse the anticoagulant effect of the pentasaccharide fondaparinux in healthy volunteers. Circulation 2002;106:2550–4.
[154] Yee AJ, Kuter DJ. Successful recovery from an overdose of argatroban. Ann Pharmacother 2006;40:446–9.

[155] Knoderer CA, Knoderer HM, Turrentine MW, et al. Lepirudin anticoagulation for heparin-induced thrombocytopenia after cardiac surgery in a pediatric patient. Pharmacotherapy 2006;26:709–12.

[156] Saxon BR, Black MD, Edgell D, et al. Pediatric heparin-induced thrombocytopenia: management with danaparoid (Orgaran). Ann Thorac Surg 1999;68:1076–8.

[157] Messmore H, Jeske W, Wehrmacher W, et al. Benefit–risk assessment of treatments for heparin-induced thrombocytopenia. Drug Saf 2003;26:625–41.

Hematol Oncol Clin N Am 21 (2007) 89–101

HEMATOLOGY/ONCOLOGY CLINICS
OF NORTH AMERICA

Anti-inflammatory Strategies and Hemostatic Agents: Old Drugs, New Ideas

Jerrold H. Levy, MD[a,b,]*

[a]Department of Anesthesiology, Emory University School of Medicine, 1364 Clifton Road N.E., Atlanta, GA 30322, USA
[b]Cardiothoracic Anesthesiology and Critical Care, Emory Healthcare, 1364 Clifton Road N.E., Atlanta, GA 30322, USA

H emostatic abnormalities occur following injury associated with both cardiac and noncardiac surgery [1,2]. These changes are part of inflammatory pathways with signaling mechanisms that link these diverse pathways [3,4]. The inflammatory response to surgery is exacerbated by allogeneic blood transfusion by enhancing intrinsic inflammatory activity and directly increasing plasma levels of inflammatory mediators [5]. Protein and cellular components likely contribute to the inflammatory properties of allogeneic blood transfusion and associated untoward outcomes [6]. Surgical patients can be preventively treated with pharmacologic agents to modulate inflammatory responses. Multiple studies have reported preventive pharmacologic therapies to reduce bleeding and the need for allogeneic transfusions in surgery [7,8]. Strategies for cardiac surgical patients during cardiopulmonary bypass (CPB) include administration of either lysine analogs, such as epsilon aminocaproic acid (Amicar) and tranexamic acid (Cyklokapron), or the serine protease inhibitor aprotinin (Trasylol) [8].

INFLAMMATION
Inflammation is the body's response to tissue injury [9,10]. Inflammatory responses are characterized by humoral and cellular interactions with many pathways resulting in the activation, generation, or expression of thrombin, complement, cytokines, neutrophils, adhesion molecules, and multiple inflammatory mediators [4,9,10]. Profound amplification of the response occurs, which results in multiorgan system dysfunction [11]. Inflammatory responses associated with cardiac surgery increase perioperative morbidity and mortality [9] and are characterized by activation of immunologic and hemostatic

*Department of Anesthesiology, Emory University School of Medicine, 1364 Clifton Road N.E., Atlanta, GA 30322. E-mail address: jerrold.levy@emoryhealthcare.org

0889-8588/07/$ – see front matter
doi:10.1016/j.hoc.2006.11.007

pathways [10]. Clinical expressions of inflammatory responses following surgery are manifested as bleeding, ischemia-reperfusion injury, respiratory failure, and vasodilatory shock [10]. Tissue injury in surgical patients activates hemostasis and the inflammatory response mediated by the release of various cytokines and chemokines [9,12] and may present as multiorgan system dysfunction. Bleeding, respiratory failure, myocardial dysfunction, renal insufficiency, and neurocognitive defects are all examples of clinical manifestation of inflammatory responses. Further, ischemia-reperfusion injury associated with ischemic episodes and revascularization procedures, mediated by cytokines, chemokines, adhesion molecules, and additional recruitment of inflammatory cells, contributes to tissue injury and multiorgan system dysfunction [13].

HEMOSTASIS AND INFLAMMATION

Hemostatic activation is linked to inflammatory responses by a network of humoral and cellular components, including proteases of the clotting and fibrinolytic cascades [4,10]. Hemostatic initiation, thrombin generation, contact activation, and other pathways amplify inflammatory responses to produce collectively end-organ damage as part of host defense mechanisms [4]. In surgical patients, tissue injury and cardiopulmonary bypass activate these processes [12]. Tissue factor, an important aspect of thrombin generation expressed following vascular injury, triggers coagulation activation and microvascular expression of plasminogen activator inhibitor (PAI)-1, which inhibits activation of fibrinolysis [4,10,14]. Thrombin generation advances by means of the tissue factor/factor VIIa route and simultaneous depression of concurrent inhibitory mechanisms by way of antithrombin III and the protein C system [15,16]. Also, altered fibrin degradation, resulting from elevated circulating levels of PAI-1, contributes to increased intravascular fibrin deposition [15–17].

Cross-talk between activation of inflammation and hemostasis occurs. Cytokines, the main contributors to inflammation-induced coagulation, activate coagulation proteases to modulate inflammation through specific cell receptors, including protease-activated receptors. Conversely, anticoagulant proteins and coagulation proteases bind specific cell receptors on mononuclear cells and endothelial cells affecting cytokine generation [10]. Strategies directed at inhibiting coagulation activation have been reported in experimental and early clinical studies, and include inhibiting tissue factor–mediated activation of coagulation or restoration of physiologic anticoagulant pathways by recombinant human activated protein C or antithrombin. In disseminated intravascular coagulation, disproportionate activation of thrombin, clotting, or both leads to bleeding complications; depletion of coagulation proteins, platelets, and endothelial dysfunction produces microvascular dysfunction and generates a thrombotic state [18].

ISCHEMIA-REPERFUSION INJURY

Vascular and cardiac surgery with cardiopulmonary bypass and cardioplegic arrest have been associated with ischemia-reperfusion injury characterized by increased vascular permeability leading to myocardial edema and cardiac dysfunction [14,19]. Cellular junctions regulate vascular permeability and endothelial barrier function [14]. Inflammatory mediators induce vascular permeability, including tumor necrosis factor, histamine, neutrophil-associated proteases, oxygen radicals, and thrombin [14]. Thrombin-mediated activation of protease-activated receptors also increases endothelial permeability [20,21]. Aprotinin prevents proteolytic activation of the thrombin protease-activated receptor [22–24]. Khan and colleagues [25] reported that aprotinin preserves myocardial cellular junctions and prevents myocardial edema in a clinically relevant animal model of regional ischemia and cardioplegic arrest (see also Ref. [19]).

MODULATING INFLAMMATION PERIOPERATIVELY

Strategies to modulate the perioperative inflammatory response include pharmacologic agents to attenuate the harmful effects of the systemic inflammatory response. Therapeutic strategies can be directed at modulating multiple aspects of the inflammatory response, including coagulation, contact activation, cytokines, neutrophils, intracellular molecular targets, and adhesion molecules [2,12,14,26,27]. Anti-inflammatory agents prevent proteolysis of the protease-activated receptor (aprotinin), inhibit complement-mediated injury (pexelizumab), or inhibit contact activation (aprotinin and selective kallikrein inhibitors). The role of anesthetic agents may also contribute in part to responses, but these seem minimal in comparison to other more potent stimuli [28].

Aprotinin inhibits trypsin, chymotrypsin, plasmin, tissue plasminogen activator, and kallikrein [29]. Aprotinin in cardiac and orthopedic surgical patients reduces blood loss and transfusion requirements [12]. Reducing allogeneic blood transfusions represent an important aspect of anti-inflammatory strategies, and aprotinin consistently reduces bleeding and transfusion requirement [30]. Although corticosteroids have been extensively examined as anti-inflammatory agents, controlled studies, including placebo-controlled studies, have not demonstrated efficacy in cardiac surgical patients [31]. Aprotinin has a different mechanism of action from corticosteroids and may attenuate other aspects of the inflammation associated with cardiopulmonary bypass, including inhibiting neutrophil adhesion and activation [32]. Aprotinin reduces bleeding and transfusion requirements in high-risk patients undergoing repeat median sternotomy [33], in patients taking aspirin [30], and in patients receiving clopidogrel [34]. Results from multicenter studies of aprotinin show no increased risk for early graft thrombosis, myocardial infarction, or renal failure in aprotinin-treated patients [30]. In repeat coronary artery surgery, the incidence of stroke was significantly lower in aprotinin-treated patients [33].

PROTEASE-ACTIVATED RECEPTORS

Aprotinin is considered to be an effective hemostatic agent, but with suggested hemostatic and antithrombotic properties [22,35,36]. Poullis [22] reported that aprotinin selectively blocks the proteolytically activated thrombin receptor on platelets and the protease-activated receptor 1 (PAR-1), while leaving other mechanisms of platelet aggregation and its other novel anti-inflammatory targets unaffected [35,36]. Aprotinin prevents leukocyte transmigration by inhibiting intercellular adhesion molecule-1 and vascular cell adhesion molecule-1, but not E-selectin and expression on tumor necrosis factor-alpha–activated endothelial cells [32,36]. Aprotinin also inhibits thrombin-induced platelet activation by preventing proteolysis of the PAR-1 receptor in vitro and in patients undergoing bypass surgery [22,23]. Platelets are protected from undesirable activation by thrombin in the bypass circuit, yet they retain their ability to take part in forming fibrin clots at wound sites as needed.

TRANSFUSION AS AN INFLAMMATORY RESPONSE

Transfusion of allogeneic blood is reported to have multiple immunomodulatory effects, including immunosuppression; to contain bioactive substances that cause febrile reactions; and to release inflammatory mediators [37]. Fransen and colleagues [5] showed that inflammatory responses to cardiac surgery are affected by giving packed red cells during surgery as displayed by neutrophil activation. Neutrophils in allogeneic cellular blood components are associated with adverse effects in the recipient [38]. In cardiac surgical patients who are already immunosuppressed by surgical trauma, added inhibition of immunomodulation may have harmful effects. One of the most life-threatening inflammatory responses from blood, however, is transfusion-related acute lung injury (TRALI). TRALI presents with acute respiratory failure manifested by bilateral pulmonary edema and hypoxemia, and hypotension [38]. The onset is following the transfusion of plasma-containing blood components, always within 1 to 6 hours, and usually within 1 to 2 hours [38,39]. Studies report that 5% to 8% of patients die of complications related to the pulmonary insult [38]. TRALI may be significantly underdiagnosed and confused with other potential problems in a multiply transfused, critically ill, surgical patient (see the article on TRALI elsewhere in this issue).

One important aspect of inflammatory responses includes platelet transfusions. Spiess and colleagues [6] reported platelet transfusions are associated with adverse outcomes associated with coronary artery bypass graft surgery (CABG). Data originally collected during double-blind placebo-controlled phase III trials for licensure of aprotinin were retrospectively analyzed for adverse patient outcomes (n = 1720). Patients who received perioperative platelet transfusion were compared with those who did not. Logistic regression analysis was used to assess the association of perioperative adverse events with platelet transfusion. Propensity scoring analysis was used to verify results of the logistic regression. Spiess noted patients receiving platelets were more likely to have prolonged hospital stays, longer surgeries, more bleeding, reoperation for bleeding, and more red blood cell (RBC) transfusions, and less likely to have full-dose aprotinin administration. Adverse events were statistically more frequent in patients who received one or more platelet transfusion. Logistic regression analysis showed that platelet transfusion was associated with infection, vasopressor use, respiratory medication use, stroke, and death. Propensity scoring analysis confirmed the risk for platelet transfusion. The authors inferred that platelet transfusion in the perioperative period of CABG was associated with increased risk for serious adverse events. Although platelet transfusion may be a surrogate marker for sicker patients and have no causal role in the outcomes noted, the direct contribution of platelet transfusion to adverse outcomes should be a consideration when evaluating the risk–benefit of platelet transfusion in the surgical patient [6].

PHARMACOLOGIC AGENTS TO REDUCE BLEEDING DURING SURGERY

Multiple meta-analyses have analyzed pharmacologic agents in surgical patients. Levi reported a meta-analysis of all randomized controlled trials of the three pharmacologic strategies most often used to decrease perioperative blood loss (aprotinin, lysine analogs [epsilon aminocaproic acid (EACA) and tranexamic acid (TXA)], and desmopressin) [40]. Studies were included if they reported at least one clinically relevant outcome (mortality, rethoracotomy, proportion of patients receiving a transfusion, or perioperative myocardial infarction) besides perioperative blood loss. In addition, a separate meta-analysis was done for studies on complicated cardiac surgery. Seventy-two trials (8409 patients) met the inclusion criteria. Treatment with aprotinin decreased mortality almost twofold (odds ratio [OR] = 0.55, 95% CI: 0.34–0.90) compared with placebo. Treatment with aprotinin and with lysine analogs decreased the frequency of surgical re-exploration (OR = 0.37, 95% CI: 0.25–0.55, and OR = 0.44, 95% CI: 0.22–0.90, respectively) compared with placebo. These two treatments also significantly decreased the proportion of patients receiving any allogeneic blood transfusion. The use of desmopressin resulted in a small decrease in perioperative blood loss but was not associated with a favorable effect on other clinical outcomes. Aprotinin and lysine analogs did not increase the risk for perioperative myocardial infarction; however, desmopressin was associated with a 2.4-fold increase in the risk for this complication [40].

From the Cochrane database, Henry and colleagues [41] reported an evaluation of the randomized controlled trials of antifibrinolytic drugs in adults scheduled for nonurgent surgery. Two reviewers independently assessed trial quality and extracted data. They found 61 trials of aprotinin (7027 participants). Aprotinin reduced the rate of RBC transfusion by a relative 30% (relative risk [RR] = 0.70, 95% CI: 0.64–0.76). The average risk reduction (ARR) was 20.4% (95% CI: 15.6%–25.3%). On average, aprotinin use saved 1.1 units of RBC (95% CI: 0.69–1.47) in those needing transfusion. Aprotinin also significantly reduced the need for reoperation because of bleeding (RR = 0.40, 95% CI: 0.25–0.66). They did not report added decrease in transfusion factors (ie, platelets), however. They also found 18 trials of TXA (1342 participants). TXA reduced the rate of RBC transfusion by a relative 34% (RR = 0.66, 95% CI: 0.54–0.81). This represented an ARR of 17.2% (95% CI: 8.7%–25.7%). TXA use resulted in a saving of 1.03 units of RBC (95% CI: 0.67–1.39) in those needing transfusion. They found four trials of EACA (208 participants). EACA use resulted in a statistically nonsignificant decrease in RBC transfusion

(RR = 0.48, 95% CI: 0.19–1.19). Eight trials made head-to-head comparisons between TXA and aprotinin. There was no significant difference between the two drugs in the rate of RBC transfusion (RR = 1.21, 95% CI: 0.83–1.76) for TXA compared with aprotinin.

Henry and colleagues [41] also provided analysis of several safety parameters. Twenty-nine trials of aprotinin reported data on reoperation for bleeding (aprotinin, 1758 patients; control, 1142 patients) and showed that aprotinin significantly reduced the need for reoperation for bleeding by a relative 60% (RR = 0.40, 95% CI: 0.25–0.66). Nine trials of TXA reported data on reoperation for bleeding (TXA, 423 patients; control, 351 patients). The relative risk for reoperation for bleeding in patients treated with TXA compared with control was not significant (RR = 0.72, 95% CI: 0.29–1.79). Five trials of EACA reported data on reoperation for bleeding (EACA, 306; control, 316). The relative risk for reoperation for bleeding in patients treated with EACA compared with control was not significant (RR = 0.32, 95% CI: 0.07–1.39). The authors also reported aprotinin did not seem to be associated with an excess risk for adverse effects, including thromboembolic events (thrombosis RR = 0.64, 95% CI: 0.31–1.31) and renal failure (RR = 1.19, 95% CI: 0.79–1.79). They noted the lack of safety data that were available for TXA and EACA. The investigators concluded that aprotinin reduces the need for red cell transfusion, and the need for reoperation because of bleeding, without serious adverse effects. Although they noted that similar trends were seen with TXA and EACA, they reported "the data were rather sparse." The evidence reviewed supported the use of aprotinin in cardiac surgery. They also suggested that further small trials of this drug are not warranted [41].

Although it is widely used, one of the problems regarding EACA is the question regarding its efficacy. A recent study evaluated the efficacy of EACA in a prospective placebo-controlled trial in 100 patients undergoing primary coronary artery bypass grafting surgery [42]. Patients received either 100 mg/kg before skin incision followed by 1 g/hour continuous infusion until chest closure, 10 g in cardiopulmonary bypass circuit, or placebo, and the efficacy was evaluated by the reduction in postoperative thoracic-drainage volume and in donor-blood transfusion up to postoperative day 12. Although thoracic-drainage volume was significantly lower in the EACA group compared with the placebo group (EACA, 649 ± 261 mL versus placebo, 940 ± 626 mL; $P = .003$), there were no significant differences between the EACA and placebo groups in the percentage of patients requiring donor RBC transfusions (EACA, 24% versus placebo, 18%; $P = .62$) or in the number of units of donor RBC transfused (EACA, 2.2 ± 0.8 U versus placebo, 1.9 ± 0.8 U; $P = .29$). EACA did not reduce the risk for donor RBC transfusions compared with placebo (OR = 1.2, 95% CI: 0.4–3.2, $P = .63$). The authors suggest prophylactic administration of EACA reduces postoperative thoracic-drainage volume by 30%, but it may not be potent enough to reduce the requirement and the risk for donor blood transfusion in cardiac surgery patients.

Aprotinin

Aprotinin is a protease inhibitor that attenuates multiple aspects of the inflammatory responses to CPB. Aprotinin has been shown to be effective in reducing bleeding and transfusion requirements in cardiac surgical patients. Sedrakyan and colleagues [30] recently evaluated clinical outcomes (mortality, myocardial infarction, renal failure, stroke, atrial fibrillation) in patients undergoing CABG who received aprotinin by performing a quantitative review of published randomized controlled trials. They evaluated MEDLINE, EMBASE, and PHARMLINE (1988–2001) and reference lists of relevant articles were searched for CABG studies. Criteria for data inclusion were as follows: (1) random allocation of study treatments, (2) placebo control, (3) enrollment only of patients undergoing CABG, (4) no combination with another experimental medication or device, and (5) prophylactic and continuous intraoperative use. Data from 35 CABG trials (n = 3879) confirmed that aprotinin reduces transfusion requirements (RR − 0.61, 95% CI: 0.58–0.66) relative to placebo, with a 39% risk reduction. Aprotinin therapy was not associated with increased or decreased mortality (RR = 0.96, 95% CI: 0.65–1.40), myocardial infarction (RR = 0.85, 95% CI: 0.63–1.14), or renal failure (RR = 1.01, 95% CI 0.55–1.83) risk, but it was associated with a reduced risk for stroke (RR = 0.53, 95% CI: 0.31–0.90) and a trend toward reduced atrial fibrillation (RR = 0.90, 95% CI: 0.78–1.03). The authors concluded that concerns that aprotinin therapy is associated with increased mortality, myocardial infarction, or renal failure risk are not supported by data from published randomized placebo-controlled clinical trials. Evidence for a reduced risk for stroke and a tendency toward reduction of atrial fibrillation occurrence was observed in patients who received aprotinin [30].

Aprotinin: The Controversy

A recent article in the New England Journal of Medicine (NEJM) has created major controversy regarding the use of aprotinin [43]. In an observational study involving 4374 patients undergoing revascularization, Mangano and colleagues [43] prospectively assessed three agents (aprotinin [1295 patients], aminocaproic acid [883], and TXA [822]) as compared with no agent (1374 patients) regarding serious outcomes using propensity and multivariable methods. They reported in propensity-adjusted, multivariable logistic regression (C-index, 0.72), use of aprotinin was associated with a doubling in the risk for renal failure requiring dialysis among patients undergoing complex coronary artery surgery (OR = 2.59, 95% CI: 1.36–4.95) or primary surgery (OR = 2.34, 95% CI: 1.27–4.31). Similarly, use of aprotinin in the latter group was associated with a 55% increase in the risk for myocardial infarction or heart failure ($P < 0.001$) and a 181% increase in the risk for stroke or encephalopathy ($P = .001$). Neither aminocaproic acid nor TXA was associated with an increased risk for renal, cardiac, or cerebral events. Adjustment according to propensity score for the use of any one of the three agents as compared with no agent yielded nearly identical findings. All the agents reduced blood loss.

The authors conclude that the association between aprotinin and serious end-organ damage indicates that continued use is not prudent, and they suggest that the less expensive generic medications aminocaproic acid and TXA are safe alternatives [43].

This report uses an observational, nonrandomized database and subjects it to extensive statistical analyses [43]. The author has commented with others regarding issues related to this report [44,45]. The underlying questions to any analysis using nonrandomized patients is *why* a patient receives a particular therapy and whether or not efficacy and safety of a particular therapy can be adequately evaluated using nonrandomized methods [46]. In observational studies, clinicians control the treatment assigned and by doing so may introduce bias, such as channeling bias, wherein drugs with similar therapeutic uses are prescribed to groups of patients with prognostic differences [47]. Notably, an FDA-approved agent that has established efficacy and safety may be administered preferentially over other nonapproved agents whose efficacy and safety may not be as well established in randomized placebo-controlled trials [44,45]. The different treatment cohorts evaluated may have large differences in their observed covariates that can affect the assessment of efficacy and safety, and these differences can lead to biased estimates about treatment effects and the incidence of potential complications [48]. Propensity scoring is created to reduce bias but may not eliminate it, and thus sicker patients may receive different treatments [48]. In fact, that is what was observed in the Mangano analysis. Patients at higher risk were unequally distributed between the treatment cohorts. If the interaction of other covariates with a specific agent or outcome needs to be assessed (ie, collinearity between these variables), then the first step should involve setting up a propensity scoring system based on a multivariate analysis of the disease state in question to identify the important risk factors for development of that disease. The reported methods suggest that these authors did not set up their propensity analysis on this basis. Aprotinin, an FDA-approved agent with a previously established safety record, is preferentially used to decrease bleeding and transfusion in the higher- and highest-risk patients who are also at high risk for other serious and life-threatening complications. The association identified by Mangano and colleagues [43] between aprotinin use and complications does not necessarily prove a cause-and-effect relationship any more than Connors and colleagues [49] established a cause-and-effect relationship in the association identified between the use of Swan-Ganz catheters in ICU patients and mortality.

The NEJM article also used complex composite endpoints (eg, CNS injury: stroke and encephalopathy; renal dysfunction: renal failure and an increase in creatinine >2.0). This practice makes comparison to any other meta-analysis of randomized prospective studies impossible because most studies do not use complex composite endpoints. Mangano and colleagues [43] do not list what variables were chosen and how they were selected (eg, randomly or by the authors' own personal criteria, which may have been biased) for the complete analysis (97 of 7500 fields were used as risk factors) and the propensity analysis

(40 of 7500 fields are mentioned but not listed). Another recently published large (n = 9080) analysis published by Karkouti and colleagues [50] identified several risk factors that were independently associated with development of acute renal failure with an exceptional overall predictive model of C-index 0.944. These risk factors included preoperative renal dysfunction (OR = 4.3), urgent surgery (OR = 2.0), atrial fibrillation (OR = 2.4), nadir hematocrit during CPB (OR = 2.3), difficulty with weaning from CPB (OR = 3.1), re-exploration (OR = 3.7), low-output syndrome (OR = 3.8), and other adverse events (OR = 5.2). In another recent analysis (n = 10,751) from the same authors, other independent risk factors for requirement of renal replacement therapy included diabetes (OR = 2.5), an ejection fraction less than 20% (OR = 2.6), previous cardiac surgery (OR = 1.7), valve repair (OR = 1.6), complex procedure (OR = 3.5), and either urgent (OR = 1.8) or emergent requirement for surgery (OR = 9.9), with a reasonable overall model discrimination (C-statistic = 0.87) [51]. Were these important risk factors used as covariates in the analysis by Mangano and colleagues (especially for propensity adjustment) and if not, could asymmetric distribution of these risk factors within the treatment groups (ie, aprotinin, EACA, TXA) account for the reported results?

The authors also neglect to comment on the negative effects of administration of either fresh frozen plasma (FFP) or platelets. FFP carried the same risk for developing renal dysfunction (OR = 2.5) yet there are no data to support either efficacy or safety of use of FFP to manage bleeding after cardiac surgery [43]. Blood products can have a substantial negative clinical impact on a subset of patients based on transmission of blood-borne infections or allergic reactions, but most importantly based on the incidence and mortality related to TRALI, which is increasingly recognized, especially with FFP. There is no mention of the Kincaid and colleagues [52] article that identifies poor renal outcomes to be related to the interaction of four factors, either separately or in combination: PRBC transfusion burden (ie, >4–6 units), higher-risk surgery, angiotensin-converting enzyme inhibitors, and aprotinin. None of the investigators who collected the data have been involved as authors on the manuscript, despite the presence of a well-defined structure in the McSPI organization that was designed specifically for this purpose.

The FDA released a public health advisory on February 8, 2006 suggesting that physicians should consider limiting Trasylol use to those situations in which the clinical benefit of reduced blood loss is essential to medical management of the patient and outweighs the potential risks. The FDA is evaluating the studies more closely, along with other scientific literature and reports submitted to the FDA to determine if labeling changes or other actions are warranted. On December 15, 2006, the Trasylol US Package Information was updated to focus use in patients who are at increased risk for blood loss and blood transfusion in association with cardiopulmonary bypass in CABG and in the operative setting where cardiopulmonary bypass can be rapidly initiated. Also, the label now states administration increases the risk for renal dysfunction and may increase the need for dialysis in the perioperative period.

Further, stronger warnings about anaphylactic reactions with a contraindication for previous aprotinin exposure during the past 12 months are stated [53]. The FDA also states, as we reviewed, that a limitation to this study was that doctors chose which patients were to receive Trasylol or another treatment. They note, "It is possible that patients treated with Trasylol may have been sicker than other patients. The studies used complex statistical methods to adjust for possible differences in patient risk factors" [53].

The risks of excessive bleeding and transfusion after cardiac surgery are well established. Aprotinin is the only FDA-approved agent to reduce the incidence of potentially life-threatening complications related to excessive bleeding with cardiac surgery and is indicated for patients at high risk for bleeding. We agree with the FDA guidelines that physicians need to discuss with patients at substantial risk for bleeding and transfusion the potential risks and benefits of using of aprotinin, the only FDA-approved drug extensively studied for safety and efficacy in extensive randomized clinical studies [30,44,45], to minimize bleeding-related complications.

SUMMARY

Cardiac surgery and cardiopulmonary bypass are risk factors for bleeding. Bleeding requires transfusion of allogeneic RBC and other hemostatic blood components and re-exploration. Bleeding occurs following cardiac surgery even in patients undergoing off-pump surgery because of bleeding producing dilutional thrombocytopenia, tissue injury, and hemostatic activation, and increasing use of irreversible antiplatelet or antithrombotic agents. Although multiple therapeutic approaches have been studied to attenuate bleeding, pharmacologic interventions are an important option to attenuate excessive bleeding and requirements for transfusion and re-exploration. Cardiac surgery provides a unique opportunity to prevent hemostatic activation with the prophylactic administration of pharmacologic agents. The agents most extensively studied have antifibrinolytic, anticoagulant, and possibly anti-inflammatory properties. Aprotinin is the most extensively studied and effective blood conservation agent with the most potent antifibrinolytic effects. Further, recent studies have also explored its anti-inflammatory effects. Other agents, including EACA and TXA, are lysine analogs with antifibrinolytic properties that have also been studied. Pharmacologic approaches to reduce bleeding, transfusions, operative times, and re-exploration rates favorably affect patient outcomes, availability of blood products, and overall health care costs as reported in studies by Miller and colleagues [54] and Smith and colleagues [55].

References
  [1] Despotis GJ, Avidan MS, Hogue CW Jr. Mechanisms and attenuation of hemostatic activation during extracorporeal circulation. Ann Thorac Surg 2001;72:S1821–31.
  [2] Dixon B, Santamaria J, Campbell D. Coagulation activation and organ dysfunction following cardiac surgery. Chest 2005;128:229–36.
  [3] Esmon CT. Inflammation and thrombosis. J Thromb Haemost 2003;1:1343–8.

[4] Esmon CT. The impact of the inflammatory response on coagulation. Thromb Res 2004;114:321–7.

[5] Fransen E, Maessen J, Dentener M, et al. Impact of blood transfusions on inflammatory mediator release in patients undergoing cardiac surgery. Chest 1999;116:1233–9.

[6] Spiess BD, Royston D, Levy JH, et al. Platelet transfusions during coronary artery bypass graft surgery are associated with serious adverse outcomes. Transfusion 2004;44:1143–8.

[7] Levy JH. Novel pharmacologic approaches to reduce bleeding. Can J Anaesth 2003;50:S26–30.

[8] Levy JH. Overview of clinical efficacy and safety of pharmacologic strategies for blood conservation. Am J Health Syst Pharm 2005;62:S15–9.

[9] Levy JH, Tanaka KA. Inflammatory response to cardiopulmonary bypass. Ann Thorac Surg 2003;75:S715–20.

[10] Levi M, van der Poll T, Buller HR. Bidirectional relation between inflammation and coagulation. Circulation 2004;109:2698–704.

[11] Johnson D, Mayers I. Multiple organ dysfunction syndrome: a narrative review. Can J Anaesth 2001;48:502–9.

[12] Mojcik CF, Levy JH. Aprotinin and the systemic inflammatory response after cardiopulmonary bypass. Ann Thorac Surg 2001;71:745–54.

[13] Carden DL, Granger DN. Pathophysiology of ischaemia-reperfusion injury. J Pathol 2000;190:255–66.

[14] Mackman N. The role of the tissue factor-thrombin pathway in cardiac ischemia-reperfusion injury. Semin Vasc Med 2003;3:193–8.

[15] Chandler WL, Velan T. Estimating the rate of thrombin and fibrin generation in vivo during cardiopulmonary bypass. Blood 2003;101:4355–62.

[16] Chandler WL, Velan T. Plasmin generation and D-dimer formation during cardiopulmonary bypass. Blood Coagul Fibrinolysis 2004;15:583–91.

[17] Chandler WL. Effects of hemodilution, blood loss, and consumption on hemostatic factor levels during cardiopulmonary bypass. J Cardiothorac Vasc Anesth 2005;19:459–67.

[18] Levi M, Ten Cate H. Disseminated intravascular coagulation. N Engl J Med 1999;341:586–92.

[19] Vinten-Johansen J. Involvement of neutrophils in the pathogenesis of lethal myocardial reperfusion injury. Cardiovasc Res 2004;61:481–97.

[20] Coughlin SR, Camerer E. Participation in inflammation. J Clin Invest 2003;111:25–7.

[21] Coughlin SR. Protease-activated receptors in hemostasis, thrombosis and vascular biology. J Thromb Haemost 2005;3:1800–14.

[22] Poullis M, Manning R, Laffan M, et al. The antithrombotic effect of aprotinin: actions mediated via the proteaseactivated receptor 1. J Thorac Cardiovasc Surg 2000;120:370–8.

[23] Day JR, Punjabi PP, Randi AM, et al. Clinical inhibition of the seven-transmembrane thrombin receptor (PAR1) by intravenous aprotinin during cardiothoracic surgery. Circulation 2004;110:2597–600.

[24] Day JR, Taylor KM, Lidington EA, et al. Aprotinin inhibits proinflammatory activation of endothelial cells by thrombin through the protease-activated receptor 1. J Thorac Cardiovasc Surg 2006;131:21–7.

[25] Khan TA, Bianchi C, Voisine P, et al. Reduction of myocardial reperfusion injury by aprotinin after regional ischemia and cardioplegic arrest. J Thorac Cardiovasc Surg 2004;128:602–8.

[26] Verrier ED, Shernan SK, Taylor KM, et al. Terminal complement blockade with pexelizumab during coronary artery bypass graft surgery requiring cardiopulmonary bypass: a randomized trial. JAMA 2004;291:2319–27.

[27] Chong AJ, Shimamoto A, Hampton CR, et al. Toll-like receptor 4 mediates ischemia/reperfusion injury of the heart. J Thorac Cardiovasc Surg 2004;128:170–9.

[28] Laffey JG, Boylan JF, Cheng DC. The systemic inflammatory response to cardiac surgery: implications for the anesthesiologist. Anesthesiology 2002;97:215–52.

[29] Levy JH. Pharmacologic preservation of the hemostatic system during cardiac surgery. Ann Thorac Surg 2001;72:S1814–20.

[30] Sedrakyan A, Treasure T, Elefteriades JA. Effect of aprotinin on clinical outcomes in coronary artery bypass graft surgery: a systematic review and meta-analysis of randomized clinical trials. J Thorac Cardiovasc Surg 2004;128:442–8.

[31] Chaney MA. Corticosteroids and cardiopulmonary bypass: a review of clinical investigations. Chest 2002;121:921–31.

[32] Asimakopoulos G, Thompson R, Nourshargh S, et al. An anti-inflammatory property of aprotinin detected at the level of leukocyte extravasation. J Thorac Cardiovasc Surg 2000;120: 361–9.

[33] Levy JH, Pifarre R, Schaff HV, et al. A multicenter, double-blind, placebo-controlled trial of aprotinin for reducing blood loss and the requirement for donor-blood transfusion in patients undergoing repeat coronary artery bypass grafting. Circulation 1995;92:2236–44.

[34] van der Linden J, Lindvall G, Sartipy U. Aprotinin decreases postoperative bleeding and number of transfusions in patients on clopidogrel undergoing coronary artery bypass graft surgery: a double-blind, placebo-controlled, randomized clinical trial. Circulation 2005; 112(Suppl 9):I276–80.

[35] Landis RC, Asimakopoulos G, Poullis M, et al. The antithrombotic and antiinflammatory mechanisms of action of aprotinin. Ann Thorac Surg 2001;72:2169–75.

[36] Landis RC, Haskard DO, Taylor KM. New antiinflammatory and platelet-preserving effects of aprotinin. Ann Thorac Surg 2001;72:S1808–13.

[37] Blajchman MA. Transfusion immunomodulation or TRIM: what does it mean clinically? Hematology 2005;10(Suppl 1):208–14.

[38] Silliman CC, Ambruso DR, Boshkov LK. Transfusion-related acute lung injury. Blood 2005;105:2266–73.

[39] Popovsky MA. Transfusion-related acute lung injury. Curr Opin Hematol 2000;7:402–7.

[40] Levi M, Cromheecke ME, de Jonge E, et al. Pharmacological strategies to decrease excessive blood loss in cardiac surgery: a meta-analysis of clinically relevant endpoints. [see comment]. Lancet 1999;354:1940–7.

[41] Henry DA, Moxey AJ, Carless PA, et al. Anti-fibrinolytic use for minimising perioperative allogeneic blood transfusion. Cochrane Database Syst Rev 2001;CD001886.

[42] Kikura M, Levy JH, Tanaka KA, et al. A double-blind, placebo-controlled trial of epsilon-aminocaproic acid for reducing blood loss in coronary artery bypass grafting surgery. J Am Coll Surg 2006;202:216–22 [quiz: A44–5].

[43] Mangano DT, Tudor IC, Dietzel C. The risk associated with aprotinin in cardiac surgery. N Engl J Med 2006;354:353–65.

[44] Levy JH, Ramsay JG, Guyton RA. Aprotinin in cardiac surgery. N Engl J Med 2006;354: 1953–7 [author reply: 1953–7].

[45] Levy JH, Despotis GJ, Spitznagel E. Should aprotinin continue to be used during cardiac surgery? Nat Clin Pract Cardiovasc Med 2006;3:360–1.

[46] D'Agostino RB Jr. Propensity score methods for bias reduction in the comparison of a treatment to a non-randomized control group. Stat Med 1998;17:2265–81.

[47] Petri H, Urquhart J. Channeling bias in the interpretation of drug effects. Stat Med 1991;10: 577–81.

[48] Byar DP. Problems with using observational databases to compare treatments. Stat Med 1991;10:663–6.

[49] Connors AF Jr, Speroff T, Dawson NV, et al. The effectiveness of right heart catheterization in the initial care of critically ill patients. SUPPORT Investigators. JAMA 1996;276:889–97.

[50] Karkouti K, Beattie WS, Dattilo KM, et al. A propensity score case-control comparison of aprotinin and tranexamic acid in high-transfusion-risk cardiac surgery. Transfusion 2006;46:327–38.

[51] Wijeysundera DN, Karkouti K, Beattie WS, et al. Improving the identification of patients at risk of postoperative renal failure after cardiac surgery. Anesthesiology 2006;104:65–72.

[52] Kincaid EH, Ashburn DA, Hoyle JR, et al. Does the combination of aprotinin and angiotensin-converting enzyme inhibitor cause renal failure after cardiac surgery? Ann Thorac Surg 2005;80:1388–93 [discussion: 1393].

[53] FDA Public Health Advisory. Available at: http://www.fda.gov/bbs/topics/news/2006/NEW01311.html. Accessed February 8, 2006.

[54] Miller BE, Tosone SR, Tam VK, et al. Hematologic and economic impact of aprotinin in reoperative pediatric cardiac operations. Ann Thorac Surg 1998;66(2):535–40, discussion 541.

[55] Smith PK, Datta SK, Muhlbaier LH, et al. Cost analysis of aprotinin for coronary artery bypass patients: analysis of the randomized trials. Ann Thorac Surg 2004;77(2):635–42, discussion 642–3.

Hematol Oncol Clin N Am 21 (2007) 103–113

HEMATOLOGY/ONCOLOGY CLINICS
OF NORTH AMERICA

ELSEVIER
SAUNDERS

Protease Activated Receptors: Clinical Relevance to Hemostasis and Inflammation

R. Clive Landis, PhD

Edmund Cohen Laboratory for Vascular Research, University of the West Indies,
Chronic Disease Research Centre, Jemmotts Lane, Barbados, West Indies

THE PROTEASE-ACTIVATED RECEPTOR FAMILY: KEEPING THE LIGAND CLOSE AT HAND

There are four members of the protease-activated receptor (PAR) family, PARs1–4, which are expressed on the major cells of the vasculature, including platelets, leukocytes, endothelial cells, and vascular smooth muscle cells [1]. The ligand for each PAR receptor is kept close at hand, hidden within the extracellular domain. It is unmasked by proteolytic cleavage with a serine protease and then autoactivates the receptor by binding to an intramolecular binding site, finally delivering G protein–coupled signals into the cell [2]. This curious autoactivation mechanism probably evolved from zymogen activation mechanisms used by other serine proteases, such as trypsin. During the zymogen activation of trypsinogen, a protonated amino group docks intramolecularly to trap the newly activated protein, now trypsin, in its active conformation [3]. Because activation of PARs by proteolytic cleavage is irreversible, cells have evolved ways to shut off signaling by internalizing the cleaved receptors [4]. In essence, PARs are disposable once activated.

The four PARs in humans can be grouped according to their activating protease: thrombin activates PARs-1, -3, and -4, whereas PAR-2 is activated by trypsin, mast cell tryptase, and factor Xa in association with tissue factor-VIIa (Table 1). The thrombin-specific PARs can be further grouped according to the presence of a hirudin-like binding site located proximal to the cleavage site; this is present in PARs-1 and -3 and confers high-affinity status on those receptors by helping to localize thrombin to the cell surface. Studies in human platelets have shown that the rate-limiting step in PAR1 activation is the binding of thrombin to PAR1, whereupon cleavage follows rapidly [5]. PAR4, which lacks the hirudinlike binding site, is the low-affinity thrombin receptor

Dr. Landis holds an equipment grant from Bayer Pharmaceuticals Corporation.

E-mail address: clandis@uwichill.edu.bb

0889-8588/07/$ – see front matter
doi:10.1016/j.hoc.2006.11.005

Table 1
Protease-activated thrombin receptors

	Coagulation protease	Hirudin-like binding site	Affinity thrombin receptor
PAR	Thrombin	Yes	High
PAR	TF-VIIa-Xa	No	—
PAR	Thrombin	Yes	High
PAR	Thrombin	No	Low

Three PAR receptors recognize thrombin as their principal ligand: PAR1, PAR3, and PAR4. PAR2 is activated by another coagulation protease, factor Xa, in association with TF-VIIa. The thrombin PAR receptors are activated by a two-step mechanism: (1) binding of thrombin to the receptor (the rate-limiting step) and (2) proteolytic cleavage of the receptor. A hirudin-like binding site present in the extracellular domain of PAR1 and PAR3 helps localize thrombin and confers high-affinity receptor status; the high-affinity receptor in humans is PAR1, whereas in rodents it is PAR3. PAR4, which lacks a hirudin-like binding site, is the low-affinity thrombin receptor in all mammal species studied thus far.
Abbreviation: PAR, protease-activated receptor.

and has evolved ways to co-opt other surface receptors to help trap thrombin, including GPIb and other high-affinity PARs, PAR1 and PAR3, through a bridging mechanism [5,6]. PAR1 is the high-affinity thrombin receptor in humans, whereas that role is taken by PAR-3 in rodents [7,8].

This two-step activation mechanism (binding of thrombin to the receptor followed by cleavage) means that therapeutic PAR1 antagonists can be developed against either step, and examples of both types of antagonist exist. Perhaps unfortunately, the recent emphasis has been on developing peptide mimetics to compete with "tethered ligand" for the ligand-binding pocket [9,10]. These need to have a high affinity and slow off rate to effectively compete with natural ligand. The alternative type of antagonist, one that blocks the hirudin-like binding site on human PAR1, is clearly effective in vitro and in vivo but has seen limited development as a therapeutic agent [11,12]. The working hypothesis is that aprotinin, discussed later as a PAR1 inhibitor, works by the latter mechanism [13].

This article focuses on the role of the thrombin PAR receptors in hemostasis and inflammation, and ways in which these pathways can be therapeutically targeted in the context of cardiothoracic surgery.

ROLE OF PROTEASE-ACTIVATED RECEPTORS IN HEMOSTASIS AND THROMBOSIS: THE KNOCK-OUT STUDIES

Thrombin promotes hemostasis and thrombosis by two main pathways: (1) by mediating fibrin formation, and (2) by mediating platelet activation by way of the PARs. Mouse knock-out studies have provided insight into the relative importance of each thrombin pathway in hemostasis and thrombosis (Fig. 1).

In hemostasis, fibrinogen knock-out mice exhibit a moderately severe phenotype, with perinatal hemorrhage, bleeding at placentation, and prolonged bleeding in a tail transection model [14]. Nevertheless, the mice grow to old age in contrast to prothrombin-deficient mice, which die spontaneously either at midgestation or by exsanguination immediately following birth [15,16].

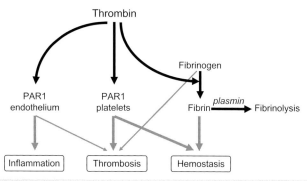

Fig. 1. Role of thrombin in inflammation, thrombosis, and hemostasis. The central platelet PAR1 axis is the main thrombotic pathway triggered by thrombin, although a contribution to clot stability is derived from fibrinogen in a cross-over from the hemostatic axis. Hemostasis receives almost equal contributions from the fibrin and platelet PAR1 axes activated by thrombin. Some of the bleeding problems in surgery may therefore be attributable to a platelet defect following desensitization of PAR1 by thrombin in the bypass circuit. Finally, PAR1 receptors on endothelium make a contribution to the inflammatory response, because PAR1 is linked to proinflammatory cytokine secretion (eg, IL-6, MCP-1) and adhesion molecule expression (eg, ICAM-1, P-selectin), promoting leukocyte diapedesis. Activation of PAR1 by thrombin also leads to von Willebrand factor expression and transudation of plasma proteins, which may indirectly amplify thrombosis through platelet attachment and contact of plasma coagulation factors with tissue factor in the subendothelium.

Some other pathway besides the fibrin pathway must play an important role in the hemostatic process. PAR4-deficient mice show no evidence for spontaneous bleeding but when challenged in the tail transection model show markedly prolonged bleeding times [17]. Double knock-out mice carrying both fibrinogen and PAR4 deletions almost exactly recapitulate the severe hemostatic defect seen in prothrombin-deficient mice, with death by exsanguination at birth [18]. Therefore, fibrin formation and platelet PAR activation each seem to play a significant and independent role in thrombin-mediated hemostasis.

PAR4 knock-out mice are strongly protected against thrombosis in an experimental thrombosis model, equally well as NF-E2–deficient mice that lack platelets altogether [19,20]. Fibrinogen-deficient mice form small thrombi, but these are unstable and readily embolize because of the absence of fibrinogen needed to stabilize the thrombus [21]. It is not possible to deduce from the knock-out studies whether fibrin formation, over and above fibrinogen, plays a part in arterial thrombosis. A dominant role for platelet PAR activation is well established in thrombin-dependent arterial thrombosis models, however. Furthermore, in higher primates, which share the human PAR1/PAR4 system of thrombin receptors on platelets, blockade of the high-affinity PAR1 receptor seems to be sufficient to deliver a therapeutic effect in experimental models of thrombosis [9,12]. Any strategy aimed at disrupting thrombin activation of platelets in humans by way of PAR1 thus is likely to exert an antithrombotic effect.

ROLE OF PROTEASE-ACTIVATED RECEPTORS
IN INFLAMMATION

In addition to a central role in platelet thrombosis, PAR receptors on endothelial cells mediate a range of inflammatory responses to thrombin (Fig. 1). Thrombin signaling is mediated primarily by way of PAR1, whereas PAR2 is responsive to the ternary coagulation complex consisting of TF-VIIa-Xa and other proteases of the trypsin family (eg, trypsin and mast cell tryptase) [22–24]. PAR1 is most probably the first receptor to respond during coagulation because it is constitutively expressed on endothelium, whereas PAR2 is up-regulated during inflammation [22,25–27]. The initial response of endothelial cells to thrombin is proinflammatory, through release of proinflammatory cytokines (IL-1, IL-6, IL-8, MCP-1) and induction of adhesion molecules on vessels (ICAM-1, P-selectin) [28–30]. These effector pathways promote diapedesis and activation of leukocytes at sites of thrombin generation and cause PAR2 up-regulation. Once PAR2 is expressed, the thrombin response becomes skewed through a novel bridging mechanism between PAR1 and PAR2 to induce cell survival (antiapoptotic) and complement protective (DAF) pathways [31]. This later response to thrombin may be important in helping endothelial cells to survive within the inflammatory wound environment. Thrombin also induces von Willebrand factor expression and enhances vascular permeability of endothelial cells, thus amplifying thrombosis indirectly by way of platelet recruitment and through contact of plasma coagulation factors with tissue factor exposed in and around the vessel wall [32,33]. Activation of endothelial PARs alone is sufficient to trigger platelet and leukocyte margination, but not the thrombotic sequelae. This response to coagulation by vascular endothelium probably evolved to allow initial inspection of sites by inflammatory leukocytes to help isolate and destroy pathogens. In the presence of other stimuli, such as endotoxin, a positive feedback loop between inflammation and coagulation may lead to hemorrhagic infarction of tissues [34].

CORONARY ARTERY BYPASS GRAFTING SURGERY:
A CHALLENGE TO THE HEMOSTATIC AND
INFLAMMATORY SYSTEMS

Coronary artery bypass graft (CABG) with cardiopulmonary bypass (CPB) creates a challenging environment for the hemostatic and inflammatory systems of the patient. Operative trauma is combined with systemic activation of the various blood components and ischemic injury to organs, especially the lung, brain, and kidneys. Overlaying all of these concerns is the possibility of thrombotic occlusion to the grafted vessels.

A central challenge for the surgeon is to control bleeding, which is exacerbated by the hyperfibrinolytic state and loss of platelet function because of thrombin activation in the bypass circuit. Antifibrinolytic agents (ϵ-amino caproic acid, tranexamic acid, and aprotinin) have been successfully used to prevent bleeding during surgery. Only aprotinin additionally preserves platelet function, however [35–38]. The issue of platelet preservation during bypass is especially important in an era of antiplatelet agents, such as aspirin and clopidogrel, which surgeons want to maintain patients on for as long as possible before surgery while not compromising the hemostatic capacity of platelets.

Inflammatory activation of blood takes place during its passage through the extracorporeal circuit [39]. The earliest system to be activated is the coagulation cascade through contact with the foreign surface. Platelets are rapidly activated by thrombin generated in linear relation to time spent on bypass [40–42], causing activation through PAR1 and return of desensitized platelets into the patient [43,44]. Neutrophils are also activated by direct adhesion to plastic surfaces and kallikrein, leading to up-regulation of activation markers and IL-8 secretion as early as 15 minutes of bypass [45,46]. Neutrophils and monocytes express complement receptors that are activated by C3a and C5a generated during bypass, thus amplifying leukocyte activation [47,48]. Monocyte activation is generally slower and is observed between 2 to 4 hours following bypass [48]. The soup of inflammatory cytokines induced during bypass, including IL-1, IL-6, IL-8, and TNFα, leads to endothelial cell activation [49]. Endothelial cells may already be primed for activation through ischemia reperfusion injury, which has been shown to induce adhesion molecule expression supportive for neutrophil diapedesis, such as P-selectin and ICAM-1 [50,51]. Endothelial PAR1, as discussed above, is also linked to various inflammatory cytokine and adhesion molecule programs in the vessel wall [28–30, 32,33]. The combined activation of blood and vascular cells causes the systemic inflammatory response to bypass. This response varies greatly in severity between patients, but of particular concern to the surgeon is injury to the ischemic lung and brain. The incidence of adult respiratory distress syndrome and frank strokes perioperatively are thankfully rare (0.5%–2.6%) in low-risk patients [52–56]. The risk for strokes may increase to 16.1% in high-risk patients [57], whereas more subtle neurocognitive defects probably occur in more than 90% of patients [58].

APROTININ: MULTIPLE BENEFITS IN CORONARY ARTERY BYPASS GRAFTING SURGERY

The surgeon has at his disposal several single target therapies aimed at improving either the bleeding or inflammatory complications to bypass, and one multi-target drug, aprotinin, which exerts simultaneous effects on fibrinolysis, platelets, and the inflammatory response to bypass (Fig. 2) [59–62].

The clinical efficacy of aprotinin in attenuating the bleeding and inflammatory complications of bypass is not in doubt [63,64]. Concerns have been expressed, however, about the mechanisms through which this can be safely achieved and on the cost–benefit of using an expensive drug [65,66]. The identification of PAR1 as a therapeutic target on platelets and endothelium has revealed an ideal mechanism for use in cardiopulmonary bypass, which combines a subtle antithrombotic yet hemostatic effect with antiinflammatory and neuroprotective properties, as explained below.

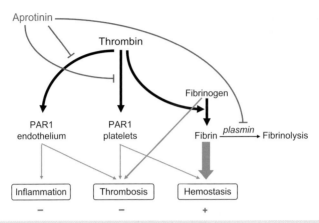

Fig. 2. Multiple targets for aprotinin in inflammation, thrombosis, and hemostasis. The best known property of aprotinin is its hemostatic effect, mediated through targeting of plasmin in the fibrinolytic pathway [59]. An antithrombotic property is mediated through preventing platelet PAR1 activation by thrombin, whereas a subsidiary hemostatic benefit may be achieved by preserving platelets from PAR1 activation in the bypass circuit. Further net antiin-flammatory and antithrombotic effects are predicted through sparing of PAR1 activation on endothelium. Other antiinflammatory effects, independent of the PAR1 axis, have been identified by targeting of soluble plasma proteins (eg, kallikrein and bradykinin) and through attenuation of leukocyte diapedesis in experimental models of inflammation [60–62]. The broad-acting serine protease inhibitor aprotinin may thus confer multiple therapeutic benefits during cardio-thoracic surgery with bypass by hitting multiple targets in the inflammatory, thrombotic, and hemostatic pathways.

PAR1 on Platelets

The high-affinity thrombin receptor, PAR1, is a unique marker for the desensitization of platelets that occurs during cardiopulmonary bypass [43]. This is because of activation of PAR1 by thrombin in the bypass circuit and the subsequent loss of receptor from the platelet surface. Not only can PAR1 loss be reversed by aprotinin clinically [67] but aprotinin also does not interfere with the hemostatic capacity of platelets in the chest cavity [68]. This is because aprotinin specifically targets proteolytic activation of PAR1 by thrombin but has no antiplatelet effects on protease-independent pathways of platelet activation, such as by collagen, ADP, or epinephrine found in the chest cavity [69]. A theoretic prediction arising from this PAR1-centric mode of action is that treatment with clopidogrel (an anti-ADP drug) before surgery ought not to interfere with the platelet-preserving properties of aprotinin, nor should it impact on the hemostatic properties of this drug. In agreement with this prediction, recent clinical trials examining the effect of aprotinin on patients maintained on clopidogrel less than 5 days before surgery showed that the hemostatic and platelet-preserving properties of aprotinin were maintained [70–72].

PAR1 targeting also led to postulation of an antithrombotic yet hemostatic paradigm governing aprotinin's mechanism of action: antithrombotic because it counteracts platelet activation by thrombin and hemostatic because it targets plasmin in the fibrinolytic pathway [73]. The antithrombotic yet hemostatic paradigm has since been confirmed and extended in a rabbit model of vascular injury [74]. This showed that vascular thrombosis in a carotid artery injury model was significantly attenuated by aprotinin through a platelet PAR mechanism, whereas its hemostatic properties in an incisional bleeding model were maintained.

PAR1 on Endothelium

The extent to which thrombin-induced PAR1 activation contributes to systemic endothelial activation during bypass is not known. In vitro, however, aprotinin exerts an identical PAR1-sparing property as observed in platelets, in which cleavage of the receptor by thrombin is prevented [75]. Aprotinin also blocked downstream inflammatory signaling pathways linked to PAR1, culminating in the inhibition of IL-6 secretion. Interleukin-6 is an acute phase inflammatory cytokine that plays a critical role in leukocytosis, thrombosis, inflammation, and neurodegeneration [76]. Plasma IL-6 levels are strongly induced at 3 to 4 hours following CPB and IL-6 was shown to be the most highly up-regulated gene (>41-fold increase) by microarray analysis of 12,625 genes in patients undergoing CPB and cardioplegic arrest [77,78]. There may also be a link between IL-6 and neurodegeneration and stroke. A gain of-function mutation in the IL-6 promoter is overrepresented in patients who have a history of ischemic stroke, and high plasma IL-6 levels are associated with neurologic worsening immediately following stroke [79,80]. Although the source of IL-6 postbypass is unclear, therapeutic blockade of endothelial PAR1 fits well as a molecular mechanism to explain, at least in part, the growing anti-stroke properties reported for aprotinin clinically [53–58].

The Anti-PAR1 Mechanism of Aprotinin

Aprotinin has clearly been shown to prevent proteolytic activation of PAR1 by thrombin, whereas nonproteolytic activation through PAR1-specific activating peptide SFLLRN remains intact [67,75]. Despite this evidence, aprotinin is not believed to inhibit the serine protease activity of thrombin directly, because its inhibitory constant (Ki) for thrombin is weak [81]. The systemic concentration of aprotinin achievable during bypass is nearly two orders of magnitude below that required to inhibit the amidolytic activity of thrombin directly. The working hypothesis is that aprotinin blocks the rate-limiting step of thrombin binding to the PAR1 receptor by preventing access of thrombin to the hirudin-like binding site on PAR1. This hypothetical mechanism is under current investigation.

SUMMARY

The human thrombin receptor PAR1 plays an important role in coordinating local coagulation and inflammatory responses to vascular injury. PAR1 may be activated systemically on platelets and vascular endothelium during cardiothoracic surgery with bypass, leading to thrombotic and inflammatory complications. The protease inhibitor aprotinin attenuates platelet and inflammatory complications by protecting PAR1 on platelets and endothelium from activation by thrombin, while maintaining a hemostatic effect through targeting of plasmin in the fibrinolytic pathway. This unique combination of targets makes it a safe and effective drug for use in cardiothoracic surgery. Other combinations of mono-targeting drugs may recapitulate the multiple benefits of aprotinin in cardiac surgery, but this possibility remains to be evaluated.

References

[1] Coughlin SR. Protease activated receptors in hemostasis, thrombosis and vascular biology. J Thromb Haemost 2005;3:1800–14.

[2] Vu TK, Hung DT, Wheaton VI, et al. Molecular cloning of a functional thrombin receptor reveals a novel proteolytic mechanism of receptor activation. Cell 1991;64:1057–68.

[3] Bode W, Schwager P, Huber R. The transition of bovine trypsinogen to a trypsin-like state upon strong ligand binding. J Mol Biol 1978;118:99–112.

[4] Hoxie JA, Ahuja M, Belmonte E, et al. Internalization and recycling of activated thrombin receptors. J Biol Chem 1993;268:13756–63.

[5] De Candia E, Hall SW, Rutella S, et al. Binding of thrombin to glycoprotein Ib accelerates the hydrolysis of PAR1 on intact platelets. J Biol Chem 2001;276:4692–8.

[6] Nakanishi-Matsui M, Zheng YW, Sulciner DJ, et al. PAR3 is a cofactor for PAR4 activation by thrombin. Nature 2000;404:609–13.

[7] Kahn ML, Zheng YW, Huang W, et al. A dual thrombin receptor system for platelet activation. Nature 1998;394:690–4.

[8] Kahn ML, Nakanishi MM, Shapiro MJ, et al. Protease-activated receptors 1 and 4 mediate activation of human platelets by thrombin. J Clin Invest 1999;103:879–87.

[9] Derian CK, Damiano BP, Addo MF, et al. Blockade of the thrombin receptor protease-activated receptor-1 with a small molecule antagonist prevents thrombus formation and vascular occlusion in non-human primates. J Pharmacol Exp Ther 2003;304:855–61.

[10] Covic L, Misra M, Badar J, et al. Pepducin-based intervention of thrombin-receptor signaling and systemic platelet activation. Nat Med 2002;8:1161–5.

[11] Brass LF, Vassallo RJ, Belmonte E, et al. Structure and function of the human platelet thrombin receptor. Studies using monoclonal antibodies directed against a defined domain within the receptor N terminus. J Biol Chem 1992;267:13795–8.

[12] Cook JJ, Sitko GR, Bednar B, et al. An antibody against the exosite of the cloned thrombin receptor inhibits experimental arterial thrombosis in the African green monkey. Circulation 1995;91:2961–71.

[13] Day JRS, Haskard DO, Taylor KM, et al. The effect of aprotinin and recombinant variants on platelet PAR1 activation. Ann Thorac Surg 2006;81:619–24.

[14] Suh TT, Holmback K, Jensen NJ, et al. Resolution of spontaneous bleeding events but failure of pregnancy in fibrinogen-deficient mice. Genes Dev 1995;9:2020–33.

[15] Sun WY, Witte DP, Degen JL, et al. Prothrombin deficiency results in embryonic and neonatal lethality in mice. Proc Natl Acad Sci U S A 1998;95:7597–602.

[16] Xue J, Wu Q, Westfield LA, et al. Incomplete embryonic lethality and fatal neonatal hemorrhage caused by prothrombin deficiency in mice. Proc Natl Acad Sci U S A 1998;95:7603–7.

[17] Sambrano GR, Weiss EJ, Zheng YW, et al. Role of thrombin signalling in platelets in hemostasis and thrombosis. Nature 2001;413:74–8.

[18] Camerer E, Duong DN, Hamilton JR, et al. Combined deficiency of protease-activated receptor-4 and fibrinogen recapitulates the hemostatic defect but not the embryonic lethality of prothrombin deficiency. Blood 2004;103:152–4.

[19] Hamilton JR, Cornelissen I, Coughlin SR. Impaired hemostasis and protection against throm-bosis in protease-activated receptor-4-deficient mice is due to lack of thrombin signaling in platelets. J Thromb Haemost 2004;2:1429–35.

[20] Shivdasani RA, Rosenblatt MF, Zucker-Franklin D, et al. Transcription factor NF-E2 is re-quired for platelet formation independent of the actions of thrombopoietin/MDGF in mega-karyocyte development. Cell 1995;81:695–704.

[21] Jirouskova M, Chereshney I, Vaananen H, et al. Antibody blockade or mutation of the fibrin-ogen gamma-chain C-terminus is more effective in inhibiting murine arterial thrombus forma-tion than complete absence of fibrinogen. Blood 2004;103:1995–2002.

[22] Molino M, Barnathan ES, Numerof R, et al. Interactions of mast cell tryptase with thrombin receptors and PAR-2. J Biol Chem 1997;272:4043–9.

[23] Camerer E, Huang W, Coughlin SR. Tissue factor- and factor X-dependent activation of pro-tease-activated receptor 2 by factor VIIa. Proc Natl Acad Sci U S A 2000;97:5255–60.

[24] Riewald M, Ruf W. Mechanistic coupling of protease signaling and initiation of coagulation by tissue factor. Proc Natl Acad Sci U S A 2001;98:7742–7.

[25] Lidington EA, Haskard DO, Mason JC. Induction of decay-accelerating factor by thrombin through a protease-activated receptor 1 and protein kinase C-dependent pathway protects vascular endothelial cells from complement-mediated injury. Blood 2000;96:2784–92.

[26] Hamilton JR, Frauman AG, Cocks TM. Increased expression of protease-activated receptor-2 (PAR2) and PAR4 in human coronary artery by inflammatory stimuli unveils endothelium-de-pendent relaxations to PAR2 and PAR4 agonists. Circ Res 2001;89:92–8.

[27] Nystedt S, Ramakrishnan V, Sundelin J. The proteinase-activated receptor 2 is induced by inflammatory mediators in human endothelial cells. Comparison with the thrombin receptor. J Biol Chem 1996;271:14910–5.

[28] Kaplanski G, Marin V, Fabrigoule M, et al. Thrombin-activated human endothelial cells sup-port monocyte adhesion in vitro following expression of intercellular adhesion molecule-1 (ICAM-1; CD54) and vascular cell adhesion molecule-1 (VCAM-1; CD106). Blood 1998; 92:1259–67.

[29] Wu SQ, Minami T, Donovan DJ, et al. The proximal serum response element in the Egr-1 pro-moter mediates response to thrombin in primary human endothelial cells. Blood 2002;100: 4454–61.

[30] Marin V, Montero-Julian FA, Gres S, et al. The IL-6-soluble IL-6Ralpha autocrine loop of en-dothelial activation as an intermediate between acute and chronic inflammation: an exper-imental model involving thrombin. J Immunol 2001;167:3435–42.

[31] Lidington EA, Steinberg R, Kinderlerer AR, et al. A role for protease-activated receptor-2 and PKCε in thrombin-mediated induction of decay accelerating factor on human endothelial cells. Am J Physiol Cell Physiol 2005;289(6):C1437–47.

[32] Hattori R, Hamilton KK, Fugate RD, et al. Stimulated secretion of endothelial von Willebrand factor is accompanied by rapid redistribution to the cell surface of the intracellular granule membrane protein GMP-140. J Biol Chem 1989;264:7768–71.

[33] Lum H, Malik AB. Regulation of vascular endothelial barrier function. Am J Physiol 1994; 267(3 Pt 1):L223–41.

[34] Pawlinski R, Pederson B, Schabbauer G, et al. Role of tissue factor and protease activated receptors in endotoxemia and sepsis. Blood 2003;101:3940–7.

[35] Wildevuur CR, Eijsman L, Roozendaal KJ, et al. Platelet preservation during cardiopulmo-nary bypass with aprotinin. Eur J Cardiothorac Surg 1989;3:533–7.

[36] Mohr R, Goor DA, Lusky A, et al. Aprotinin prevent cardiopulmonary bypass-induced plate-let dysfunction: a scanning electron microscope study. Circulation 1992;86:II-405–9.

[37] Blauhut B, Harringer W, Bettelheim P, et al. Comparison of the effects of aprotinin and tra-nexamic acid on blood loss and related variables after cardiopulmonary bypass. J Thorac Cardiovasc Surg 1994;108:1083–91.

[38] Bradfield JE, Bode AP. Aprotinin restores the adhesive capacity of dysfunctional platelets. Thromb Res 2003;109:181–8.

[39] Edmonds LH Jr. Cardiopulmonary bypass and blood. In: Roque, editor. Blood conservation with aprotinin. Philadelphia: Hanley and Belfus Inc; 1995. p. 45–66.

[40] Rinder CS, Bohnert J, Rinder HM, et al. Platelet activation and aggregation during cardiopulmonary bypass. Anesthesiology 1991;75:388–93.

[41] Boisclar MD, Lane DA, Philippou H, et al. Thrombin production, inactivation and expression during open heart surgery measured by assays for activation fragments including new ELISA for prothrombin fragment F1 + 2. Thromb Haemost 1993;70:253–8.

[42] Brister SJ, Ofosu FA, Buchanan MR. Thrombin generation during cardiac surgery: is heparin the ideal anticoagulant? Thromb Haemost 1993;70:259–62.

[43] Ferraris VA, Ferraris SP, Singh A, et al. The platelet thrombin receptor and postoperative bleeding. Ann Thorac Surg 1998;65:352–8.

[44] Landis RC, Haskard DO, Taylor KM. New antiinflammatory and platelet-preserving effects of aprotinin. Ann Thorac Surg 2001;72:S1808–13.

[45] Wachtfogel YT, Kucich U, Hack CE, et al. Aprotinin inhibits the contact, neutrophil, and platelet activation systems during simulated extracorporeal perfusion. J Thorac Cardiovasc Surg 1993;106:1–10.

[46] Hill GE, Alonso A, Spurzem JR, et al. Aprotinin and methylprednisolone equally blunt neutrophil cardiopulmonary bypass-induced inflammation in humans. J Thorac Cardiovasc Surg 1995;110:1658–62.

[47] Rinder CS, Rinder HM, Smith BR, et al. Blockade of C5a and C5b-9 generation inhibits leukocyte and platelet activation during extracorporeal circulation. J Clin Invest 1995;96:1564–72.

[48] Rinder CS, Rinder HM, Johnson K, et al. Role of C3 cleavage in monocyte activation during extracorporeal circulation. Circulation 1999;100:553–8.

[49] Bevilaqua MP, Pober JS, Majeau GR, et al. Recombinant tumor necrosis factor induces procoagulant activity in cultured human vascular endothelium: characterization and comparison with the actions of interleukin 1. Proc Natl Acad Sci U S A 1986;83:4533–7.

[50] Horgan MJ, Ge M, Gu J, et al. Role of ICAM-1 in neutrophil-mediated lung vascular injury after occlusion and reperfusion. Am J Physiol 1991;261:H1578–84.

[51] Naka Y, Toda K, Kayano K, et al. Failure to express the P-selectin gene or P-selectin blockade confers early pulmonary protection after lung ischemia or transplantation. Proc Natl Acad Sci U S A 1997;94:757–61.

[52] Asimakopoulos G, Smith PL, Ratnatunga CP, et al. Lung injury and acute respiratory distress syndrome after cardiopulmonary bypass. Ann Thorac Surg 1999;68:1107–15.

[53] Levy JH, Pifarre R, Schaff HV, et al. A multicenter, double-blind, placebo-controlled trial of aprotinin for reducing blood loss and the requirement for donor-blood transfusion in patients undergoing repeat coronary artery bypass grafting. Circulation 1995;92:2236–44.

[54] Smith PK, Muhlbaier LH. Aprotinin: safe and effective only with the full-dose regimen. Ann Thorac Surg 1996;62:1575–7.

[55] Murkin JM. Attenuation of neurologic injury during cardiac surgery. Ann Thorac Surg 2001;72:S1838–44.

[56] Sedrakyan A, Treasure T, Elefteriades JA. Effect of aprotinin on clinical outcomes in coronary artery bypass graft surgery: a systematic review and meta-analysis of randomized clinical trials. J Thorac Cardiovasc Surg 2004;128:442–8.

[57] Frumento RJ, O'Malley CMN, Bennett-Guerrero E. Stroke after cardiac surgery: a retrospective analysis of the effect of aprotinin dosing regimens. Ann Thorac Surg 2003;75:479–84.

[58] Harmon DC, Ghori KG, Eustace NP, et al. Aprotinin decreases the incidence of cognitive deficit following CABG and cardiopulmonary bypass: a pilot randomized controlled study. Can J Anaesth 2004;51:1002–7.

[59] Berghoff von A, Glatzel U. [Inhibition of the fibrinolytic potential by Trasylol]. Med Klin 1963;12:476–8 [in German].

[60] Werle E, Trautschold I. Kallikrein, kallidin and kallikrein inhibitors. Ann N Y Acad Sci 1963;104:117–29.

[61] Kamiya T, Katayama Y, Kashiwagi F, et al. The role of bradykinin in mediating ischemic brain edema in rats. Stroke 1993;24:571–5.

[62] Asimakopoulos G, Thompson R, Nourshargh S, et al. An anti-inflammatory property of aprotinin discovered at the level of leukocyte extravasation. J Thorac Cardiovasc Surg 2000; 120:361–9.

[63] Royston D, Bidstrup BP, Taylor KM, et al. Effect of aprotinin on need for blood transfusion after repeat open heart surgery. Lancet 1987;2:1289–92.

[64] Bidstrup BP, Royston D, Sapsford RN, et al. Reduction in blood loss after cardiopulmonary bypass using high dose aprotinin (Trasylol). J Thorac Cardiovasc Surg 1989;97: 364–72.

[65] Mangano DT, Tudor IC, Dietzel C, et al. The risk associated with aprotinin in cardiac surgery. N Engl J Med 2006;354:353–65.

[66] Gott JP, Cooper WA, Schmidt FE Jr, et al. Modifying risk for extracorporeal circulation: trial of four antiinflammatory strategies. Ann Thorac Surg 1998;66:747–53.

[67] Day JRS, Punjabi PP, Haskard DO, et al. Clinical inhibition of the seven-transmembrane thrombin receptor (PAR1) by intravenous aprotinin during cardiothoracic surgery. Circulation 2004;110:2597–600.

[68] Maquelin KN, Nieuwland R, Lentjes EG, et al. Aprotinin administration in the pericardial cavity does not prevent platelet activation. J Thorac Cardiovasc Surg 2000;120:552–7.

[69] Poullis M, Manning R, Laffan M, et al. The anti-thrombotic effect of aprotinin: actions mediated through the protease-activated receptor 1. J Thorac Cardiovasc Surg 2000;120: 370–8.

[70] Lindvall G, Sartipy U, van der Linden J. Aprotinin reduces bleeding and blood product use in patients treated with clopidogrel before coronary artery bypass grafting. Ann Thorac Surg 2005;80:922–7.

[71] van der Linden J, Lindvall G, Sartipy U. Aprotinin decreases postoperative bleeding and number of transfusions in patients on clopidogrel undergoing coronary artery bypass graft surgery: a double-blind, placebo-controlled, randomized clinical trial. Circulation 2005; 112(9 Suppl):I276–80.

[72] Akowuah E, Shrivastava V, Jamnadas B, et al. Comparison of two strategies for the management of antiplatelet therapy during urgent surgery. Ann Thorac Surg 2005;80:149–52.

[73] Landis RC, Asimakopoulos G, Poullis M, et al. The antithrombotic and antiinflammatory mechanisms of action of aprotinin. Ann Thorac Surg 2001;72:2169–75.

[74] Khan TA, Bianchi C, Voisine P, et al. Aprotinin inhibits protease-dependent platelet aggregation and thrombosis. Ann Thorac Surg 2005;79:1545–50.

[75] Day JRS, Taylor KM, Haskard DO, et al. Aprotinin inhibits proinflammatory activation of endothelial cells by thrombin via the protease-activated receptor 1. J Throac Cardiovasc Surg 2006;131:21–7.

[76] Kerr R, Sterlin D, Ludlam CA. Interleukin-6 and haemostasis. Br J Haematol 2001;115: 3–12.

[77] Steinberg JB, Kapelanski DP, Olson JD, et al. Cytokine and complement levels in patients undergoing cardiopulmonary bypass. J Thorac Cardiovasc Surg 1993;106:1008–16.

[78] Voisine P, Ruel M, Khan TA, et al. Differences in gene expression profiles of diabetic and non-diabetic patients undergoing cardiopulmonary bypass and cardioplegic arrest. Circulation 2004;110:II280–6.

[79] Pola R, Flex A, Gaetani E, et al. Synergistic effect of -174 G/C polymorphism of the interleukin-6 gene promoter and 469 E/K polymorphism of the intercellular adhesion molecule-1 gene in Italian patients with history of ischemic stroke. Stroke 2003;34: 881–5.

[80] Vila N, Castillo J, Davalos A, et al. Levels of anti-inflammatory cytokines and neurological worsening in acute ischemic stroke. Stroke 2003;34:671–5.

[81] Pintigny D, Dachary-Prigent J. Aprotinin can inhibit the proteolytic activity of thrombin. A fluorescence and an enzymatic study. Eur J Biochem 1992;207(1):89–95.

Hematol Oncol Clin N Am 21 (2007) 115–121

HEMATOLOGY/ONCOLOGY CLINICS
OF NORTH AMERICA

Platelets as Mediators of Inflammation

Steven R. Steinhubl, MD

Division of Cardiology, University of Kentucky, 900 South Limestone Avenue,
326 Charles T. Wellington Building, Lexington, KY 40536-0200, USA

It is now well-recognized that atherosclerosis is an inflammatory disease [1]. It is equally well-established that platelets play a central role in the development, progression, and clinical stability of atherosclerotic disease [2]. What is less well-appreciated is the role of the platelet as an inflammatory cell. Understanding that the platelet evolved from single circulatory cells, the hemocyte, that were critical in hemostasis, inflammation, and oxygen transport [3], it is perhaps easier to realize how the platelet does much more than just serve as a passive accomplice in the thrombotic response to vascular injury. The association between the platelet and inflammatory diseases is highlighted by the number of inflammatory disease processes shown to be associated with platelet activation (Box 1).

When a platelet undergoes activation, over 300 proteins are released [4]. Only a relatively small proportion of these proteins have been identified, but clearly a significant proportion are known inflammatory mediators (Fig. 1). Although much still needs to be learned about the role of most of the components of the releasate of an activated platelet, a number of the proinflammatory molecules–CD40 ligand (CD40L), P-selectin, IL-1β, platelet factor 4, and RANTES–have been well-established in the progression and stability of atherosclerotic disease [5].

No inflammatory marker better establishes the important association between platelet activation, thrombosis, and inflammation than does CD40L (also known as CD154). CD40L is a primarily platelet-based immunomodulator of the tumor necrosis factor family that has only recently been shown to be expressed by activated platelets [6]. Following platelet surface expression of CD40L, it is cleaved over a period of minutes to hours, and can be measured in plasma as soluble CD40L. Once thought to be primarily limited to lymphocytes, it is now know that activated platelets secrete more than 90% of the circulating CD40L [6], which is responsible for antibody class switching, apoptosis, coagulation, and stimulation of proinflammatory cytokines and COX-2 prostaglandins. The release of stored CD40L on platelet activation leads to stimulation of vascular endothelial cells to produce cytokines, such

E-mail address: steinhubl@uky.edu

0889-8588/07/$ – see front matter
doi:10.1016/j.hoc.2006.11.015

Box 1: Inflammatory conditions, other than atherosclerosis, associated with platelet activation

Systemic lupus erythematosus

Rheumatoid arthritis

Psoriasis

Inflammatory bowel disease

Sepsis

Migraine headaches

Coronary artery bypass grafting

as IL-1 and IL-18, and increased thrombotic activity [7]. CD40L appears to be directly involved in the inflammatory response of the vessel wall, activating vascular endothelial cells to secrete many chemokines that attract leukocytes to the site of injury and induce expression of tissue factor. CD40L has also been shown to promote the formation of thrombi by binding the glycoprotein

Inflammation Modulating Factors Released By Activated Platelets

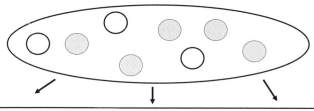

P-selectin	Thromboxane A2
CD40 ligand (CD 154)	Neutrophil Activating Peptide 2
Platelet Factor 4	Sphigosine1-phosphate
TGF- β1	LIGHT
Macrophage Inflammatory Protein-1α	IL-7
12-HETE	Monocyte Chemotactic Protein 3
Nitric Oxide	Epithelial Neutrophil Activating Prot. 78
Histamine	Growth-Regulating Oncogene-α
Serotonin	High Mobility Group Box 1
RANTES	IL-1β
Platelet Activating Factor	

Fig. 1. Factors released by activated platelets know to be involved in inflammation. HETE, hydroxyeicosatetrenoate; IL, interleukin; LIGHT, derived from "homologous to lymphotoxins, exhibits inducible expression, and competes with herpes simplex virus (HSV) glycoprotein D for herpes virus entry mediator (HVEM/TR2), a receptor expressed by T lymphocytes"; RANTES, regulated on activation, normal T expressed and secreted; TGF, transforming growth factor.

(GP) IIb/IIIa receptor [8]. In several animal models, inhibiting CD40L leads to stabilization of atherosclerotic lesions [9,10]. Consistent with its role in inflammatory disease states, several models of chronic inflammatory conditions, including arthritis, can be blocked or substantially relieved by inhibiting the binding of CD40L to its receptor [11,12].

Platelet activation also leads to surface expression of P-selectin (CD62), which binds to P-selectin glycoprotein ligand-1 (PSGL-1) on leukocytes, promoting the formation of platelet-leukocyte complexes [13,14]. The resulting leukocyte activation leads to surface expression of the β2 integrin Mac-1 [15], another receptor for platelet-leukocyte interaction. P-selectin expression also results in monocyte expression of tissue factor, and causes monocytes to release inflammatory cytokines [16]. In several animal models, selective blockade of P-selectin has been shown to limit infarct size following coronary ischemia and reperfusion [17]. Patients who have acute myocardial infarction (MI) show increased P-selectin–mediated platelet-leukocyte adhesion [18], whereas those who have non-ST-segment elevation acute coronary syndromes (ACS) show sustained P-selectin expression after the ischemic event [19].

DO ANTIPLATELET AGENTS INFLUENCE INFLAMMATION?
Aspirin
Aspirin is commonly thought of as an anti-inflammatory agent, and at doses of approximately 1300 mg a day, it clearly is. What is less clear is if doses commonly used for the prevention and treatment of cardiovascular disease (75 mg to 325 mg daily) have any direct anti-inflammatory effects. In one early study, 300 mg of aspirin daily was found to reduce C-reactive protein (CRP) and IL-6 levels in patients who had chronic stable angina [20]; however, these findings have not been supported by other recent studies. In a randomized, double-blind study in healthy men, changes in CRP levels produced by exercise were measured at baseline and after 7 days' treatment with acetylsalicylic acid (ASA)–81 or 325 mg/day [21]. This study found no significant effect of aspirin on CRP levels, either at rest or post-exercise. Similarly, in a placebo-controlled trial in 57 healthy male and female volunteers, 31 days' treatment with ASA 81 mg, a regimen that potently inhibited platelet cyclooxygenase activity, produced no significant reduction in the level of high-sensitivity CRP [22].

Evidence for a role of ASA in the prevention of inflammation-induced endothelial dysfunction has been reported from a study that used *Salmonella typhi* vaccination to generate an inflammatory response [23]. The protective effect of ASA was postulated to occur via modulation of the cytokine cascade; however, the ASA dose used (single oral dose of ASA 1.2 g) was much higher than that used clinically.

Clopidogrel
Several studies have also evaluated the ability of clopidogrel to decrease levels of measured systemic markers of inflammation. In a study of patients undergoing a percutaneous coronary intervention (PCI), clopidogrel pretreatment, like

aspirin, was associated with a reduction in ADP-induced expression of platelet CD40L immediately after the intervention, as well as reductions in ADP- and TRAP-induced expression of platelet P-selectin [24]. In another observational study of nearly 900 patients undergoing a PCI, clopidogrel pretreated patients experienced a significantly lower increase in CRP levels following the procedure than those patients not pretreated [25].

In a study of patients who had a non-ST-segment elevation ACS, platelet-leukocyte conjugates were significantly reduced at 24 hours after administration of a 300 mg clopidogrel loading dose (also in addition to aspirin) [26]. These effects were accompanied by significant reductions in platelet surface CD40L, and circulating levels of soluble P-selectin and soluble CD40L in plasma.

In a third study involving patients who had suffered an acute ischemic stroke, the influence of treatment with clopidogrel on top of ASA for 7 days was compared with those of aspirin alone [27]. In the clopidogrel group, both P-selectin expression and plasma levels of CRP were significantly reduced at 7 days post-stroke. Interestingly, these improvements in inflammatory biomarkers correlated with clinical improvement, as assessed by the National Institutes of Health (NIH) stroke scale score.

The data regarding whether treatment with clopidogrel in addition to aspirin has any influence on inflammatory markers compared with aspirin alone are not entirely consistent, though. In a sub-study of the Clopidogrel in Unstable Angina to Prevent Recurrent Events (CURE) trial, in which patients who had ACS were randomized to clopidogrel plus aspirin versus aspirin alone, randomization to clopidogrel did not influence the mean plasma P-selectin levels after 7 and 30 days of treatment [28]. Similar results have been presented from the CURE trial, although not yet published, for CRP levels at 7 and 30 days, with again no difference in patients treated with clopidogrel and aspirin compared with aspirin alone.

DOES INFLAMMATION INFLUENCE THE BENEFIT OF ANTIPLATELET AGENTS?

Although the data are not convincing that antiplatelet therapies decrease plasma levels of inflammatory biomarkers, limited data do suggest that the level of inflammatory biomarkers, in particular CRP, are associated with the clinical benefit of the antiplatelet agents clopidogrel and aspirin.

One of the first studies to suggest that a patient's CRP level may be predictive of his risk of future thrombotic events was a case-control analysis from the Physicians Health Study, in which primarily healthy males were randomized to 325 mg of aspirin every other day or placebo [29]. The analysis found that increasing quartiles of CRP were associated with a significant increase in risk for an MI in patients randomized to placebo. On the other hand, patients randomized to aspirin experienced a blunting of the risk associated with an elevation in baseline CRP, with the greatest relative risk reduction from aspirin in those who had the highest baseline levels of CRP.

Similar data suggest that clopidogrel in addition to aspirin may be particularly beneficial compared with aspirin alone in patients who have higher levels of inflammation. In an initial study in PCI patients, clopidogrel pretreatment on a background of ASA therapy was shown to reduce the increased 30-day risk of death or MI associated with elevated baseline levels of CRP [30]. A post hoc analysis of the Clopidogrel for Reduction of Events During Observation (CREDO) trial has also analyzed the benefit of clopidogrel according to baseline level of high-sensitivity CRP. In this analysis, the combined risk of death, MI, or stroke at 12 months was significantly correlated with increasing tertiles of CRP among patients in the control arm. Long-term clopidogrel therapy was associated with a statistically significant 44% relative risk reduction for this end point in patients in the highest tertile of CRP, whereas randomized therapy had no obvious impact on clinical outcomes among individuals in the lowest tertile of CRP. Importantly, this benefit of clopidogrel was achieved not only early following the PCI, but had its most marked effect with prolonged treatment from 28 days and 1 year.

Whether the clinical benefit of aspirin and the thienopyridines can be determined based on a patient's baseline inflammatory levels requires validation in a prospective trial. In the meantime, the inflammation sub-study of the Clopidogrel for High Atherothrombotic Risk and Ischemic Stabilization, Management and Avoidance (CHARISMA) trial, which studied clopidogrel plus aspirin versus aspirin alone in over 15,000 patients, will provide more important data regarding the association between inflammation and the clinical benefit of antiplatelet agents.

SUMMARY

An expanding body of evidence continues to build upon the central role of inflammation in the progression and clinical manifestations of atherosclerosis. Platelets, long thought to play only a reactionary role at the time of endothelial disruption, are now recognized as important mediators of the inflammatory process. Although compelling evidence is lacking that antiplatelet therapies directly lower markers of inflammation, there are intriguing, although preliminary, data suggesting that markers of inflammation predict the clinical benefit of antiplatelet therapies.

Improving our understanding of the platelet as an inflammatory cell and how various therapies influence it will likely lead to significant improvements in the treatment and prevention of atherosclerotic diseases.

References
[1] Ross RS. Atherosclerosis: an inflammatory disease. N Engl J Med 1999;340:115–26.
[2] Steinhubl SR, Moliterno DJ. The role of the platelet in the pathogenesis of atherothrombosis. Am J Cardiovasc Drugs 2005;5(6):399–408.
[3] Iwanaga S. Primitive coagulation systems and their message to modern biology. Thromb Haemost 1993;70(1):48–55.
[4] Coppinger JA, Cagney G, Toomey S, et al. Characterization of the proteins released from activated platelets leads to localization of novel platelet proteins in human atherosclerotic lesions. Blood 2004;103(6):2096–104.

[5] Wagner DD, Burger PC. Platelets in inflammation and thrombosis. Arterioscler Thromb Vasc Biol 2003;23(12):2131–37.

[6] Henn V, Slupsky JR, Grafe M, et al. CD40 ligand on activated platelets triggers an inflammatory reaction of endothelial cells. Nature 1998;391(6667):591–4.

[7] Schonbeck U, Libby P. CD40 signaling and plaque instability. Circ Res 2001;89(12): 1092–103.

[8] May AE, Kalsch T, Massberg S, et al. Engagement of glycoprotein IIb/IIIa (alpha(IIb)beta3) on platelets upregulates CD40L and triggers CD40L-dependent matrix degradation by endothelial cells. Circulation 2002;106(16):2111–7.

[9] Lutgens E, Cleutjens KB, Heeneman S, et al. Both early and delayed anti-CD40L antibody treatment induces a stable plaque phenotype. Proc Natl Acad Sci USA 2000;97(13): 7464–9.

[10] Schonbeck U, Sukhova GK, Shimizu K, et al. Inhibition of CD40 signaling limits evolution of established atherosclerosis in mice. Proc Natl Acad Sci USA 2000;97(13):7458–63.

[11] Durie FH, Aruffo A, Ledbetter J, et al. Antibody to the ligand of CD40, gp39, blocks the occurrence of the acute and chronic forms of graft-vs-host disease. J Clin Invest 1994;94(3): 1333–8.

[12] Durie FH, Fava RA, Foy TM, et al. Prevention of collagen-induced arthritis with an antibody to gp39, the ligand for CD40. Science 1993;261(5126):1328–30.

[13] Rinder HM, Bonan JL, Rinder CS, et al. Activated and unactivated platelet adhesion to monocytes and neutrophils. Blood 1991;78(7):1760–9.

[14] Rinder HM, Bonan JL, Rinder CS, et al. Dynamics of leukocyte-platelet adhesion in whole blood. Blood 1991;78(7):1730–7.

[15] Neumann FJ, Zohlnhofer D, Fakhoury L, et al. Effect of glycoprotein IIb/IIIa receptor blockade on platelet-leukocyte interaction and surface expression of the leukocyte integrin Mac-1 in acute myocardial infarction. J Am Coll Cardiol 1999;34(5):1420–6.

[16] Huo Y, Ley KF. Role of platelets in the development of atherosclerosis. Trends Cardiovasc Med 2004;14(1):18–22.

[17] Wang K, Zhou X, Zhou Z, et al. Recombinant soluble P-selectin glycoprotein ligand-Ig (rPSGL-Ig) attenuates infarct size and myeloperoxidase activity in a canine model of ischemia-reperfusion. Thromb Haemost 2002;88(1):149–54.

[18] Neumann FJ, Marx N, Gawaz M, et al. Induction of cytokine expression in leukocytes by binding of thrombin-stimulated platelets. Circulation 1997;95(10):2387–94.

[19] Ault KA, Cannon CP, Mitchell J, et al. Platelet activation in patients after an acute coronary syndrome: results from the TIMI-12 trial. J Am Coll Cardiol 1999;33:634–9.

[20] Ikonomidis I, Andreotti F, Economou E, et al. Increased proinflammatory cytokines in patients with chronic stable angina and their reduction by aspirin. Circulation 1999; 100(8):793–8.

[21] Feng D, Tracy RP, Lipinska I, et al. Effect of short-term aspirin use on C-reactive protein. J Thromb Thrombolysis 2000;9(1):37–41.

[22] Feldman M, Jialal I, Devaraj S, et al. Effects of low-dose aspirin on serum C-reactive protein and thromboxane B2 concentrations: a placebo-controlled study using a highly sensitive C-reactive protein assay. J Am Coll Cardiol 2001;37(8):2036–41.

[23] Kharbanda RK, Walton B, Allen M, et al. Prevention of inflammation-induced endothelial dysfunction: a novel vasculo-protective action of aspirin. Circulation 2002;105(22): 2600–4.

[24] Quinn MJ, Bhatt DL, Zidar F, et al. Effect of clopidogrel pretreatment on inflammatory marker expression in patients undergoing percutaneous coronary intervention. Am J Cardiol 2004;93(6):679–84.

[25] Vivekananthan DP, Bhatt DL, Chew DP, et al. Effect of clopidogrel pretreatment on periprocedural rise in C-reactive protein after percutaneous coronary intervention. Am J Cardiol 2004;94(3):358–60.

[26] Xiao Z, Theroux P. Clopidogrel inhibits platelet-leukocyte interactions and thrombin receptor agonist peptide-induced platelet activation in patients with an acute coronary syndrome. J Am Coll Cardiol 2004;43(11):1982–88.

[27] Cha JK, Jeong MH, Lee KM, et al. Changes in platelet P-selectin and in plasma C-reactive protein in acute atherosclerotic ischemic stroke treated with a loading dose of clopidogrel. J Thromb Thrombolysis 2002;14(2):145–50.

[28] Eikelboom JW, Weitz JI, Budaj A, et al. Clopidogrel does not suppress blood markers of coagulation activation in aspirin-treated patients with non-ST-elevation acute coronary syndromes. Eur Heart J 2002;23(22):1771–9.

[29] Ridker PM, Cushman M, Stampfer MJ, et al. Inflammation, aspirin, and the risk of cardiovascular disease in apparently healthy men. N Engl J Med 1997;336(14):973–9.

[30] Chew DP, Bhatt DL, Robbins MA, et al. Effect of clopidogrel added to aspirin before percutaneous coronary intervention on the risk associated with C-reactive protein. Am J Cardiol 2001;88:672–4.

Hematol Oncol Clin N Am 21 (2007) 123–145

HEMATOLOGY/ONCOLOGY CLINICS
OF NORTH AMERICA

Inflammation, Proinflammatory Mediators and Myocardial Ischemia–reperfusion Injury

Jakob Vinten-Johansen, PhD[a],[*], Rong Jiang, MD, PhD[a],
James G. Reeves, MD[b], James Mykytenko, MD[b],
Jeremiah Deneve, MD[a], Lynetta J. Jobe, DVM, PhD[c]

[a]Department of Surgery (Cardiothoracic), Cardiothoracic Research Laboratory, Carlyle Fraser Heart Center of Emory Crawford Long Hospital, Emory University, 550 Peachtree Street NE, Atlanta, GA 30308-2225, USA
[b]Department of Surgery, Emory University School of Medicine, Atlanta, GA, USA
[c]Department of Physiology, Mercer University College of Pharmacy and Health Sciences, Atlanta, GA, USA

THE PATHOPHYSIOLOGY OF MYOCARDIAL ISCHEMIA—REPERFUSION INJURY

In 2002, there were over 3,480,000 heart attacks in the United States alone. There were 1,121,000 angioplasties performed in the United States; this number is estimated to increase to 2.4 million in 2004 to 2005. Angioplasty is the primary approach to achieving reperfusion and is the definitive treatment for coronary occlusive disease to reduce the extent of myocardial infarction. Without reperfusion, the entire area at risk involved in a coronary occlusion will become necrotic.

In the 1970s, investigations sought to describe the determinants of myocardial infarction so that appropriate therapies could be strategically developed to reduce infarct size. In 1977, Reimer and colleagues [1] described the time course of infarction resulting from coronary artery occlusion (regional ischemia) as an advancing "wavefront" whereby the necrotic edges extended toward the epicardial surface with increasing durations of coronary artery occlusion. The implication was that the advancing necrotic wavefront within the area at risk myocardium could be limited by initiating reperfusion as early as possible after the onset of ischemia. The study by DeWood and colleagues [2] demonstrating that acute myocardial infarction was precipitated by intracoronary thrombus was the genesis of thrombolysis as a therapeutic approach to initiating timely

This study was supported in part by a grant from the National Heart Lung and Blood Institute of the National Institutes of Health to JV-J (HL069487).

*Corresponding author. E-mail address: jvinten@emory.edu (J. Vinten-Johansen).

0889-8588/07/$ – see front matter
doi:10.1016/j.hoc.2006.11.010

reperfusion—an approach that remains the cornerstone of myocardial reperfusion therapeutics and salvage today [3]. Reperfusion of ischemic myocardium was further advanced by primary percutaneous coronary intervention including angioplasty and deployment of stents. Currently, the principle treatments for acute myocardial infarction are acetylsalicylic acid, thrombolysis using streptokinase or tissue plasminogen activators, or primary percutaneous coronary intervention—the latter combined with platelet glycoprotein IIb/IIIa inhibitors. This approach is focused on restoring blood flow as quickly and as completely as possible to reduce the duration of ischemia that predetermines infarct size.

Although timely reperfusion of epicardial vessels successfully restores blood flow (TIMI grade 3) in 30% to 95% of cases and thereby limits infarct size by reducing the duration of occlusion, there is substantial evidence that the process of reperfusion contributes to the ultimate extent of postischemic myocardial injury [4–11]. An entire issue of Cardiovascular Research has been devoted to the topic of reperfusion injury (Volume 61, February 2004). Reperfusion injury is expressed in many ways, including 1) dysfunction of the area at risk (either the area at risk or the entire left ventricle if global ischemia is induced [eg, in cardiac surgery]), 2) endothelial dysfunction, 3) microvascular blood flow defects, 4) metabolic defects, 5) cellular necrosis, and 6) apoptosis [12]. In 1960, Jennings and colleagues [13] first described the deleterious changes observed after reperfusion of ischemic myocardium. They suggested, however, that reperfusion hastened the demise of cells that were already injured by ischemia; reperfusion was not thought to induce cell death in cells that were viable at the end of ischemia. "While reperfusion ... relieves or at least greatly reduces myocardial ischemia, it also results in a complex group of phenomena, some of which may initially appear to be deleterious...[These deleterious phenomena] ... include the hastening of the necrotic process of irreversibly injured myocytes." [14]. It was not until later that reperfusion was viewed as instigating irreversible cell death by either necrosis or apoptosis. The postischemic events and their physiologic manifestations are collectively termed "reperfusion injury" [9,12,15]. Reperfusion injury in its various manifestations has been observed in most experimental models and, to one degree or another, in humans [16–18]. Cardiac surgeons have long recognized that reperfusion of postischemic hearts was associated with morbid consequences such as edema, contractile dysfunction (the extreme of which is the "stone heart" [19]), metabolic abnormalities, and myocardial necrosis, pathophysiological events which have long been suspected of contributing significantly to the overall morbidity and mortality of cardiac surgery [20].

The hypothesis was put forth by early experimentation in surgical myocardial protection that reperfusion was a potential contributor to lethal injury of previously ischemic myocardium [21]. "If this is so, then it might be expected that protective pharmacologic agents administered during the reperfusion phase should be capable of limiting tissue necrosis..." [14], which was demonstrated by some early experimental evidence in nonsurgical models of coronary artery occlusion–reperfusion [22,23] as well as surgical models of myocardial protection (ie, cardioplegia compositions) [24–26]. Bulkley and Hutchins [27], reporting in 1977 on the manifestation of necrosis after successful surgical re-vascularization of acute myocardial infarction, concluded that "...prevention of intraoperative myocardial injury must also focus on characteristics of the phase of myocardial reperfusion." Indeed, seminal research established that reperfusion injury could be attenuated by both mechanical and pharmacologic strategies applied at or just before the onset of reperfusion. Mechanical interventions applied at the time of reperfusion have shown an impressive reduction in postischemic injury. Hypothermia [28,29] and gradual reperfusion [30–32] are examples of mechanical interventions applied at the time of reperfusion that have reduced infarct size and other manifestations of postischemic injury. One of the most recent mechanical interventions to show reductions in postischemic injury after coronary artery occlusion is "postconditioning" [33,34], also called "stutter" reperfusion [35]. The ability of these interventions to reduce postischemic injury indirectly supports the existence of reperfusion injury.

Reperfusion "syndrome" or injury has been observed clinically after thrombolysis or primary angioplasty as an additional elevation of ST segment by 25% to 50% [36–43]. Some clinical investigators have reported a significant increase in cardiac enzymes, used as a surrogate measure of infarct size, upon reperfusion [16,18]. However, the full extent of morphologic injury (eg, infarction, apoptosis) attributable to reperfusion events is currently unknown in clinical populations but has been estimated to range from 25% to over 50% [18,44]. This increase in myocardial injury upon reperfusion over and above that observed at the end of ischemia implies that (1) reperfusion injury offsets to some (unknown) extent the salvage of myocardium achieved with reperfusion; (2) myocardial injury (ie, infarct size, endothelial dysfunction and left ventricular systolic and diastolic dysfunction) may be reduced by therapies applied at the onset of reperfusion using strategies targeting the numerous mechanisms of reperfusion injury [7,12,10,45,11].

Nature demonstrates its proclivity to redundancy and complexity in the multiplicity of contributors to reperfusion injury in the myocardium. The major causes of reperfusion injury in postischemic myocardium are summarized (see later discussion).

Rapid and Persistent Generation of Reactive Oxygen Species

The generation of reactive oxygen species (ROS) has been associated with myocardial contracture and the release of intracellular enzymes through a disrupted cell membrane. This series of events has been termed the "oxygen paradox", a term coined by David Hearse and associates. ROS generation has been observed to a limited extent during ischemia, but with a marked respiratory burst occurring within the first minutes [46] and even seconds [47] of reperfusion. The primary species of oxygen radicals include superoxide anions, hydrogen peroxide, and hydroxyl radicals. These ROS will damage cell membranes by peroxidation of the membrane polyunsaturated lipids. Myocardial infarction resulting from ROS generation can be reduced by scavengers

administered during reperfusion [48]. For effective reduction of these endogenously generated oxidants, the oxidant therapy must be in place during the first
minutes of reperfusion [6]. ROS are generated by activated neutrophils [5,49],
cardiomyocytes, activated vascular endothelium, and to a minor extent perivascular tissue. Neutrophils generate ROS principally through the reduced nicotin-
amide adenine dinucleotide phosphate (NADPH) oxidase system. Neutrophils
may be activated by cytokines, platelet activating factor [50], and complement
to produce ROS in a respiratory burst within the first minutes of reperfusion
[5]. However, neutrophils may also be involved in a lower level of ROS generation that exceeds baseline values. Superoxide radical generation has been
observed 3 or more hours after the onset of reperfusion in both large [51]
and small [52] animal models of coronary artery occlusion–reperfusion. In addition, neutrophils generate hypochlorous acid through the enzyme myeloperoxidase that degrades membrane components. However, neutrophils are not
the only source of ROS (or other deleterious substances for that matter) during
stress or reperfusion because ROS are detected in neutrophil-free crystalloid
buffer perfusates [53] and in whole blood [5,54].

The neutrophil response during reperfusion involves specific interactions between neutrophils and coronary artery and venous endothelial cells in the early
moments of reperfusion. Neutrophils are recruited to the reperfused myocardium during the early minutes of reperfusion by proinflammatory (TNF-α,
IL-6, platelet activating factor, complement, LTB$_4$) [55–58] and chemotactic
factors (IL-8) released by the myocardium. The first interaction is a tethering
or "rolling" of neutrophils along the endothelial surface [59–64], which is mediated by P-selectin on the endothelium and a sialylated glycoprotein on the
neutrophil, most likely sialyl Lewis^x or the sialomucin P-selectin glycoprotein
ligand-1 [65,66]. Two to 4 hours later, platelet activating factor and LTB$_4$ in
the microenvironment can increase the surface expression of CD11/CD18 on
neutrophils, whereas IL-1 and TNF-α increase ICAM-1 expression on the endothelium, which then initiates a firm adherence to the endothelium. The initial
loose adherence step is obligatory for later firm adherence mediated by the
CD11/CD18 complex on neutrophils and ICAM-1 on endothelial cells and is
critical in the pathogenesis of myocardial infarction, microvascular injury,
and apoptosis. A link has been established between the accumulation of neutrophils and the development of reperfusion injury during the early reperfusion
period [67]. This link has been substantiated by several studies investigating
the time course of neutrophil accumulation and progression of injury [55,68].
The inflammatory response induced by cardiopulmonary bypass may syner-
gize with the local inflammatory response to myocardial ischemia–reperfusion,
leading to an exaggerated activation of neutrophils [69–79]. Furthermore, the
intermittent ischemia that occurs with multidose delivery of cardioplegia may
add an ischemic stimulus to the global heart in addition to any local ischemia
for which the patient is being revascularized.

Vascular endothelial cells have several enzyme systems that generate ROS,
including the endothelial NAD(P)H oxidase system that generates superoxide

anions [80], and xanthine oxidase that generates superoxide anions from xan-thine and hypoxanthine. The endothelial nitric oxide synthase can generate superoxide anions under conditions of oxygen deprivation, which may be irrel-evant to reperfusion. Therefore, one must appreciate that there is an integrated oxidative response at reperfusion involving many cell types, not just cardiomyocytes. Reperfusion injury can occur in the absence of neutrophils because reperfusion injury can occur in tissues perfused with crystalloid solu-tions; in these circumstances the ROS and other noxious substances released by other cells are the sources of damage. Hence, reperfusion injury can be thought of as having neutrophil-related (eg, ROS, cytokines, hypochlorous acid, proteases) and neutrophil-independent causes.

Activation of the Sodium-Hydrogen Exchanger

The conversion of the cardiomyocyte from aerobic to anaerobic metabolism during ischemia promotes the accumulation of protons (H^+) and rapidly depletes adenosine triphosphate (ATP), which attenuates the actions of several energy-requiring mechanisms. Hence, during ischemia, there is a build-up of both Na^+ and H^+ inside the cell. This H^+ accumulation stimulates the Na^+/H^+ exchange type 1 (NHE-1) system, which transports one H^+ out in an elec-troneutral exchange for one Na^+ moving into the cell, thereby leading to a net accumulation of intracellular Na^+. The Na^+ accumulation is usually normal-ized by the Na^+–potassium (K^+) adenosine triphosphatase pump, but there is insufficient ATP to power this system, and $Na+$ accumulates within the cell. The net intracellular accumulation of Na^+ in turn attenuates or reverses the direction of the Na^+/Ca^{2+} exchange system located on the sarcolemma, thereby allowing the influx of Ca^{2+} into the cell in exchange for Na^+ efflux. The net effect of this reversal of the Na^+/Ca^{2+} is an accumulation of intracel-lular Ca^{2+}. Intracellular Ca^{2+} accumulation has been associated with a de-crease in mitochondrial ATP production and opening of the mitochondrial transition pore (see later discussion). There is some controversy whether the NHE is active [81] only during ischemia or is active primarily during reperfu-sion. The former is supported by data showing a reduction of infarct size when NHE-1 inhibitors are given as a pretreatment before ischemia; there is lit-tle reduction in infarct size when administered only at the onset of reperfusion [82–84]. However, some studies show that the NHE-1 is activated during the early moments of reperfusion [81], and such reperfusion activation would be consistent with an infarct sparing effect of NHE inhibitors administered at or just before the onset of reperfusion [85].

Calcium Overload and Calcium Overload-Induced Myocardial Contracture

Cells exquisitely regulate their intracellular calcium concentration, which is lower than the surrounding environment by two orders of magnitude. With the loss of ATP supplies and other calcium-regulating mechanisms, calcium may accumulate during ischemia and certainly an enhanced accumulation during reperfusion would occur. Intracellular calcium accumulation will compromise the metabolic function of mitochondria. In addition, high intracellular calcium concentrations may lead to hypercontracture (ie, a sustained shortening and stiffening of the myocardium) observed to occur during the early moments of reperfusion. This event has been linked to the pathogenesis of necrosis [86–89]. High intracellular calcium concentrations have also been shown to trigger opening of the mitochondrial permeability transition pore (see later discussion).

Opening of the Mitochondrial Permeability Transition Pore

A nonspecific pore localized in the mitochondrial inner membrane opens under conditions of stress including ischemia–reperfusion. Opening of this mitochondrial permeability transition pore alters the permeability characteristics of the membrane, favoring the influx of water and normally impermeable peptides with subsequent mitochondrial swelling and a breakdown in the proton gradient and uncoupling of oxidative phosphorylation. The opening of the mitochondrial permeability transition pore (mPTP), which occurs in the early minutes of reperfusion, is accompanied by the release of pro-apoptotic substances such as cytochrome C, which has been linked to the development of both necrosis and apoptosis. Thus opening of the mPTP may be a key factor in the transition from reversible to irreversible cell injury [90,91]. Opening of the mPTP is triggered by mitochondrial calcium overload and oxidative stress (ROS generation), both events of which have been observed during the early moments of reperfusion.

The Local Inflammatory Response to Reperfusion as a Component of Postischemic Injury

The response of the myocardium to reperfusion is similar to inflammatory responses induced by cardiopulmonary bypass, sepsis, and circulatory shock. Proinflammatory cytokines such as TNFα [92,93], IL-6, and IL-8, as well as complement [94,95] are released during ischemia–reperfusion. Complement is activated by ischemia–reperfusion through the antibody-dependent classical pathway, the alternative pathway, and the mannose-binding lectin (MBL)-MBL-associated serine proteases (MASP) pathway. The complement fragment C5a is the most potent of the anaphylatoxins stimulated by direct complement activation. C5a will directly stimulate neutrophil activation and recruitment to the ischemic–reperfused myocardium. In addition, C5b is important in the formation of the terminal membrane attack complex that causes formation of pores in the cell membrane leading to cell death.

Cytokines and complement will activate neutrophils and endothelial cells, thereby promoting their interaction, which may be a critical event that initiates the inflammatory component of reperfusion injury [8,67]. The mere presence of these proinflammatory mediators during reperfusion does not imply an active role in the pathogenesis of reperfusion injury. However, a causal role is suggested by studies in which inhibitors have been administered at the time of reperfusion with a resultant decrease in infarct size as a measure of myocardial injury.

Time Course of Reperfusion Events

Many of the events described are observed to take place in the early moments of reperfusion [89,96] and have been linked directly to the pathogenesis of both reversible and irreversible myocardial injury. In addition, several events listed also trigger a cascade of responses that continue later in the course of reperfusion injury; these events ultimately contribute to cell injury and irreversible cell death even 72 hours after reperfusion, [97] and therefore represent a permanent injury. The rationale for initiating treatment at onset of reperfusion in the currently advocated strategy of reperfusion therapeutics is embodied in a statement by Piper and Schafer [96]: "What comes first must be treated first, as otherwise the opportunity for specific treatment is lost." This axiom is further supported by observations in the postconditioning (see later definition) literature that even a brief delay in initiating treatment at the onset of reperfusion will fail to protect the previously ischemic myocardium, whereas immediate application will protect the myocardium [52,98]. Indeed, the opportunity to salvage myocardium and vascular function are lost by delaying treatment for even a few moments [52,99].

The Tissue Factor–Thrombin Pathway and Protease Activated Receptors in Reperfusion Injury

Protease activated receptors (PARs) belong to a subfamily of G protein–coupled receptors with the characteristic seven transmembrane domain, with an extracellular N-terminus and an intracellular carboxy-terminus. The PARs are activated through proteolytic cleavage of their N-terminus, which unmasks an amino acid sequence that acts as a tethered ligand to bind to the self-same receptor [100]. Of the four members of the PAR family, only PAR1, PAR3, and PAR4 are receptors cleaved at the N-terminus by the serine protease thrombin. PAR1 is the primary receptor for thrombin. PAR2, although not cleaved directly by thrombin, can be activated by other proteases, including trypsin, mast cell tryptase, Factor VIIa, and Factor Xa. Factors VIIa and Xa are cofactors that complex with tissue factor to form the prothrombinase complex that converts prothrombin to thrombin. Both PAR1 and PAR2 are constitutively expressed in endothelial cells and cardiomyocytes [101]. Expression of PAR2 is up-regulated in endothelial cells by proinflammatory stimuli (TNF-α, IL-1β and LPS) and ischemia–reperfusion itself [102]. PAR 2 is also highly expressed in human coronary atherosclerotic lesions [103]. PAR1 activation induces monocyte chemoattractant protein-1 and alters vascular permeability.

Recent studies suggest that proteases contribute to reperfusion injury by stimulating a proinflammatory state [104]. Serine proteases such as Factor VIIa, Factor Xa, and thrombin are increased in reperfused myocardium concomitant with an increased expression of tissue factor in reperfused myocardium [105]. Thrombin is a direct activator of P-selectin, which ultimately recruits neutrophils to the endothelial surface, thereby initiating neutrophil–endothelial cell interactions and inflammation. This process is mediated by thrombin PAR1 interaction [106]. The tissue factor (TF)–thrombin pathway has also been implicated in the pathogenesis of myocardial necrosis (AJ Chong, TH Pohlman, CR Hampton, unpublished data, 2004) and postischemic blood flow defects [107], which implicates a functional role for PAR1 receptors in reperfusion injury. The following evidence suggests that the TF–thrombin pathway and PAR1 activation are involved in the pathogenesis of myocardial infarction:

TF is expressed during ischemia–reperfusion. Golino and colleagues [107] reported an increased expression of TF and TF mRNA in the area at risk myocardium in ischemic–reperfused rabbit hearts, primarily localized in the coronary circulation. The expression of TF protein and mRNA was stimulated by reactive oxygen species that are generated at early reperfusion [5,108,53] and that were inhibited by oxygen radical scavengers.

Blockade of the TF/FVIIa/FX complex at reperfusion reduces infarct size. In a rabbit model of 30 minutes and 5.5 hours of reperfusion, Golino and colleagues [109] showed that human recombinant site-blocked activated factor VII (rhFVIIai), which blocks formation and activity of the TF/FVIIa/FX complex, administered intravenously at the onset of reperfusion reduced infarct size and the size of the no-reflow zone.

TF is expressed in area at risk myocardium during reperfusion. Erlich and colleagues [110,111] reported that TF antigen and mRNA were expressed on myocytes after ischemia–reperfusion, thereby providing a basis for local generation of thrombin in the area at risk myocardium after I-R. Data from the authors' laboratory showed that TF and the prothrombinase complex are expressed in myocardium and endothelium primarily during reperfusion [105].

Thrombin is linked to postischemic injury. Cirino and colleagues [104] suggest that thrombin has a direct proinflammatory effect by promoting degranulation of mast cells and release of bioactive amines such as histamine, thereby causing an increase in vascular permeability, edema, and the no-reflow phenomenon. Thrombin also amplifies the stimulation of proinflammatory TF [112]. A recent study by Mirabet and colleagues [113] showed that the presence of thrombin during simulated ischemia–reperfusion increases cardiomyocyte cell death by a mechanism that involves activation of PAR1 receptors and which is independent of coagulation cascade. Furthermore, Gurevitch and colleagues [114] showed that inhibition of the PAR1 receptor with aprotinin during reperfusion improved postischemic contractile function independent of inflammatory cell types.

In addition to thrombin, other proteases such as cathepsin G and elastase, present in azurophilic granules of neutrophils and monocytes, are released during reperfusion by activated neutrophils and contribute to myocardial injury by degrading the integrity of the basement membrane [115] These proteases thereby facilitate transendothelial migration of neutrophils out of the vascular compartment and into tissue parenchyma. The transmigration of neutrophils has been linked to the pathogenesis of both necrosis and apoptosis [55–57,116–118]. Elastase induces apoptosis in human lung epithelial cells by way of PAR1 activation. PAR1 activation by agonist peptides also induces lung epithelial cell apoptosis [119]. In summary, activation of the PAR1 by

proteases has been linked to ischemia–reperfusion injury, which is supported by data (see later discussion) that inhibition of protease stimulation of PAR1 is a therapeutic target.

ATTENUATING REPERFUSION INJURY IN ACUTE MYOCARDIAL ISCHEMIA WITH REPERFUSION THERAPEUTICS: GOING BEYOND RESTORING BLOOD FLOW

The questions must be asked: (1) whether infarct size and other manifestations of postischemic damage can be reduced by therapies applied at reperfusion, and (2) is it important to limit infarct size in the setting of percutaneous coronary intervention or cardiac surgery? Acute myocardial ischemia is used here instead of acute myocardial infarction because reperfusion contributes to the ultimate infarct size (and other injuries), and therefore there is the *potential* for infarction depending on *how* reperfusion is restored. Infarct size limitation is important in patients who have acute myocardial infarction because for patients who do not die of out-of-hospital arrhythmias, the prognosis of survival is dependent on the amount of myocardium that is salvaged [120,121]. Although reducing time to transport to the catheterization laboratory has been a primary focus of new modifications to first responder measures, "...it [is] unlikely that additional substantive improvements in morbidity and mortality can be achieved by reperfusion therapy without the development of new adjunctive therapies" [122]. In addition, heart failure is an increasingly common outcome of myocardial infarction and a frequent cause of cardiovascular morbidity and mortality, with approximately 400,000 new cases reported annually in the United States alone [123–125]. Survival 5 years after the diagnosis of heart failure is poor, ranging as low as 25% to 35% [126]. The treatment of heart failure represents a major health care expense. Infarct size limitation may be an important approach to limiting the incidence and severity of heart failure secondary to acute myocardial infarction. It seems that the limitation of unfavorable left ventricular remodeling is an unspecific consequence of infarct size limitation [127]. This is in agreement with clinical reports indicating that peak plasma creatine kinase values, a surrogate marker for infarct size, is an independent predictor of left ventricular remodeling [128]. Hence, limitation of infarct size has major ramifications on health as well as the financial burden of health care.

However, limiting the complex determinants of reperfusion injury directly is not addressed by the paradigms and strategies used currently in percutaneous coronary interventions [3]. In addition, the "new generation" of early adjunctive therapy including beta blockers, glucose–insulin–potassium, and platelet inhibitors do not target the many causes of reperfusion injury and therefore would not be expected to be effective when delivered after the percutaneous coronary intervention procedure (ie, at reperfusion). Experimental studies have shown that the first minutes of reperfusion are absolutely critical for the effective introduction of reperfusion therapy [33,129,52,51]. Therefore, therapy to attenuate reperfusion injury would have to be initiated immediately at the onset of reflow, or the window for therapy will be lost [6,8,52,96].

Therapies have been identified from preclinical experiments that reduce reperfusion-induced injury when delivered just before or at the onset of reperfusion. Such drugs, including adenosine and related analogs, nitric oxide, anti-inflammatory agents (targeted against cytokines, complement), oxygen radical inhibitors and scavengers, neutrophil and platelet inhibitors, Na^+/H^+ exchange inhibitors, and contraction uncouplers, have all been shown to attenuate various aspects of reperfusion injury in preclinical studies. By attenuating postischemic injury when given only at the onset of reperfusion, these studies provide indirect proof that reperfusion injury contributes to postischemic injury. In addition, these studies provide an extensive menu of therapies that may be applied at reperfusion for treatment of reperfusion injury in the clinical setting. However, many of these agents have vasoactive or cytotoxic effects when administered systemically by intravenous route. This can be overcome by delivering the drugs locally by intracoronary catheter. Although some drugs can be delivered through the lumen of non-rapid exchange catheters, technologies are not currently available to locally deliver adjunctive therapies that embrace the integrated strategies of *controlled reperfusion* (ie, exerting control over the conditions and the compositional attributes of coronary perfusion being delivered to the target myocardium undergoing reperfusion). The concept of controlled reperfusion, first developed and applied in the strategic delivery of cardioplegia solutions in cardiac surgery, advocates controlling the pressure and temperature at which intracoronary perfusates are delivered, as well as modulating the composition of the perfusate to combat specific aspects of reperfusion injury. The strategy of controlled reperfusion also provides for the local delivery of drugs to the heart in effective concentrations. The concentrations of many of these drugs are associated with significant side effects, such as hypotension, anginal-like pain, hepatotoxicity, and increased propensity to bleeding. Certainly, this is the case with adenosine and nitric oxide, both of which are potent anti-infarct drugs but which cannot be systemically administered because of propensity of hypotension. These drugs therefore are not used clinically on a routine basis for adjunctive reperfusion therapies in the setting of percutaneous coronary intervention [3]. Technologies to deliver reperfusion therapeutics locally as an adjunct to percutaneous coronary intervention will be important for the treatment of reperfusion injury following acute myocardial infarction.

NEW ANTI-INFLAMMATORY THERAPIES TO ATTENUATE REPERFUSION INJURY

Nitric Oxide Therapy

Numerous experimental studies have tested agents with anti-inflammatory properties delivered at the time of reperfusion as a therapeutic approach. Nitric oxide [130], nitric oxide donor agents [131], and the physiologic precursor L-arginine [132,133] have been effective at reducing postischemic injury by reducing neutrophil activation, accumulation, superoxide anion generation, and endothelial cell activation. Nitric oxide has also been used in cardioplegia solutions to protect hearts from injury resulting from ischemia, intentional ischemia as part of the cardioplegia interval, and reperfusion [134–136]. Nitric oxide also has cardioprotective effects independent of neutrophils and inflammatory effects [137], perhaps reflecting the effects of increased intracellular cyclic guanosine monophosphate.

Adenosine Therapy

Adenosine is another agent that has been rigorously explored for its cardioprotective properties when delivered at reperfusion. Adenosine has been shown to attenuate the activation of neutrophils and associated generation of superoxide anions and release of proinflammatory mediators [138–141]. In addition, adenosine inhibits the activation of the vascular endothelium and therefore inhibits neutrophil–endothelial cell interactions that may contribute to postischemic injury [142]. Accordingly, adenosine delivered at reperfusion reduces infarct size and other manifestations of postischemic injury in experimental models [143–145].

Inhibition of PAR1 Activity by Aprotinin

The participation of serine proteases such as thrombin in postischemic injury suggests that inhibition of the PAR1–thrombin (or other serine protease) component during reperfusion may attenuate reperfusion injury. Aprotinin is a naturally occurring, 58-amino acid nonspecific serine protease inhibitor currently derived from bovine lungs. It is used in cardiac surgery to reduce postoperative blood loss and the need for blood transfusions [146]. Pruefer and colleagues [147] recently reported that aprotinin administered systemically before reperfusion decreased neutrophil accumulation in regionally ischemic–reperfused myocardium, reduced infarct size assessed by creatine kinase release, and reduced apoptosis. As a potential mechanism, aprotinin also inhibits inflammatory cytokines. In addition, aprotinin inhibits neutrophil elastase release [148] and superoxide anion formation [149], and inhibits leukocyte–endothelial cell interactions [150] as potential mediators to reperfusion injury [8]. Aprotinin is a potent inhibitor of serine protease activity used in blood conservation. Serine proteases such as tissue factor, factor Xa, elastase, and thrombin may be involved in the pathogenesis of ischemia–reperfusion injury in part by initiating local inflammatory responses. A study in the authors' laboratory [151] tested the hypothesis that intravenous aprotinin administered during reperfusion attenuates endothelial activation and neutrophil accumulation in the area at risk and reduces infarct size. In an anesthetized closed-chest pig model of LAD occlusion (75 minutes) using an angioplasty balloon catheter followed by 3 hours of reperfusion, treatment 30 minutes before the onset of reperfusion was randomly assigned to saline (vehicle, n = 8), low-dose aprotinin (7,000 KIU/kg, n = 9), or high-dose aprotinin (30,000 KIU/kg, n = 6). In vitro IL-8–stimulated neutrophil chemotaxis was reduced by aprotinin in a dose-dependent manner within the range of 400 to 1600 KIU/mL. Balloon-induced occlusion reduced subendocardial blood flow in the area at risk (15 μm microspheres, mL/min/g) from 1.02 ± 0.33 to 0.01 ± 0.01 in vehicle, from 0.80 ± 0.11 to 0.03 ± 0.02 in the low-dose aprotinin group, and from 0.78 ± 0.21

to 0.02 ± 0.01 in the high-dose aprotinin group ($P < .01$ versus baseline; $P > .10$ versus groups). The area at risk was comparable among the three groups (vehicle: 38 ± 2; low-dose: 34 ± 2; high-dose: 35 ± 2, $P = .3$). Low-dose aprotinin did not significantly reduce infarct size (triphenyltetrazolium chloride staining, $42 \pm 1\%$) relative to the vehicle group ($48 \pm 4\%$). In contrast, high-dose aprotinin at reperfusion significantly ($P < .05$) reduced infarct size ($20 \pm 5\%$) by 60% of that in the vehicle group. P-selectin and vWF expression were significantly attenuated in the low-dose and high-dose aprotinin groups compared with vehicle. Neutrophil accumulation in area at risk was reduced in the high-dose aprotinin group assessed by either direct histochemical quantification of CD18-positive cells (vehicle: 1350 ± 182PMNs/slide; low-dose aprotinin 485 ± 235 PMNs/slide; high-dose aprotinin 120 ± 13 PMNs/slide, $P < .05$). This study suggested that serine proteases contribute to the pathogenesis of endothelial activation and infarct size upon reperfusion, and that this injury can be attenuated by a serine protease inhibitor administered at reperfusion.

Stimulation of PAR2 Activity

The PAR2 represents an endogenous force opposing proinflammatory effects of the PAR1. The cardioprotective effects of PAR2 was first reported by Napoli and colleagues [102]. A selective PAR2 agonist peptide SLIGRL-NH2 decreased postischemic myocardial dysfunction and decreased the incidence of ventricular arrhythmias in an ex vivo rat model of myocardial ischemia–reperfusion [102]. The cardioprotective effects of PAR2 activation have been attributed by McLean and colleagues [152] to PAR2-dependent regulation of coronary vascular tone. PAR2 agonists promote coronary vasodilation, leading to improved perfusion of the compromised ventricle. However, improved blood flow is not tightly linked to reduction in postischemic injury [31,132,153]. For example, the isolated perfused heart preparation does not include neutrophils, platelets, and plasma-borne lipid mediators that contribute to reperfusion injury by enhancing the release of oxidants [5], cytokines, and lipid mediators that amplify the injury process [154,155]. The participation of PAR2 activation in vivo by endogenous stimulating factors during reperfusion is unknown. Recently, a study by Feistritzer and associates [156] indicated that PAR2 activation can reduce thrombin-induced hyperpermeability in endothelial cells, but little is known whether PAR2 stimulation can have similar protection in coronary endothelium during ischemia–reperfusion. Preliminary data from the authors' laboratory suggest that stimulation of the PAR2 receptor using the selective agonist peptide SLIGRL administered 5 minutes before the onset of reperfusion reduces infarct size in an in vivo rat model of ischemia–reperfusion. Hence, PAR2 represents a promising therapeutic target to influence the pathogenesis of in vivo ischemia–reperfusion injuries.

Postconditioning to Attenuate Reperfusion Injury

Postconditioning, introduced by Zhao and colleagues [51] in 2003, is the term used to describe a series of alternating cycles of reperfusion and ischemia applied at the immediate onset of reperfusion (Fig. 1) [33,51]. This mechanical

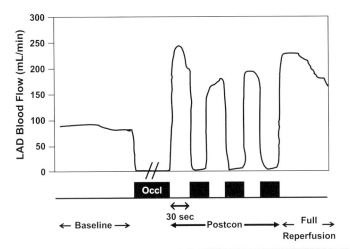

Fig. 1. Mean blood flow in the canine left anterior descending (LAD) coronary artery during baseline, LAD occlusion, and reperfusion with postconditioning (Postcon) (*lower figure*). Black-boxes in the lower figure represent balloon occlusion in the experimental porcine model. Note the three cycles of coronary blood flow alternating with complete cessation of blood flow due to controlled coronary occlusion. The representation of the duration of LAD occlusion (60 minutes) has been shortened (*hatch marks*).

maneuver lasts only from 1 to 6 minutes in total intervention time, depending on whether the model is one of small animals, or large animals or humans, respectively. Postconditioning has reduced postischemic coronary artery endothelial dysfunction (expressed as vasorelaxant responses to incremental concentrations of acetylcholine, in vitro neutrophil adherence to coronary artery endothelium, superoxide anion generation detected by chemiluminescence), myocardial blood flow defects, tissue superoxide anion generation, edema, infarct size (Fig. 2), and apoptosis. The early application of this intervention is critical to its cardioprotection due to applying the reperfusion–reocclusion algorithm after the initial minutes of reperfusion rather than immediately at the onset abrogates protection [52,98]. These studies have shown the importance of the early minutes of reperfusion as a trigger of postischemic injury and have put forth the concept of immediate application of reperfusion therapeutics to capture the cardioprotective window. This point was made in discussing the mechanisms of reperfusion injury that many of the contributors are activated during the early phase of reperfusion. Which contributors are attenuated directly and indirectly by postconditioning still remains to be elucidated. However, it is important that postconditioned hearts generate less oxygen radicals (dihydroethidium staining) [33,51,52], less TNF-α, and accumulate fewer neutrophils. Hence, the authors hypothesize that postconditioning attenuates the integrated inflammatory response to reperfusion [11,45].

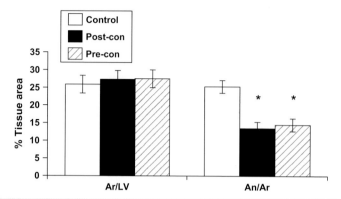

Fig. 2. Infarct size [area necrosis (An) relative to area at risk (Ar)] in a canine model of left anterior descending occlusion reperfusion is reduced by postconditioning (Post-con) in the first 3 minutes of reperfusion. Infarct reduction is comparable to that of classical ischemic preconditioning (Pre-con), the "gold standard" of protection in ischemic myocardium. *P<.05 versus control.

To support a role of attenuating proinflammatory mediators in reperfusion, the authors tested whether postconditioning could reduce reperfusion injury by inhibiting the TF–thrombin pathway in a closed-chest porcine model of ischemia–reperfusion that simulated closely a patient who had evolving acute myocardial infarction and was treated in the catheterization laboratory. In closed-chest anesthetized pigs, the left anterior descending coronary artery was occluded for 75 minutes by fluoroscopically-guided angioplasty balloon catheter followed by 3 hours of reperfusion with abrupt reperfusion (control) or with postconditioning, defined as 30 seconds reperfusion, 30 seconds reocclusion by reinflating the angioplasty balloon, repeated for 3 cycles applied at the onset of reperfusion. Postconditioning significantly reduced infarct size (triphenyltetrazolium chloride stain) compared with control ($12\% \pm 4\%$ versus $45\% \pm 5\%$ necrotic/area at risk ratio, $P < .05$). TF protein expression (Western blot) in the nonischemic zone of the left ventricle was not different between control and postconditioning groups. However, TF protein density in the nonnecrotic zone of the area at risk was significantly less in postconditioned hearts versus untreated control hearts ($10,155 \pm 3095$ versus $18,447 \pm 1080$ densitometry units, $P < .05$). Thrombin activity in the area at risk myocardium quantified by chromogenic assay was lower in postconditioned versus control hearts (0.79 ± 0.27 versus 3.05 ± 0.63 U/mg protein, $P<.05$). The expression of P-selectin (immunohistochemistry) was visually increased along the endothelial surface of vessels in the area at risk myocardium of controls, whereas there was less P-selectin immunoreactivity in vascular endothelium in the area at risk myocardium in postconditioned hearts. This study suggests that the down-regulation of TF expression and inhibition of local thrombin generation in area at risk myocardium may be a mechanism by which postconditioning reduces the inflammatory response to reperfusion.

SUMMARY

Although ischemic myocardium must be reperfused to survive, there is a cost to reperfusion that offsets the intended clinical benefits of minimizing infarct size, postischemic blood flow defects, and contractile dysfunction. There is a multiplicity of contributors to reperfusion injury. Proinflammatory mediators and inflammatory cells play an integral part by not only triggering deleterious responses but also by amplifying ongoing responses to build a cascade of injury. This cascade may be triggered as early as within the first few minutes of onset of reperfusion. This early onset defines a window of therapy that if missed, may predetermine the failure or reduced benefit of that therapy. An integrated strategy of reducing reperfusion injury in the catheterization laboratory setting involves controlling the conditions of reperfusion (intracoronary pressure, flow rate, temperature, pulsativity) as well as the composition of the reperfusate. Mechanical interventions such as gradually restoring blood flow or applying postconditioning may be used independently in or conjunction with cardioprotective pharmaceuticals in an integrated strategy of reperfusion therapeutics.

Acknowledgments

The authors thank the Carlyle Fraser Heart Center Foundation for their continued support of the research effort.

References

[1] Reimer KA, Lowe JE, Rasmussen MM, et al. The wavefront phenomenon of ischemic cell death. 1. Myocardial infarct size vs duration of coronary occlusion in dogs. Circulation 1977;56:786–94.

[2] DeWood MA, Spores J, Notske R. Prevalence of total coronary occlusion during the early hours of transmural myocardial infarction. N Engl J Med 1980;303:897–902.

[3] Kloner RA, Rezkalla SH. Cardiac protection during acute myocardial infarction: where do we stand in 2004? J Am Coll Cardiol 2004;44:276–86.

[4] Becker LC, Ambrosio G. Myocardial consequences of reperfusion. Prog Cardiovasc Dis 1987;30:23–44.

[5] Duilio C, Ambrosio G, Kuppusamy P, et al. Neutrophils are primary source of O_2 radicals during reperfusion after prolonged myocardial ischemia. Am J Physiol Heart Circ Physiol 2001;280:H2649–57.

[6] Lucchesi BR. Myocardial reperfusion injury-role of free radicals and mediators of inflammation. In: Sperelakis N, Kurachi Y, Terzic A, et al, editors. Heart physiology and pathophysiology. 4th edition. San Diego (CA): Academic Press; 2001. p. 1181–210.

[7] Quintana M, Kahan T, Hjemdahl P. Pharmacological prevention of reperfusion injury in acute myocardial infarction a potential role for adenosine as a therapeutic agent. Am J Cardiovasc Drugs 2004;4:159–67.

[8] Vinten-Johansen J. Involvement of neutrophils in the pathogenesis of lethal myocardial reperfusion injury. Cardiovasc Res 2004;61:481–97.

[9] Vinten-Johansen J, Johnston WE, Mills SA, et al. Reperfusion injury after temporary coronary occlusion. J Thorac Cardiovasc Surg 1988;95:960–8.

[10] Vinten-Johansen J, Yellon DM, Opie LH. A simple, clinically applicable procedure to improve revascularization in acute myocardial infarction. Circulation 2005;112: 2085–8.

[11] Vinten-Johansen J, Zhao Z-Q, Jiang R, et al. Myocardial protection in reperfusion with post-conditioning. Expert Rev Cardiovasc Ther 2005;3:1035–45.

[12] Moens AL, Claeys MJ, Timmermans JP, et al. Myocardial ischemia/reperfusion-injury, a clinical view on a complex pathophysiological process. Int J Cardiol 2005;100: 179–90.

[13] Jennings RB, Sommers HM, Smyth GA, et al. Myocardial necrosis induced by temporary occlusion of a coronary artery in the dog. Arch Pathol Lab Med 1960;70:68–78.

[14] Braunwald E, Kloner RA. Myocardial reperfusion: a double-edged sword? J Clin Invest 1985;76:1713–9.

[15] Vinten-Johansen J. Reperfusion injury: idle curiosity or therapeutic vector? J Thromb Thrombolysis 1997;4:59–61.

[16] Cobbaert C, Hermens WT, Kint PP, et al. Thrombolysis-induced coronary reperfusion causes acute and massive interstitial release of cardiac muscle cell proteins. Cardiovasc Res 1997;33:147–55.

[17] Kloner RA. Does reperfusion injury exist in humans? [review]. J Am Coll Cardiol 1993;21: 537–45.

[18] Staat P, Rioufol G, Piot C, et al. Postconditioning the human heart. Circulation 2005;112: 2143–8.

[19] Cooley DA, Ruel GJ, Wukasch DC. Ischemic contracture of the heart: "Stone Heart". Am J Cardiol 1972;29:575–7.

[20] Weman SM, Karhunen PJ, Penttila A, et al. Reperfusion injury associated with one-fourth of deaths after coronary artery bypass grafting. Ann Thorac Surg 2000;70: 807–12.

[21] Buckberg GD. Strategies and logic of cardioplegic delivery to prevent, avoid, and reverse ischemic and reperfusion damage. J Thorac Cardiovasc Surg 1987;93:127–39.

[22] Powell WJ Jr, DiBona DR, Flores J, et al. The protective effect of hyperosmotic mannitol in myocardial ischemia and necrosis. Circulation 1976;54:603–15.

[23] Reynolds RD, Burmeister WE, Gorczynski RJ, et al. Effects of propranolol on myocardial infarct size with and without coronary artery reperfusion in the dog. Cardiovasc Res 1981;15:411–20.

[24] Follette DM, Fey K, Buckberg GD, et al. Reducing postischemic damage by temporary modification of reperfusate calcium, potassium, pH, and osmolarity. J Thorac Cardiovasc Surg 1981;82:221–38.

[25] Follette DM, Mulder DG, Maloney JV Jr, et al. Advantages of blood cardioplegia over continuous coronary perfusion and intermittent ischemia. J Thorac Cardiovasc Surg 1978;76: 604–17.

[26] Vinten-Johansen J, Edgerton TA, Howe HR, et al. Immediate functional recovery and avoidance of reperfusion injury with surgical revascularization of short-term coronary occlusion. Circulation 1985;72:431–9.

[27] Bulkley BH, Hutchins GM. Myocardial consequences of coronary artery bypass graft surgery. The paradox of necrosis in areas of revascularization. Circulation 1977;56: 906–13.

[28] Miki T, Liu GS, Cohen MV, et al. Mild hypothermia reduces infarct size in the beating rabbit heart: a practical intervention for acute myocardial infarction. Basic Res Cardiol 1998;93: 372–83.

[29] Schwartz DS, Bremner RM, Baker CJ, et al. Regional topical hypothermia of the beating heart: preservation of function and tissue. Ann Thorac Surg 2001;73:804–9.

[30] Pisarenko OI, Shulzhenko VS, Studneva IM, et al. Effects of gradual reperfusion on postischemic metabolism and functional recovery of isolated guinea pig heart. Biochem Med Metab Biol 1993;50:127–34.

[31] Sato H, Jordan JE, Zhao Z-Q, et al. Gradual reperfusion reduces infarct size and endothelial injury but augments neutrophil accumulation. Ann Thorac Surg 1997;64:1099–107.

[32] Vinten-Johansen J, Lefer DJ, Nakanishi K, et al. Controlled coronary hydrodynamics at the time of reperfusion reduces postischemic injury. Coron Artery Dis 1992;3:1081–93.

[33] Halkos ME, Kerendi F, Corvera JS, et al. Myocardial protection with postconditioning is not enhanced by ischemic preconditioning. Ann Thorac Surg 2004;78:961–9.

[34] Zhao Z-Q, Corvera JS, Wang N-P, et al. Reduction in infarct size and preservation of endothelial function by ischemic postconditioning: comparison with ischemic preconditioning [abstract]. Circulation 2002;106(19):II314.

[35] Darling CE, Jiang R, Maynard M, et al. Postconditioning via stuttering reperfusion limits myocardial infarct size in rabbit hearts: role of ERK1/2. Am J Physiol Heart Circ Physiol 2005;289:H1618–26.

[36] Laskey WK. Brief repetitive balloon occlusions enhance reperfusion during percutaneous coronary intervention for acute myocardial infarction: a pilot study. Catheter Cardiovasc Interv 2005;65:361–7.

[37] Dissmann R, Goerke M, von Ameln H, et al. Detection of early reperfusion and prediction of left ventricular damage from the course of increased ST values in acute myocardial infarct with thrombolysis [in German]. Z Kardiol 1993;82:271–8.

[38] Feldman LJ, Himbert D, Juliard J-M, et al. Reperfusion syndrome: relationship of coronary blood flow reserve to left ventricular function and infarct size. J Am Coll Cardiol 2000;35:1162–9.

[39] Ito H, Tomooka T, Sakai N, et al. Time course of functional improvement in stunned myocardium in risk area in patients with reperfused anterior infarction [see comments]. Circulation 1993;87:355–62.

[40] Kobayashi N, Ohmura N, Nakada I, et al. Further ST elevation at reperfusion by direct percutaneous transluminal coronary angioplasty predicts poor recovery of left ventricular systolic function in anterior wall AMI. Am J Cardiol 1997;79:862–6.

[41] Ochiai M, Isshiki T, Takeshita S, et al. Relation of duration of ST re-elevation at reperfusion and improvement of left ventricular function after successful primary angioplasty of the left anterior descending coronary artery in anterior wall acute myocardial infarction. Am J Cardiol 1997;79:1667–70.

[42] Shah A, Wagner GS, Granger CB, et al. Prognostic implications of TIMI flow grade in the infarct related artery compared with continuous 12-lead ST-segment resolution analysis. Reexamining the ''gold standard'' for myocardial reperfusion assessment. J Am Coll Cardiol 2000;35:666–72.

[43] Ito H, Okamura A, Iwakura K, et al. Myocardial perfusion patterns related to thrombolysis in myocardial infarction perfusion grades after coronary angioplasty in patients with acute anterior wall myocardial infarction. Circulation 1996;93:1993–9.

[44] Yellon DM, Baxter GF. Protecting the ischaemic and reperfused myocardium in acute myocardial infarction: distant dream or near reality? Heart 2000;83:381–7.

[45] Vinten-Johansen J, Zhao ZQ, Kerendi F, et al. Postconditioning: a new link in nature's armor against ischemia-reperfusion injury [abstract]. J Mol Cell Cardiol 2004;36(4):637.

[46] Kevin LG, Camara AKS, Riess ML, et al. Ischemic preconditioning alters real-time measure of O_2 radicals in intact hearts with ischemia and reperfusion. Am J Physiol Heart Circ Physiol 2003;284:H566–74.

[47] Ambrosio G, Zweier JL, Flaherty JT. The relationship between oxygen radical generation and impairment of myocardial energy metabolism following post-ischemic reperfusion. J Mol Cell Cardiol 1991;23:1359–74.

[48] Jolly SR, Kane WJ, Bailie MB, et al. Canine myocardial reperfusion injury: its reduction by the combined administration of superoxide dismutase and catalase. Circ Res 1984;54:277–85.

[49] Bagchi D, Das DK, Engelman RM, et al. Polymorphonuclear leukocytes as potential source of free radicals in the ischaemic-reperfused myocardium. Eur Heart J 1990;11:800–13.

[50] Ko W, Hawes AS, Lazenby WD, et al. Myocardial reperfusion injury. Platelet-activating factor stimulates polymorphonuclear leukocyte hydrogen peroxide production during myocardial reperfusion. J Thorac Cardiovasc Surg 1991;102:297–308.

[51] Zhao Z-Q, Corvera JS, Halkos ME, et al. Inhibition of myocardial injury by ischemic postconditioning during reperfusion: comparison with ischemic preconditioning. Am J Physiol Heart Circ Physiol 2003;285:579–88.

[52] Kin H, Zhao Z-Q, Sun H-Y, et al. Postconditioning attenuates myocardial ischemia-reperfusion injury by inhibiting events in the early minutes of reperfusion. Cardiovasc Res 2004;62:74–85.

[53] Zweier JL, Flaherty JT, Weisfeldt ML. Direct measurement of free radicals generated following reperfusion of ischemic myocardium. Proc Natl Acad Sci U S A 1987;84: 1404–7.

[54] Bolli R, Jeroudi MO, Patel BS, et al. Marked reduction of free radical generation and contractile dysfunction by antioxidant therapy begun at the time of reperfusion: evidence that myocardial "stunning" is a manifestation of reperfusion injury. Circ Res 1989;65: 607–22.

[55] Dreyer WJ, Michael LH, West MW, et al. Neutrophil accumulation in ischemic canine myocardium: insights into time course, distribution, and mechanism of localization during early reperfusion. Circulation 1991;84:400–11.

[56] Dreyer WJ, Smith CW, Michael LH, et al. Canine neutrophil activation by cardiac lymph obtained during reperfusion of ischemic myocardium. Circ Res 1989;65: 1751–62.

[57] Entman ML, Michael L, Rossen RD, et al. Inflammation in the course of early myocardial ischemia. FASEB J 1991;5:2529–37.

[58] Lefer AM, Lefer DJ. Pharmacology of the endothelium in ischemia-reperfusion and circulatory shock. Annu Rev Pharmacol Toxicol 1993;33:71–90.

[59] Davenpeck KL, Gauthier TW, Albertine KH, et al. Role of P-selectin in microvascular leukocyte-endothelial interaction in splanchnic ischemia-reperfusion. Am J Physiol 1994;267: H622–30.

[60] Kubes P, Jutila M, Payne D. Therapeutic potential of inhibiting leukocyte rolling in ischemia/reperfusion. J Clin Invest 1995;95:2510–9.

[61] Kubes P, Kurose I, Granger DN. NO donors prevent integrin induced leukocyte adhesion but not P- selectin-dependent rolling in postischemic venules. Am J Physiol 1994;267: H931–7.

[62] Ley K. Molecular mechanisms of leukocyte rolling and adhesion to microvascular endothelium [review]. Eur Heart J 1993;14(Suppl I):68–73.

[63] Ley K, Tangelder GJ, von Andrian UH. Modulation of leukocyte rolling in vivo. In: Granger DN, Schmid–Schönbein GW, editors. Physiology and pathophysiology of leukocyte adhesion. New York: Oxford University Press; 1995. p. 217–40.

[64] Ley K, Tedder TF. Leukocyte interactions with vascular endothelium. New insights into selectin-mediated attachment and rolling. J Immunol 1995;155:525–8.

[65] McEver RP, Cummings RD. Role of PSGL-1 binding to selectins in leukocyte recruitment. J Clin Invest 1997;100:485–92.

[66] Moore KL, Patel KD, Bruehl RE, et al. P-selectin glycoprotein ligand-1 mediates rolling of human neutrophils on p-selectin. J Cell Biol 1995;128:661–71.

[67] Lefer AM, Ma X-L, Weyrich A, et al. Endothelial dysfunction and neutrophil adherence as critical events in the development of reperfusion injury. Agents Actions Suppl 1993;41: 127–35.

[68] Albertine KH, Weyrich AS, Ma X-L, et al. Quantification of neutrophil migration following myocardial ischemia and reperfusion in cats and dogs. J Leukoc Biol 1994;55: 557–66.

[69] Boyle EM, Pohlman TH, Johnson MC, et al. Endothelial cell injury in cardiovascular surgery: the systemic inflammatory response. Ann Thorac Surg 1997;63:277–84.

[70] Dreyer WJ, Michael LH, Millman EE, et al. Neutrophil activation and adhesion molecule expression in a canine model of open heart surgery with cardiopulmonary bypass. Cardiovasc Res 1995;29:775–81.

[71] Dreyer WJ, Smith CW, Entman ML. Invited letter concerning: neutrophil activation during cardiopulmonary bypass. J Thorac Cardiovasc Surg 1991;102:318–20.

[72] Gillinov AM, Bator JM, Zehr KJ, et al. Neutrophil adhesion molecule expression during cardiopulmonary bypass with bubble and membrane oxygenators. Ann Thorac Surg 1993;56:847–53.

[73] Gillinov AM, DeValeria PA, Winkelstein JA, et al. Complement inhibition with soluble complement receptor type 1 in cardiopulmonary bypass. Ann Thorac Surg 1993;55:619–24.

[74] Gillinov AM, Redmond JM, Winkelstein JA, et al. Complement and neutrophil activation during cardiopulmonary bypass: a study in the complement-deficient dog. Ann Thorac Surg 1994;57:345–52.

[75] Gillinov AM, Redmond JM, Zehr KJ, et al. Inhibition of neutrophil adhesion during cardiopulmonary bypass. Ann Thorac Surg 1994;57:126–33.

[76] Kawamura T, Wakusawa R, Okada K, et al. Elevation of cytokines during open heart surgery with cardiopulmonary bypass: participation of interleukin 8 and 6 in reperfusion injury [see comments]. Can J Anaesth 1993;40:1016–21.

[77] Levy JH, Kelly AB. Inflammation and cardiopulmonary bypass [editorial; comment]. Can J Anaesth 1993;40:1009–15.

[78] Prasad K, Kalra J, Bharadwaj B, et al. Increased oxygen free radical activity in patients on cardiopulmonary bypass undergoing aortocoronary bypass surgery. Am Heart J 1992;123:37–45.

[79] Wilson I, Gillinov AM, Curtis WE, et al. Inhibition of neutrophil adherence improves postischemic ventricular performance of the neonatal heart. Circulation 1993;88:II372–9.

[80] Mohazzab KM, Kaminski PM, Wolin MS. NADH oxidoreductase is a major source of superoxide anion in bovine coronary artery endothelium. Am J Physiol 1994;266:H2568–72.

[81] Allen DG, Xiao X-H. Role of the cardiac Na^+/H^+ exchanger during ischemia and reperfusion. Cardiovasc Res 2003;57:934–41.

[82] Gross GJ, Gumina RJ. Cardioprotective effects of Na+/H+ exchange inhibitors. Drugs of the Future 2001;26:253–60.

[83] Gumina RJ, Auchampach JA, Wang R, et al. Na^+/H^+ exchange inhibition-induced cardioprotection in dogs: effects on neutrophils versus cardiomyocytes. Am J Physiol Heart Circ Physiol 2000;279:H1563–70.

[84] Klein HH, Pich S, Bohle RM, et al. Na^+/H^+ exchange inhibitor cariporide attenuates cell injury predominantly during ischemia and not at onset of reperfusion in porcine hearts with low residual blood flow. Circulation 2000;102:1977–82.

[85] Hurtado C, Pierce GN. Sodium-hydrogen exchange inhibition: pre- versus post-ischemic treatment. Basic Res Cardiol 2001;96:312–7.

[86] Garcia-Dorado D, Gonzalez MA, Barrabes JA, et al. Prevention of ischemic rigor contracture during coronary occlusion by inhibition of Na+/H+ exchange. Cardiovasc Res 1997;35:80–9.

[87] Piper HM. Energy deficiency, calcium overload or oxidative stress: possible causes of irreversible ischemic myocardial injury. Klin Wochenschr 1989;67:465–76.

[88] Piper HM, Garcia-Dorado D. Prime cause of rapid cardiomyocyte death during reperfusion. Ann Thorac Surg 1999;68:1913–9.

[89] Piper HM, Garcia-Dorado D, Ovize M. A fresh look at reperfusion injury. Cardiovasc Res 1998;38:291–300.

[90] Crompton M. The mitochondrial permeability transition pore and its role in cell death. Biochem J 1999;341:233–49.

[91] Halestrap AP, Kerr PM, Javadov S, et al. Elucidating the molecular mechanism of the permeability transition pore and its role in reperfusion injury of the heart. Biochim Biophys Acta 1998;1366:79–94.

[92] Cain BS, Meldrum DR, Dinarello CA, et al. Adenosine reduces cardiac TNF-alpha production and human myocardial injury following ischemia-reperfusion. J Surg Res 1998;76(2): 117–23.

[93] Meldrum DR. Tumor necrosis factor in the heart. Am J Physiol 1998;274:R577–95.

[94] Lucchesi BR. Complement activation, neutrophils, and oxygen radicals in reperfusion injury. Stroke 1993;24:I-41–I-47.

[95] Lucchesi BR. Complement, neutrophils and free radicals: mediators of reperfusion injury [review]. Arzneim-Forsch/Drug Res 1994;44:420–32.

[96] Piper HM, Schafer AC. The first minutes of reperfusion: a window of opportunity for cardioprotection. Cardiovasc Res 2004;61:365–71.

[97] Zhao Z-Q, Nakamura M, Wang N-P, et al. Dynamic progression of contractile and endothelial dysfunction and infarct extension in the late phase of reperfusion. J Surg Res 2000;94:1–12.

[98] Philipp SD, Downey JM, Cohen MV. Postconditioning must be initiated in less than 1 minute following reperfusion and is dependent on adenosine receptors and P13-kinase [abstract]. Circulation 2004;110(17):III-168.

[99] Yang X-M, Proctor JB, Cui L, et al. Multiple, brief coronary occlusions during early reperfusion protect rabbit hearts by targeting cell signaling pathways. J Am Coll Cardiol 2004;44:1103–10.

[100] Coughlin SR. Thrombin signaling and protease-activated receptors. Nature 2000;407: 258–64.

[101] Sabri A, Muske G, Zhang H, et al. Signaling properties and functions of two distinct cardiomyocyte protease-activated receptors. Circ Res 2000;86:1054–61.

[102] Napoli C, Cicala C, Wallace JL, et al. Protease-activated receptor-2 modulates myocardial ischemia-reperfusion injury in the rat heart. Proc Natl Acad Sci U S A 2000;97: 3678–83.

[103] Napoli C, De Nigris F, Wallace JL, et al. Evidence that protease activated receptor 2 expression is enhanced in human coronary atherosclerotic lesions. J Clin Pathol 2004;57: 513–6.

[104] Cirino G, Cicala C, Bucci MR, et al. Thrombin functions as an inflammatory mediator through activation of its receptor. J Exp Med 1996;183:821–7.

[105] Jobe LJ, Jiang R, Wang N-P, et al. Tissue factor, factors VIIa and Xa expression and local generation of thrombin in at risk myocardium occurs specifically during reperfusion. Circulation 2004;110(17):III-297.

[106] Fu J, Naren AP, Gao X, et al. Protease-activated receptor-1 activation of endothelial cells induces protein kinase Cα-dependent phosphorylation of syntaxin 4 and Munc18c. J Biol Chem 2005;280:3178–84.

[107] Golino P, Ragni M, Cirillo P, et al. Effects of tissue factor induced by oxygen free radicals on coronary flow during reperfusion. Nat Med 1996;2:35–40.

[108] Grill HP, Zweier JL, Kuppusamy P, et al. Direct measurement of myocardial free radical generation in an in vivo model: effects of postischemic reperfusion and treatment with human recombinant superoxide dismutase. J Am Coll Cardiol 1992;20:1604–11.

[109] Golino P, Ragni M, Cirillo P, et al. Recombinanat human, active site-blocked factor VIIa reduces infarct size and the no-reflow phenomenon in rabbits. Am J Physiol Heart Circ Physiol 2000;278:H1507–16.

[110] Erlich JH, Boyle EM, Santucci RA, et al. Tissue factor upregulation in cardiomyocytes after ischemia/reperfusion [abstract]. Am J Pathol 2000;147:37.

[111] Erlich JH, Boyle EM, Labriola J, et al. Inhibition of the tissue factor-thrombin pathway limits infarct size after myocardial ischemia-reperfusion injury by reducing inflammation. Am J Pathol 2000;157:1849–62.

[112] Liu Y, Pelekanakis K, Woolkalis MJ. Thrombin and tumor necrosis factor α synergistically stimulate tissue factor expression in human endothelial cells. J Biol Chem 2004;279: 36142–7.

[113] Mirabet M, Garcia-Dorado D, Ruiz-Meana M, et al. Thrombin increases cardiomyocyte acute cell death after ischemia and reperfusion. J Mol Cell Cardiol 2005;39:277–83.

[114] Gurevitch J, Barak J, Hochhauser E, et al. Aprotinin improves myocardial recovery after ischemia and reperfusion. Effects of the drug on isolated rat hearts. J Thorac Cardiovasc Surg 1994;108:109–18.

[115] Zimmerman BJ, Granger N. Reperfusion-induced leukocyte infiltration: role of elastase. Am J Physiol 1990;259:H390–4.

[116] Hansen PR, Stawski G. Neutrophil mediated damage to isolated myocytes after anoxia and reoxygenation. Cardiovasc Res 1994;28:565–9.

[117] Sabri A, Alcott SG, Elouardighi H, et al. Neutrophil cathepsin G promotes detachment-induced cardiomyocyte apoptosis via a protease-activated receptor-independent mechanism. J Biol Chem 2003;278:23944–54.

[118] Vinten-Johansen J, Thourani VH, Ronson RS, et al. Broad-spectrum cardioprotection with adenosine. Ann Thorac Surg 1999;68:1942–8.

[119] Suzuki T, Moraes TJ, Vachon E, et al. Proteinase-activated receptor-1 mediates elastase-induced apoptosis of human lung epithelial cells. Am J Respir Cell Mol Biol 2005;33: 231–47.

[120] Miller TD, Christian TF, Hopfenspirger MR, et al. Infarct size after acute myocardial infarction measured by quantitative tomographic 99mTc sestamibi imaging predicts subsequent mortality. Circulation 1995;92:334–41.

[121] Pfetter MA, Braunwald E. Ventricular remodeling after myocardial intarction. Experimental observation and clinical implications. Circulation 1990;81:1161–72.

[122] Bolli R, Becker L, Gross G, et al. Myocardial protection at a crossroads: the need for translation into clinical therapy. Circ Res 2004;95:125–34.

[123] Gheorghiade M, Bonow RO. Chronic heart failure in the United States. A manifestation of coronary artery disease. Circulation 1998;97:282–9.

[124] Massie BM, Shah NB. Evolving trends in the epidemiologic factors of heart failure: rational for preventive strategies and comprehensive disease management. Am Heart J 1997;133:703–12.

[125] Sharpe N, Doughty R. Epidemiology of heart failure and ventricular dysfunction. Lancet 1998;352:3–7.

[126] Ho KK, Anderson KM, Kannel WB, et al. Survival after the onset of congestive heart failure in Framingham heart study subjects. Circulation 1993;88:107–15.

[127] Yang F, Liu YH, Yang XP, et al. Myocardial infarction and cardiac remodeling in mice. Exp Physiol 2002;87:547–55.

[128] Bolognese L, Neskovic AN, Parodi G, et al. Left ventricular remodeling after primary coronary angioplasty: patterns of left ventricular dilation and long-term prognostic implications. Circulation 2002;106:2351–7.

[129] Kin H, Zatta AJ, Lofye MT, et al. Postconditioning reduces infarct size via adenosine receptor activation by endogenous adenosine. Cardiovasc Res 2005;67:124–33.

[130] Johnson G III, Tsao PS, Mulloy D, et al. Cardioprotective effects of acidified sodium nitrite in myocardial ischemia with reperfusion. J Pharmacol Exp Ther 1990;252:35–41.

[131] Lefer DJ, Nakanishi K, Johnston WE, et al. Anti-neutrophil and myocardial protecting action of SPM-5185, a novel nitric oxide (NO) donor, following acute myocardial ischemia and reperfusion in dogs. Circulation 1993;88:2337–50.

[132] Nakanishi K, Vinten-Johansen J, Lefer DJ, et al. Intracoronary L-arginine during reperfusion improves endothelial function and reduces infarct size. Am J Physiol 1992;263: H1650–8.

[133] Weyrich AS, Ma X-L, Lefer AM. The role of L-arginine in ameliorating reperfusion injury after myocardial ischemia in the cat. Circulation 1992;86:279–88.

[134] Engelman DT, Watanabe M, Maulik N, et al. Critical timing of nitric oxide supplementation in cardioplegic arrest and reperfusion. Circulation 1996;94:II-407–II-411.

[135] Ihnken K. Myocardial protection in hypoxic immature hearts. Thorac Cardiovasc Surg 2000;48:46–54.

[136] Nakanishi K, Zhao Z-Q, Vinten-Johansen J, et al. Blood cardioplegia enhanced with nitric oxide donor SPM-5185 counteracts postischemic endothelial and ventricular dysfunction. J Thorac Cardiovasc Surg 1995;109:1146–54.

[137] Beresewicz A, Karwatowska-Prokopczuk E, Lewartowski B, et al. A protective role of nitric oxide in isolated ischaemic reperfused rat heart. Cardiovasc Res 1995;30:1001–8.

[138] Cronstein BN. Adenosine, an endogenous anti-inflammatory agent. J Appl Physiol 1994;76:5–13.

[139] Cronstein BN, Kramer SB, Weissmann G, et al. Adenosine: a physiological modulator of superoxide anion generation by human neutrophils. J Exp Med 1983;158:1160–77.

[140] Jordan JE, Thourani VH, Auchampach JA, et al. A_3 adenosine receptor activation attenuates neutrophil function and neutrophil-mediated reperfusion injury. Am J Physiol 1999;277:H1895–905.

[141] Jordan JE, Zhao Z-Q, Sato H, et al. Adenosine A_2 receptor activation attenuates reperfusion injury by inhibiting neutrophil accumulation, superoxide generation and coronary endothelial adherence. J Pharmacol Exp Ther 1997;280:301–9.

[142] Zhao Z-Q, Sato H, Williams MW, et al. Adenosine A_2-receptor activation inhibits neutrophil-mediated injury to coronary endothelium. Am J Physiol 1996;271:H1456–64.

[143] Babbitt DG, Virmani R, Vildibill HD Jr, et al. Intracoronary adenosine administration during reperfusion following 3 hours of ischemia: effects on infarct size, ventricular function, and regional myocardial blood flow. Am Heart J 1990;120:808–18.

[144] Muraki S, Morris CD, Budde JM, et al. Experimental off-pump coronary artery revascularization with adenosine-enhanced reperfusion. J Thorac Cardiovasc Surg 2001;121:570–9.

[145] Olafsson B, Forman MB, Puett DW, et al. Reduction of reperfusion injury in the canine preparation by intracoronary adenosine: importance of the endothelium and the no-reflow phenomenon. Circulation 1987;76:1135–45.

[146] Royston D, Bidstrup BP, Taylor KM, et al. Effect of aprotinin on need for blood transfusion after repeat open-heart surgery. Lancet 1987;2:1289–91.

[147] Pruefer D, Buerke U, Khalili M, et al. Cardioprotective effects of the serine protease inhibitor aprotinin after regional ischemia and reperfusion on the beating heart. J Thorac Cardiovasc Surg 2002;124:942–9.

[148] van Oeveren W, Jansen NJG, Bidstrup B, et al. Effects of aprotinin on hemostatic mechanisms during cardiopulmonary bypass. Ann Thorac Surg 1987;44:640–5.

[149] Lord RA, Roath OS, Thompson JF, et al. Effect of aprotinin on neutrophil function after major vascular surgery. Br J Surg 1992;79:517–21.

[150] Pruefer D, Makowski J, Dahm M, et al. Aprotinin inhibits leukocyte-endothelial cell interactions after hemorrhage and reperfusion. Ann Thorac Surg 2003;75:210–5.

[151] Reeves JG, Mykytenko J, Jiang R, et al. Inhibition of serine protease activity at reperfusion attenuates reperfusion injury [abstract]. J Mol Cell Cardiol 2005;38:830.

[152] McLean PG, Aston D, Sarkar D, et al. Protease-activated receptor-2 activation causes EDHF-like coronary vasodilation selective preservation in ischemia/reperfusion injury: involvement of lipoxygenase products, VR1 receptors, and C-fibers. Circ Res 2002;90:465–72.

[153] Lefer DJ, Nakanishi K, Vinten-Johansen J. Endothelial and myocardial cell protection by a cysteine-containing nitric oxide donor after myocardial ischemia and reperfusion. J Cardiovasc Pharmacol 1993;22(Suppl 7):S34–43.

[154] Lefer DJ, Shandelya SM, Serrano CV Jr, et al. Cardioprotective actions of a monoclonal antibody against CD-18 in myocardial ischemia-reperfusion injury. Circulation 1993;88:1779–87.

[155] Ziegelstein RC, Corda S, Pili R, et al. Initial contact and subsequent adhesion of human neutrophils or monocytes to human aortic endothelial cells releases an endothelial intracellular calcium store. Circulation 1994;90:1899–907.

[156] Feistritzer C, Lenta R, Riewald M. Protease-activated receptors-1 and -2 can mediate endothelial barrier protection: role in factor Xa signaling. J Thromb Haemost 2005;3: 2798–805.

Hematol Oncol Clin N Am 21 (2007) 147–161

HEMATOLOGY/ONCOLOGY CLINICS
OF NORTH AMERICA

ELSEVIER
SAUNDERS

Transfusion Risks and Transfusion-related Pro-inflammatory Responses

George John Despotis, MD[a,b,*], Lini Zhang, MD[a],
Douglas M. Lublin, MD, PhD[b]

[a]Department of Anesthesiology, Box 8054, Washington University School of Medicine,
660 South Euclid Avenue, St. Louis, MO 63110, USA
[b]Department of Pathology and Immunology, Box 8118, Washington University School
of Medicine, 660 South Euclid Avenue, St. Louis, MO 63110, USA

Approximately 14.2 million red cell units and 1.6 million platelet transfusions (>80% single donor apheresis platelet units and the rest pools of usually six random donor platelet units) are administered in the United States each year [1,2,3]. Transfusion-related adverse events can occur with 10% of transfusions, and serious adverse events have been estimated to less than 0.5% of transfusions. Early estimates indicated that transfusion-associated adverse events could lead to a short-term (ie, not including disease transmission-related deaths) mortality of 1 to 1.2 deaths per 100,000 patients, or approximately 35 transfusion-related deaths/year in the United States [1,2]. More recent estimates suggest transfusion-related deaths are under-reported, and that long-term or total (ie, including disease transmission-related deaths) mortality is probably closer to one death per every 37,000 platelet or 130,000 red cell units administered, or approximately 220 transfusion-related deaths per year in the United States [1]. Even these estimates, however, may be underestimating transfusion-related mortality. For example, there were only 21 transfusion-related acute lung injury (TRALI)-related fatalities reported in 2003 [4], while projections based on an incidence of 1:5,000 transfusions with a 6% mortality rate indicate that this syndrome can account for at least 300 deaths annually in the United States. With respect to the leading causes of death, reports to the Food and Drug Administration (FDA) from 2001 to 2003 indicated that TRALI (16% to 22%), ABO Blood Group hemolytic transfusion reactions (12% to 15%), and bacterial contamination of platelets (11% to 18%) accounted for 40% to 50% of all transfusion-related deaths [5].

*Corresponding author. Department of Pathology and Immunology, Box 8118, Washington University School of Medicine, 660 South Euclid Avenue, St. Louis, MO 63110. *E-mail address:* gdespotis@path.wustl.edu (G.J. Despotis).

0889-8588/07/$ – see front matter
doi:10.1016/j.hoc.2006.11.002

The composite risk of transmission of lipid-enveloped viruses such as HIV (1:1,400,000 to 2,400,000 U), human T-lymphotropic virus HTLV-I/II (1:250,000 to 2,000,000 U), hepatitis B (1:58,000 to 1: 149,000 U), hepatitis C (1:872,000 to 1,700,000 U) is estimated to be 1:83,000 U [2]. A substantial decline in the risk for transfusion-related viral transmission has occurred over the past 15 years related to implementation of donor screening and test strategies. This improvement came from immunoassays of increased sensitivity, and more recently from nucleic acid testing procedures that can detect viral RNA/DNA during the window period.

Fifty percent of patients who acquire the hepatitis C virus (HCV) develop liver disease (although symptoms can be apparent within 2 weeks to 6 months, most patients are asymptomatic); 20% develop cirrhosis within 20 years, and 1% to 5% subsequently develop hepatocellular carcinoma. In contrast, transmission of hepatitis A or E, both enteric forms of hepatitis, is rare, and not associated with chronic infection. Other blood-borne, infectious diseases such as syphilis, Epstein-Barr virus, leishmaniasis, Lyme disease, brucellosis, B-19 parvovirus (increased prevalence in hemophiliacs), tick-borne encephalitis virus, Colorado tick fever virus, severe acute respiratory syndrome (SARS), West Nile virus, human herpes viruses, parasitic diseases (eg, malaria, babesiosis, toxoplasmosis, and Chagas' disease), and variant Creutzfeldt–Jakob disease (vCJD) can be transmitted by means of transfusion, although many of these agents are rare in blood donors in the United States.

Febrile, nonhemolytic transfusion reactions (NHTR) consisting of fever (>1°C) with a transfusion, occurs with 0.5% to 1.5% of red cell transfusions and can be related to one of several potential mechanisms. Preformed cytokines within the stored unit and host antibodies to donor (ie, graft) lymphocytes are generally self-limiting. The incidence of febrile NHTR may decrease by perhaps 50% with the use of prestorage leukoreduced blood components, and these reactions often can be prevented by pretreatment with acetaminophen.

Although the estimated death rate related to HIV and hepatitis is declining, death related to transfusion caused by sepsis secondary to bacterial contamination of platelets is estimated to be at 20 deaths per million units of transfused platelets [2]. This is concerning, based on the substantially increased use of platelet transfusions in the United States to support cardiac surgery, oncology, and peripheral blood stem cell (PBSC) transplantation programs. The infusion of bacterially contaminated blood is an uncommon cause (0.0002% to 0.05%) of febrile transfusion reactions, occurring with 0.0001% to 0.002% of red blood cell (RBC) products stored at 4°C (the organism is often *Yersinia enterocolitica*) and at a much higher frequency with platelets stored at 20°C (ie, 0.05%) [1,2]. It, however, can lead to sepsis in 17% to 25% of patients transfused with contaminated blood, with an associated mortality rate of 26% [1]. Additionally, it accounts for at least 16% of transfusion-related fatalities previously reported to the FDA [6].

Bacterial growth more commonly occurs in components stored at room temperature (1:2,000 per apheresis platelet unit), especially if the storage interval is greater than 5 days, which has led to the current FDA limit for platelet out-date of 5 days. Very recently, the FDA licensed systems for storage of apheresis platelets for up to 7 days when bacterial cultures are performed on the product before release. Some form of bacterial quality control screening is performed for all platelet products, but it is not required that the method be as sensitive as culture systems. Transfusion of bacterially contaminated blood should be suspected when patients manifest one or more of the following symptoms or complications: high fever, chills, hemodynamic perturbations (eg, tachycardia, hypotension, shock), gastrointestinal (GI) symptoms (eg, emesis, diarrhea), hemoglobinuria, disseminated intravascular coagulation (DIC), or oliguria. Before transfusion, units should be examined for signs of bacterial contamination (eg, discoloration or dark color, bubbles).

Transfusion-associated respiratory distress can be related to one of the following in order of decreasing frequency: fluid overload (transfusion-associated circulatory overload or TACO), allergic reactions, or TRALI. Although the exact incidence of circulatory overload related to transfusion is unknown (eg, 1 in every 200 to 10,000 U) [7], it is more likely in older patients with a history of congestive heart failure. Estimated prevalence rates of TRALI range from 1 in 432 U to 1 in 88,000 U of transfused platelets and 1 in 4,000 U to 1 in 557,000 U of red blood cells [8]. These ranges for transfusion associated circulatory overload (TACO) and TRALI reflect the clinical difficulty of diagnosis and the under-reporting of these transfusion reactions. TRALI can occur when anti-HLA (human leukocyte antigen) or anti-HNA (human neutrophil antigen) antibodies (more commonly observed in units from multiparous donors) and possibly neutrophil-activating lipid mediators within transfused units attack circulating and pulmonary leukocytes and stimulate complement activation and pulmonary injury [7]. This hypothesis, however, cannot explain all cases of TRALI, and a two-hit hypothesis was proposed previously [9]. The first event involves priming of neutrophils by some underlying condition (eg, trauma, infection, or surgery), which is followed by the infusion of substances by transfusion (eg, anti-HLA or anti-HNA antibodies, biologically active lipids). This leads to TRALI. This syndrome is characterized by acute (<6 hours after transfusion) onset of severe hypoxemia, bilateral noncardiogenic pulmonary edema, tachycardia/hypotension, and fever [10,11]. With ventilatory and hemodynamic supportive management, most patients recover within 48 to 96 hours. The prevalence of TRALI or development of acute respiratory compromise during or after transfusion has been advocated to be much more common in a recent Canadian consensus meeting [4]. In fact, with increased reporting to the FDA, the incidence of TRALI-related deaths (5% to 25% of patients who develop this syndrome) may be much higher than previously thought (as high as 18% of all deaths reported between 2001 and 2003), which places it close to the other leading causes of death (ie, acute hemolytic reactions, or bacterial contamination of platelets) [5,12,13]. Analysis of recent publications indicates that this syndrome is under-reported, because there were only 21 fatalities reported in 2003 [4], while low-end projections (ie, incidence of 1:5,000 transfusions with a 6% mortality rate) indicate that this syndrome can account for as many as

300 deaths annually in the United States. In addition, if TRALI is not diagnosed correctly, treatment of these patients with therapy designed to manage cardiogenic pulmonary edema (ie, diuretic administration) can lead to adverse outcomes [10]. The pathophysiology of TRALI is still being elucidated, and it is uncertain whether the mechanisms will expand beyond anti-HLA and anti-HNA antibodies and lipid mediators [14]. The understanding of the exact role of transfusion in the development of acute lung injury in susceptible patients with endothelial dysfunction (eg, trauma, cardiac surgery, sepsis) who also develop other end-organ dysfunction as part of multiorgan system failure is evolving.

Hemolytic transfusion reactions can be immediate and life-threatening or delayed with minimal resulting clinical consequences (eg, serologic conversion). Current estimates indicate that the wrong unit of blood is administered 1 in every 14,000 U, of which transfusion of 1:33,000 U involves ABO incompatibility [2,15,16]. Catastrophic, acute hemolytic transfusion reactions (HTRs) are rare (ie, 1 in every 33,000 U to 1 in every 500,000 to 1,500,000 U). They can be fatal in 2% to 6% [1,2,6,15] of cases, however, and they account for at least (ie, these events are probably under-reported) 16 deaths every year (ie, 1:800,000 U transfused) in the United States [2,6]. Based on transfusion of 14.2 million units of red cells annually in the United States, there are approximately 1,000 nonfatal and 20 to 60 fatal mis-identification errors each year. This is in contrast to the 131 deaths (or 37% of the total deaths) related to ABO-incompatible transfusion reported between 1976 and 1985 [6,15]. Data from the United Kingdom for serious hazards of transfusion (SHOT) between 1996 and 2003 revealed that there were 2087 errors (1:11,000 transfusions), of which 24% resulted in major morbidity or death [15,16]. This report also revealed that in 50% of these events there were multiple errors in the process, that 70% of the errors occurred in clinical areas, and that the most frequent error (27% in 2003) involved a failure to link the unit to the patient at the bedside [16].

Catastrophic acute HTR initiates a sequence of responses, including complement and hemostatic system activation and neuroendocrine responses, which occur predominantly when host antibodies attach to red cell antigens on incompatible donor red cells. Generally, catastrophic acute HTR involves preformed IgM antibodies to ABO antigens, which lead to hemolysis by means of complement fixation and formation of immune complexes. As little as 10 to 15 mL of ABO-incompatible blood can initiate symptoms consistent with a severe, acute HTR such as:

- Fever in 48% (cytokine-related)
- Hypotension in 15% (secondary to bradykinin, mast cell histamine/serotonin and other vasoactive amines)
- Diffuse microvascular bleeding (secondary to hemostatic system activation or DIC)
- Complement-mediated acute intravascular hemolysis (eg, acute anemia, hemoglobinemia/hemoglobinuria in 87%)

- Acute renal insufficiency secondary to alpha-adrenergic vasoconstriction or deposition of antibody-coated stroma within the renal vasculature [17]

The diagnosis can be confirmed with detection of free hemoglobin within the blood and urine in the setting of a positive direct antiglobulin test (DAT) with a mixed-field pattern on post-transfusion but not pretransfusion specimens. Additional tests that should be ordered include:

- Repeat ABO/Rhesus (Rh) testing of the unit
- Repeat cross-match and antibody detection on the patient's pre- and postreaction samples and on blood from the unit
- Haptoglobin
- LDH
- Serial hemoglobin/hematocrit on patient specimens
- Examination of the blood remaining in the unit for hemolysis [18]

Treatment is generally supportive and involves resuscitation to maintain organ perfusion using volume and vasopressor, which preferably do not vasoconstrict the renal bed (eg, low dose dopamine), maintenance of good renal urine output (>100 mL/h × 24 hours) with intravenous crystalloids and diuretics, and on occasion transfusion support with hemostatic blood products in the setting of DIC and clinical bleeding.

In contrast, most reactions to non-ABO antigens involve IgG-mediated extravascular clearance within the reticuloendothelial system (RES). They often are delayed (ie, 2 to 10 days), and they are not detected by pretransfusion testing, because they represent an anamnestic response. An exception to this pattern is Kidd antibodies, which are strong complement activators that can result in acute intravascular HTR. Finally, nonimmune HTR also can occur related to temperature (eg, overwarming with blood warmers, use of microwave ovens), use of hypotonic solutions for dilution of packed red blood cells (PRBCs), and mechanical issues during administration (ie, pressure infusion pumps, pressure cuffs, and small-bore needles). In addition, normal saline should be used to dilute the red cell units (calcium-containing solutions should be avoided), and units should be examined for large clots before transfusion.

Because clerical or misidentification errors, which occur 1 in every 14,000 U, cause most immediate immune-mediated HTR [19], this potentially lethal complication can be prevented by diligent confirmation of patient and unit identification by individuals who initiate transfusion intraoperatively (ie, the anesthesiologist and circulating nurse). First, the blood bank confirms that the unit identification number and the ABO/Rh type on the unit of blood match the label attached to the unit. Most importantly, two clinical transfusionists must confirm that three pieces of patient identification (eg, patient name, hospital identification number, birth date, or social security number) on the hospital identification band or surrogate (eg, patient name plate imprint on the anesthesia record) needs to match the respective parameters on the unit of blood.

To obtain a thorough understanding of hemolytic reactions, red cell antigen systems and serologic diagnostic tests are reviewed. Red cell antigen systems include the ABO and related carbohydrate antigens (ie, H, P, I, and Lewis blood groups), the 48 Rh system antigens (including RhD) and over 200 other non-ABO/Rh antigens. The ABO carbohydrate and Rh polypeptide molecules reside on the surface of red blood cells with a US population frequency distribution (O: 44%, A: 43%, B: 9%, AB: 4%; RhD+: 84%). ABO molecules express specific antigenic activity after individual sugar moieties are added to short sugar chains (ie, oligosaccharides) by several genetically determined glycosyltransferase enzymes. The ABO antigens are linked to cells (ie, red cells and other cells) by means of their association with membrane-bound proteins (ie, glycoproteins) or ceramide residues (ie, glycosphingolipids). Antibodies to the A and B antigens generally are thought to form as a result of exposure to other sources of antigen (ie, on bacteria) after the first few months of life. Blood group A and B individuals produce predominantly IgM antibodies (ie, anti-B and anti-A, respectively), whereas blood group O individuals produce both anti-B and anti-A IgG/IgM antibodies. Antibodies to Lewis and P1 antigens are generally clinically insignificant.

Although there are 49 identified Rh antigens, the five principal antigens, D, C, E, c and e, and corresponding antibodies account for more than 99% of clinical issues involving the Rh system. The Rh system antigens are nonglycosylated, fatty-acylated polypeptides that traverse the red cell membrane 12 times. Although individuals who lack the D antigen do not form antibodies without blood exposure, the D antigen is highly immunogenic, and 80% of individuals who lack the D antigen will form anti-D once exposed through transfusion, or, at a lower frequency of approximately 15% through pregnancy.

Over 200 other non-ABO/Rh, glycoprotein antigens can be identified on red cells, and some of these antigens also are expressed on other cells and body fluids. These non-ABO/Rh antigens frequently are subdivided into common (ie, MNS, Kell, Duffy, and Kidd systems) and uncommon antigen systems (eg, Lutheran, Diego, Yt, Xg, and Scianna). Antibodies to most of the common antigens can cause both clinically significant immediate and delayed HTR, but do not usually result in catastrophic, complement-mediated hemolysis, although this can occur with Kidd, Duffy, and S antibodies. Severe delayed HTRs are particularly common with anti-Kidd antibodies. Another important factor is the relative immunogenicity (ie, antibody formation), which can vary substantially between non-ABO antigens (eg, anti-D in 80%, anti-K in 10%, and anti-Fy^a in 1% of exposures).

Several blood bank procedures (type, screen, and cross-match) are employed routinely to ensure transfusion of compatible blood. Patient ABO type is determined using direct agglutination of red cells and involves use of forward (ie, using the patient's red cells with anti-A and anti-B reagents) and reverse (using the patient's sera with reagent A1 and B cells) typing. Only forward typing is accurate in newborns or infants younger than 4 to 6 months based on transfer of maternal IgG molecules and lack of anti-A or anti-B production before 4 to 6 months of age. An antibody screen (ie, indirect antiglobulin or Coombs test) determines whether unexpected antibodies against common non-ABO red cell antigens are present, These antibodies are found in 0.2% to 0.6% of the general population [20], 1% to 2% of hospitalized patients, or in 8.3% of surgical patients. The antibody screen is performed using reagent red cells (ie, two or three screening cells) and a cross-linking antibody (rabbit/mouse antihuman globulin or Coombs reagent) that enhances the IgG-mediated agglutination of red cells. Sera is tested routinely only for antibodies to the common antigens, because the uncommon non-ABO antigens infrequently (ie, <0.01%) result in cross-match incompatibility of ABO compatible units. In the setting of a negative result on the antibody screen, the final cross-match can be done by a Coombs test, an immediate spin cross-match, or an electronic cross-match. The latter two procedures simply confirm the ABO compatibility of the donor unit and require less time. An elective procedure for which a type and screen or cross-matched blood has been requested should never commence until the antibody screen has been determined to be negative, or in the setting of a positive antibody screen, with antibodies and cross-matched compatible blood identified.

Because availability of blood for same-day and urgent surgery is of critical importance, understanding a generally applicable timetable is important [20]. O negative (in some settings O positive for males) RBCs are generally immediately (<5 minutes) available, whereas type-specific RBCs are available within 15 minutes after receipt of the patient specimen. Cross-matched RBCs are generally available within 45 to 60 minutes by means of a type and cross-match (T&C) procedure using an immediate spin cross-match, which can be done if no antibodies are detected during the antibody screen. With a positive antibody screen, additional time (1 to several hours or even days) may be required to determine the antibodies and identify and cross-match blood that is antigen-negative. In the event that antibodies are detected from the screen, the probability of finding compatible units can be calculated from the frequency of antigens for those preformed antibodies (eg, an A+ individual with anti-c, anti-Fy^a antibodies will be compatible with $0.18 \times 0.34 = 0.06$ or 6 of 100 A+ units in the blood bank). Accordingly, obtaining cross-match compatible blood is also difficult when a patient has antibodies to a very common antigen (eg, k, in which case only 1 in 500 units is compatible). Clinicians also may be faced with an inability to obtain cross-match compatible blood in patients who have a warm auto-antibody. In this setting, more extensive serologic analysis using absorption techniques is required to identify alloantibodies; alternatively, if the patient has not been transfused recently, the partial phenotype can be determined to provide antigen-negative red cells.

Single-donor, apheresis platelets (which now constitute >80% of platelet transfusions) are generally available immediately, whereas pooled platelet concentrates may take 10 to 15 minutes to process. The time required to obtain plasma or cryoprecipitate varies from 5 minutes to 30 minutes and is dependent on whether an inventory of thawed plasma units is maintained and the availability of a rapid thawing system.

Mild urticarial symptoms (eg, rash, hives, or itching) occur with 1% of transfusions [21]. They are generally self-limiting and may improve with or be prevented by antihistamine prophylaxis. More significant allergic transfusion reactions can occur with 0.1% to 0.3% units and are most likely related to reactions to other soluble transfusion constituents (eg, complement or other plasma proteins, drugs, or soluble allergens). Severe anaphylactic reactions, which occur infrequently (ie, 0.005% to 0.0007%), may be accompanied by IgE-mediated symptoms involving the respiratory (eg, dyspnea, bronchospasm), GI (eg, nausea, diarrhea, cramps) or circulatory (eg, arrhythmias, hypotension, or syncope) systems. IgA deficiency, which occurs in 1 of every 800 patients (only 30% of whom have preformed anti-IgA), is an uncommon cause of transfusion-associated anaphylaxis, and this diagnosis should be considered in any patient exhibiting anaphylaxis. Other potential causes of hemodynamic perturbations during or after a transfusion include:

- Citrate-related hypocalcemia (ie, with rapid infusion)
- Inadvertent intravenous air embolus (particularly with autologous blood recovery and reinfusion)
- Cytokine-mediated effects
- Bradykinin activation by leukoreduction filters, which may be aggravated by inadequate clearance in patients on angiotensin-converting enzyme inhibitors (80 reports to the FDA)

Metabolic consequences of transfusion include coagulopathy, hypothermia (ie, with inadequate warming of refrigerated PRBC units) and hyperkalemia, because potassium concentration increases with the storage interval of PRBC units (eg, 42 mEq/L at 42 days of storage, or approximately 6 mEq total in a unit of PRBCs).

In addition to development of alloantibodies to red cell antigens, several other immune-related phenomena can occur subsequent to transfusion. Antigens of the HLA system are determined by genes on the major histocompatibility complex on the short arm of chromosome 6. HLA gene products are cell–surface glycoproteins on all cells except mature red cells (class I comprised of HLA-A, B, or C antigens) or on B lymphocytes and cells of monocyte/macrophage lineage (class II comprised of HLA-DR, DQ, or DP gene cluster codes). Because they contribute to the recognition of self versus non-self, they are important with respect to rejection of transplanted tissue and long-term survival after solid organ and bone marrow transplantation. Alloimmunization to HLA antigens, which occurs commonly (ie, 20% to 70% of the time) in transfused and multiparous patients, can lead to immune-mediated platelet refractoriness (ie, insignificant or inadequate rise in platelet count not related to DIC, amphotericin, or splenomegaly), and febrile NHTR. Alloimmunization can be associated with development of autoantibodies, leading to autoimmune hemolytic anemia and development of post-transfusion purpura (ie, severe thrombocytopenia secondary to platelet-specific antibodies, usually anti-HPA-1a/PLA1 antibodies) 5 to 10 days after transfusion. Transfusion-associated immune system modulation has been shown to have beneficial effects, including improved renal allograft survival, reduced risk of recurrent spontaneous abortion, and reduced severity of autoimmune diseases such as rheumatoid arthritis. Proposed detrimental effects of transfusion-associated immune system modulation include increased cancer recurrence, perioperative infections, multiorgan system failure, and overall mortality, but these effects are controversial [22]. Transfusion, however, potentially can attenuate the immune response based on one of several potential mechanisms, including:

- a reduction in CD8 suppressor T cell function and number
- CD4 T helper cell number
- NK cell number and function
- Macrophage number and function,
- MLC response
- Response to mitogen,
- Cell-mediated cytotoxicity [23]

Although several studies have demonstrated an independent effect (ie, using multivariate statistical models) of transfusion on increased perioperative infection ratesfour to five times) in numerous different surgical populations (ie, trauma [24–27], hip arthroplasty [25,28], spinal [29], colorectal [30–36] and cardiac [37–39]), the immune–modulatory effect of transfusion on the incidence of perioperative infection remains controversial. In addition, a recent meta-analysis involving review of 20 peer-reviewed articles and 13,152 patients revealed that transfusion was associated with perioperative infection (odds ratio of 3.45, range 1.43 to 15.15) [27]. Accordingly, four recent studies have demonstrated that administration of leukoreduced units may reduce perioperative infection in patients undergoing either colorectal [31] or GI, [10], or cardiac surgery [41,42], This has not been confirmed by other studies, however [43–45]. Another recent retrospective analysis demonstrated a reduction in perioperative complications and mortality when leukoreduced units were used [44–46]. Rarely, transfusion-associated graft-versus-host disease, a syndrome manifested by several symptoms (ie, fever, dermatitis or erythroderma, hepatitis/enterocolitis, diarrhea, pancytopenia, or hypocellular bone marrow) may occur and be secondary to transfusion of cellular blood components that contain HLA-compatible T-lymphocytes, This occurs more frequently with transfusions from related individuals, and it can be prevented by standard irradiation of the blood product.

Several recent studies have demonstrated that transfusion has an association with multiorgan system failure (MOSF) in the perioperative setting [47–49]. Although the exact mechanisms of the potential effect of transfusion on the incidence of this complication have not been elucidated, it is postulated that in patients who are at high risk (eg, trauma, long CPB intervals) for developing endothelial dysfunction, that either white cell lytic enzymes or other cellular debris injure an already dysfunctional endothelium. These studies also have demonstrated that there is an effect imposed by the age of the PRBC units and a load effect (ie, a direct relationship between the number of PRBCs units administered and MOSF rates). The prevalence of TRALI is expanding, in part based on improved reporting and potential overlap between the diagnoses of TRALI versus MOSF in the high-risk patients. In addition, a recent study by van de Watering [41] demonstrated that mortality related to MOSF was reduced by 90% when patients undergoing cardiac surgery received leukoreduced PRBC units.

Excessive bleeding requiring transfusion to correct anemia or hemostatic defects also may result in other complications such as stroke and may affect long-term mortality. In a large (n = 16,000), recently published analysis [50], transfusion of more than 4 U of PRBC was the strongest (odds ratio = 5) independent predictor with respect to perioperative stroke; it is not clear from this analysis whether transfusion support was a causative factor versus a predictor [50]. Another recent publication demonstrated a strong relationship between perioperative platelet transfusion and both stroke and death [51]. This was supported by another recent retrospective analysis that demonstrated that the death rate in a large series of patients undergoing cardiac surgery was much higher in patients who received platelets using multivariate statistical modeling [52]. Accordingly, a retrospective analysis demonstrated that long-term mortality may be doubled in patients who receive transfusion [53]. Because of their retrospective design, these studies cannot definitively link transfusion of either PRBC or platelet components with stroke or increased mortality, which may be reflecting colinearity or a statistical passenger effect with other comorbidities such as excessive bleeding. These studies, however, do help explain why agents such as aprotinin, which has been shown to reduce blood loss and transfusion by 50% to 90% and re-exploration rates by 70% in several large, randomized, placebo-controlled trials [54–57], also is associated with a 60% to 70% reduction in perioperative stroke [58] and reduced mortality [59]. Whether the beneficial effects of this agent are related to a reduction in the incidence of anemia and hypoperfusion related to bleeding in patients who also receive multicomponent transfusion or if they are the indirect effects of this agent on reducing transfusion in the bleeding patient with a concomitant reduction in transfusion-related sequelae remains unclear. Iron overload (ie, accumulation and deposition of iron within the vital organs) can occur in chronically transfused individuals such as patients with hemoglobinopathies and other susceptible patients.

Emerging techniques to reduce disease transmission and hemolytic transfusion reactions are under active investigation and implementation. The introduction of nucleic acid technology (NAT) testing procedures can minimize blood-borne disease transmission by detecting viral RNA/DNA during the serologic window period. Inactivation of viral and bacterial RNA/DNA by photochemicals (eg, psoralen) with UVB irradiation is under investigation. Other techniques to reduce hemolytic transfusion reactions are under investigation such as conversion of A, B, or AB red cell units to O by means of enzymatic digestion of A and B antigens or generation of AB equivalent plasma by means of adsorption of anti-A and anti-B from plasma. In addition, new patient identification systems (eg, bar coding of identification bands and blood and the Bloodloc Safety System [Novatek Medical, Effingham, Illinois]) are being implemented to reduce transfusion of incompatible blood, in part based on a recent Joint Commission on Accreditation of Healthcare Organizations high-priority directive to enhance patient safety by means of improved patient identification.

Although the on-going interface between transfusion medicine and perioperative services is an important topic, it is reviewed only briefly. The transfusion medicine service can provide assistance with respect to patients with unique clinical problems (eg, patients with cold agglutinin disease), use of specialized blood components, and implementation and monitoring of one of several non-pharmacologic blood conservation strategies such as preautologous donation [60,61], normovolemic hemodilution and cell salvage techniques [62], and other technical blood conservation methods [63]. Several pharmacologic agents (eg, tranexamic acid, epsilon amino caproic acid, or aprotinin) can be used to reduce bleeding and transfusion after cardiac, orthopedic, and liver transplantation procedures. Aprotinin, however, is the only agent that is FDA-approved for patients undergoing cardiac revascularization. This is also the only agent with established efficacy and safety based on multiple prospective, randomized (placebo-controlled) trials [54–57].

Other important interactions between transfusion medicine and perioperative services include establishment and monitoring of standardized transfusion protocols for red cells, hemostatic components, and emerging and off-label indications for factor concentrates (eg, factor VIIa) as important blood management strategies. Although several case reports have indicated that off-label use of activated factor VII can reverse life-threatening bleeding, cost and risk of thrombosis preclude routine use. Because any factor concentrate potentially can lead to life-threatening thrombotic complications in a subset of high-risk patients (ie, patients with congenital or acquired thrombotic disorders or systemic activation of the hemostatic system such as with DIC or after cardiac surgery), large clinical trials evaluating the efficacy and safety of rFVIIa are needed before any widespread use can be recommended [64].

Use of point-of-care or laboratory-based coagulation results when coupled to a standardized approach (ie, algorithm) for managing bleeding after cardiac surgery has been shown to result in a 50% reduction in total donor exposures in all but one [65] of eight published studies [66–72]. Other studies also have demonstrated that certain patient subgroups may benefit from off-label use of DDAVP with respect to reduced bleeding and transfusion such as patients who have:

- Type I von Willebrand's disease
- Uremia-induced platelet dysfunction
- A platelet defect after cardiac surgery as identified using point-of-care platelet function tests [73,74]

Use and monitoring of point-of-care diagnostics to guide transfusion and pharmacologic management of bleeding also can be enhanced by means of a collaborative approach with the transfusion medicine service with respect to implementation, quality control monitoring, and regulatory compliance (eg, Joint Commission or College of American Pathologists). Future availability of blood substitutes may be critical in unique clinical situations such as in patients with multiple antibodies, with Jehovah's Witness patients, and in trauma settings. These agents also may enhance blood conservation techniques or organ preservation because of their ability to enhance tissue oxygenation.

Despite improvements in blood screening and administration techniques, serious adverse events related to transfusion continue to occur, albeit at a much lower incidence. In addition to the development and implementation of new screening and blood purification/modification techniques, the incidence and consequences of transfusion reactions can be reduced by a basic understanding of transfusion-related complications. Although acute hemolytic transfusion reactions, transfusion-associated anaphylaxis, sepsis, and TRALI occur infrequently, diligence in administration of blood and monitoring for development of respective signs/symptoms can minimize the severity of these potentially life-threatening complications. In addition, emerging blood banking techniques such as psoralen-UV inactivation of pathogens and use of patient identification systems may attenuate the incidence of adverse events related to transfusion. With respect to optimizing blood management by means of pharmacologic and nonpharmacologic strategies, the ability to reduce use of blood products and to decrease operative time or re-exploration rates has important implications for not only disease prevention, but also for blood inventory and costs and overall health care costs.

References

[1] Goodnough LT, Brecher ME, Kanter MH, et al. Transfusion medicine: blood transfusion. N Engl J Med 1999;340:438–47.
[2] Goodnough LT, Shander A, Brecher ME. Transfusion medicine: looking to the future. Lancet 2003;361(9352):161–9.
[3] Whitaker BI, Sullivan M. 2005 nationwide blood collection and utilization survey report. Rockville (MD): Department of Health and Human Services; 2006.
[4] Toy P, Popovsky MA, Abraham E, et al. Transfusion-related acute lung injury: definition and review. Crit Care Med 2005;33:721–6.
[5] Goldman M, Webert KE, Arnold DM, et al. Proceedings of a consensus conference: towards an understanding of TRALI. Transfus Med Rev 2005;19:2–31.
[6] Sazama K. Reports of 355 transfusion-associated deaths: 1976 through 1985. Transfusion 1990;30:583–90.
[7] McCullough J. Complications of transfusion. In: McCullough J, editor. Transfusion medicine. New York: McGraw-Hill; 1999. p. 337–59.
[8] Kleinman S, Caulfield T, Chan P, et al. Toward an understanding of transfusion-related acute lung injury: statement of a consensus panel. Transfusion 2004;44:1774–89.
[9] Silliman CC, Paterson AJ, Dickey WO, et al. The association of biologically active lipids with the development of transfusion-related acute lung injury: a retrospective study. Transfusion 1997;37:719–26.
[10] Looney MR, Gropper MA, Matthay MA. Transfusion-related acute lung injury: a review. Chest 2004;126(1):249–58.
[11] Silliman CC, Boshkov LK, Mehdizadehkashi Z, et al. Transfusion-related acute lung injury: epidemiology and a prospective analysis of etiologic factors. Blood 2003;101(2):454–62.
[12] Holness L, Knippen MA, Simmons L, et al. Fatalities caused by TRALI. Transfus Med Rev 2004;18(3):184–8.
[13] Kopko PM, Marshall CS, MacKenzie MR, et al. Transfusion-related acute lung injury: report of a clinical look-back investigation. JAMA 2002;287(15):1968–71.

[14] Zallen G, Moore EE, Ciesla DJ, et al. Stored red blood cells selectively activate human neutrophils to release IL-8 and secretory PLA2. Shock 2000;13(1):29–33.

[15] Stainsby D, Russell J, Cohen H, et al. Reducing adverse events in blood transfusion. Br J Haematol 2005;131:8–12.

[16] Stainsby D. Errors in transfusion medicine. Anesthesiol Clin North America 2005;23: 253–61.

[17] Pineda AA, Brzica SM Jr, Taswell HF. Hemolytic transfusion reaction. Recent experience in a large blood bank. Mayo Clin Proc 1978;53:378–90.

[18] Noninfectious complications of blood transfusion. In: Brecher ME, editor. Technical manual. Bethesda (MA): American Association of Blood Banks; 2002. p. 585–609.

[19] Linden JV, Paul B, Dressler KP. A report of 104 transfusion errors in New York State. Transfusion 1992;32:601–6.

[20] Shulman IA, Spence RK, Petz LD. Surgical blood ordering, blood shortage situations, and emergency transfusions. In: Petz LD, Swisher SN, Kleinman S, et al, editors. Clinical practice of transfusion medicine. New York: Churchill Livingstone; 1996. p. 509–19.

[21] Firestone DT. Adverse effects of blood transfusion. In: Rudman SV, editor. Textbook of blood banking and transfusion medicine. Philadelphia: WB Saunders Co; 1995. p. 406–33.

[22] Landers DF, Hill GE, Wong KC, et al. Blood transfusion-induced immunomodulation. Anesth Analg 1996;82:187–204.

[23] Blumberg N, Heal JM. Immunomodulation by blood transfusion: an evolving scientific and clinical challenge. Am J Med 1996;101:299–308.

[24] Edna TH, Bjerkeset T. Association between blood transfusion and infection in injured patients. J Trauma 1992;33(5):659–61.

[25] Agarwal N, Murphy JG, Cayten CG, et al. Blood transfusion increases the risk of infection after trauma. Arch Surg 1993;128(2):171–6.

[26] Claridge JA, Sawyer RG, Schulman AM, et al. Blood transfusions correlate with infections in trauma patients in a dose-dependent manner. Am Surg 2002;68:566–72.

[27] Hill GE, Frawley WH, Griffith KE, et al. Allogeneic blood transfusion increases the risk of postoperative bacterial infection: a meta-analysis. J Trauma 2003;54:908–14.

[28] Murphy P, Heal JM, Blumberg N. Infection or suspected infection after hip replacement surgery with autologous or homologous blood transfusions. Transfusion 1991;31: 212–7.

[29] Esposito RA, Culliford AT, Colvin SB, et al. The role of the activated clotting time in heparin administration and neutralization for cardiopulmonary bypass. J Thorac Cardiovasc Surg 1983;85(2):174–85.

[30] Jensen LS, Andersen AJ, Christiansen PM, et al. Postoperative infection and natural killer cell function following blood transfusion in patients undergoing elective colorectal surgery. Br J Surg 1992;79(6):513–6.

[31] Jensen LS, Kissmeyer-Nielsen P, Wolff B, et al. Randomised comparison of leucocyte-depleted versus buffy-coat-poor blood transfusion and complications after colorectal surgery. Lancet 1996;348(9031):841–5.

[32] Edna TH, Bjerkeset T. Association between transfusion of stored blood and infective bacterial complications after resection for colorectal cancer. Eur J Surg 1998;164(6):449–56.

[33] Tartter PI. The association of perioperative blood transfusion with colorectal cancer recurrence. Ann Surg 1992;216(6):633–8.

[34] Tartter PI. Blood transfusion and infectious complications following colorectal cancer surgery. Br J Surg 1988;75(8):789–92.

[35] Vignali A, Braga M, Dionigi P, et al. Impact of a programme of autologous blood donation on the incidence of infection in patients with colorectal cancer. Eur J Surg 1995;161(7): 487–92.

[36] Houbiers JG, van de Velde CJ, van de Watering LM, et al. Transfusion of red cells is associated with increased incidence of bacterial infection after colorectal surgery: a prospective study. Transfusion 1997;37(2):126–34.

[37] Murphy PJ, Connery C, Hicks GL Jr, et al. Homologous blood transfusion as a risk factor for postoperative infection after coronary artery bypass graft operations. J Thorac Cardiovasc Surg 1992;104(4):1092–9.

[38] Chelemer SB, Prato BS, Cox PM Jr, et al. Association of bacterial infection and red blood cell transfusion after coronary artery bypass surgery. Ann Thorac Surg 2002;73(1): 138–42.

[39] Vamvakas EC, Carven JH. Transfusion and postoperative pneumonia in coronary artery bypass graft surgery: effect of the length of storage of transfused red cells. Transfusion 1999;39:701–10.

[40] Tartter PI, Mohandas K, Azar P, et al. Randomized trial comparing packed red cell blood transfusion with and without leukocyte depletion for gastrointestinal surgery. Am J Surg 1998;176(5):462–6.

[41] van de Watering LM, Hermans J, Houbiers JG, et al. Beneficial effects of leukocyte depletion of transfused blood on postoperative complications in patients undergoing cardiac surgery: a randomized clinical trial. Circulation 1998;97:562–8.

[42] Bilgin YM, van de Watering LM, Eijsman L, et al. Double-blind, randomized controlled trial on the effect of leukocyte-depleted erythrocyte transfusions in cardiac valve surgery. Circulation 2004;109:2755–60.

[43] Baron JF, Gourdin M, Bertrand M, et al. The effect of universal leukodepletion of packed red blood cells on postoperative infections in high-risk patients undergoing abdominal aortic surgery. Anesth Analg 2002;94(3):529–37.

[44] Titlestad IL, Ebbesen LS, Ainsworth AP, et al. Leukocyte depletion of blood components does not significantly reduce the risk of infectious complications. Results of a double-blinded, randomized study. Int J Colorectal Dis 2001;16(3):147–53.

[45] Wallis JP, Chapman CE, Orr KE, et al. Effect of WBC reduction of transfused RBCs on postoperative infection rates in cardiac surgery. Transfusion 2002;42(9):1127–34.

[46] Blumberg N, Heal JM, Cowles JW, et al. Leukocyte-reduced transfusions in cardiac surgery: results of an implementation trial. Am J Clin Pathol 2002;118:376–81.

[47] Sauaia A, Moore FA, Moore EE, et al. Multiple organ failure can be predicted as early as 12 hours after injury. J Trauma 1998;45(2):291–301.

[48] Moore FA, Moore EE, Sauaia A. Blood transfusion. An independent risk factor for postinjury multiple organ failure. Arch Surg 1997;132(6):620–4.

[49] Sauaia A, Moore FA, Moore EE, et al. Early predictors of postinjury multiple organ failure. Arch Surg 1994;129(1):39–45.

[50] Bucerius J, Gummert JF, Borger MA, et al. Stroke after cardiac surgery: a risk factor analysis of 16,184 consecutive adult patients. Ann Thorac Surg 2003;75(2):472–8.

[51] Mangano DT. Aspirin and mortality from coronary bypass surgery. N Engl J Med 2002; 347(17):1309–17.

[52] Greendyke RM. Cost analysis. Bedside blood glucose testing. Am J Clin Pathol 1992;97(1): 106–7.

[53] Engoren MC, Habib RH, Zacharias A, et al. Effect of blood transfusion on long-term survival after cardiac operation. Ann Thorac Surg 2002;74(4):1180–6.

[54] Lemmer JH Jr, Stanford W, Bonney SL, et al. Aprotinin for coronary bypass operations: efficacy, safety, and influence on early saphenous vein graft patency. A multicenter, randomized, double-blind, placebo-controlled study. J Thorac Cardiovasc Surg 1994;107(2): 543–53.

[55] Lemmer JH, Dilling EW, Morton JR, et al. Aprotinin for primary coronary artery bypass grafting: a multicenter trial of three dose regimens. Ann Thorac Surg 1996;62:1659–67.

[56] Levy JH, Pifarre R, Schaff HV, et al. A multicenter, double-blind, placebo-controlled trial of aprotinin for reducing blood loss and the requirement for donor–blood transfusion in patients undergoing repeat coronary artery bypass grafting. Circulation 1995;92:2236–44.

[57] Alderman EL, Levy JH, Rich JB, et al. Analyses of coronary graft patency after aprotinin use: results from the International Multicenter Aprotinin Graft Patency Experience (IMAGE) trial. J Thorac Cardiovasc Surg 1998;116(5):716–30.

[58] Smith PK. Aprotinin: safe and effective only with the full-dose regimen. Ann Thorac Surg 1996;62:1575–7.

[59] Levi M, Cromheecke ME, de Jonge E, et al. Pharmacological strategies to decrease excessive blood loss in cardiac surgery: a meta-analysis of clinically relevant endpoints. Lancet 1999;354(9194):1940–7.

[60] Goodnough LT. Autologous blood donation. Anesthesiol Clin North America 2005;23: 263–70.

[61] Sonnenberg FA, Gregory P, Yomtovian R, et al. The cost-effectiveness of autologous transfusion revisited: implications of an increased risk of bacterial infection with allogeneic transfusion. Transfusion 1999;39:808–17.

[62] Goodnough LT, Shander A, Spence R. Bloodless medicine: clinical care without allogeneic blood transfusion. Transfusion 2003;43(5):668–76.

[63] Helm RE, Rosengart TK, Gomez M, et al. Comprehensive multimodality blood conservation: 100 consecutive CABG operations without transfusion. Ann Thorac Surg 1998;65: 125–36.

[64] Despotis G, Avidan M, Lublin DM. Off-label use of recombinant factor VIIA concentrates after cardiac surgery. Ann Thorac Surg 2005;80:3–5.

[65] Capraro L, Kuitunen A, Salmenpera M, et al. On-site coagulation monitoring does not affect hemostatic outcome after cardiac surgery. Acta Anaesthesiol Scand 2001;45(2): 200–6.

[66] Despotis GJ, Santoro SA, Spitznagel E, et al. Prospective evaluation and clinical utility of on-site monitoring of coagulation in patients undergoing cardiac operation. J Thorac Cardiovasc Surg 1994;107(1):271–9.

[67] Spiess BD, Gillies BS, Chandler W, et al. Changes in transfusion therapy and re-exploration rate after institution of a blood management program in cardiac surgical patients. J Cardiothorac Vasc Anesth 1995;9:168–73.

[68] Shore-Lesserson L, Manspeizer HE, DePerio M, et al. Thromboelastography-guided transfusion algorithm reduces transfusions in complex cardiac surgery. Anesth Analg 1999;88: 312–9.

[69] Nuttall GA, Oliver WC, Santrach PJ, et al. Efficacy of a simple intraoperative transfusion algorithm for nonerythrocyte component utilization after cardiopulmonary bypass. Anesthesiology 2001;94(5):773–81.

[70] Royston D, von Kier S. Reduced haemostatic factor transfusion using heparinase-modified thrombelastography during cardiopulmonary bypass. Br J Anaesth 2001;86: 575–8.

[71] Avidan MS, Alcock EL, Da Fonseca J, et al. Comparison of structured use of routine laboratory tests or near-patient assessment with clinical judgment in the management of bleeding after cardiac surgery. Br J Anaesth 2004;92(2):178–86.

[72] Chen L, Bracey AW, Radovancevic R, et al. Clopidogrel and bleeding in patients undergoing elective coronary artery bypass grafting. J Thorac Cardiovasc Surg 2004;128: 425–31.

[73] Despotis GJ, Levine V, Saleem R, et al. Use of point-of-care test in identification of patients who can benefit from desmopressin during cardiac surgery: a randomised controlled trial. Lancet 1999;354(9173):106–10.

[74] Mongan PD, Hosking MP. The role of desmopressin acetate in patients undergoing coronary artery bypass surgery. A controlled clinical trial with thromboelastographic risk stratification. Anesthesiology 1992;77(1):38–46.

Hematol Oncol Clin N Am 21 (2007) 163–176

HEMATOLOGY/ONCOLOGY CLINICS
OF NORTH AMERICA

Transfusion-related Acute Lung Injury

Chelsea A. Sheppard, MD[a], Lennart E. Lögdberg, MD, PhD[a],
James C. Zimring, MD, PhD[a], Christopher D. Hillyer, MD[b],*

[a]Department of Pathology and Laboratory Medicine, Room D-655, Emory University School
of Medicine, 1364 Clifton Road, NE, Atlanta, GA 30322, USA
[b]Department of Pathology and Laboratory Medicine, Transfusion Medicine Program,
Room D-655, Emory University Hospital, 1364 Clifton Road, NE, Atlanta, GA 30322, USA

Transfusion carries a variety of inherent risks to the recipient. These can be divided into infectious and noninfectious hazards, and they can manifest either during or with delay after the transfusion. During the last decades of the twentieth century, substantial scientific and lay press attention was focused on infectious risks including transfusion-associated hepatitis B and C, HIV, West Nile Virus and Variant Creutzfeldt-Jakob disease. With the addition of heightened donor screening and antibody, antigen, and/or nucleic acid testing, many of the concerns regarding transfusion transmission of infectious diseases have been well addressed and largely mitigated or eliminated. For example, the risk of acquiring HIV or hepatitis C virus has fallen by approximately 99.99% in developed countries [1–3] likely approaching a residual risk for transfusion-transmitted HIV of 1 in 5 to 8 million screening units (United States). These dramatic improvements in infectious risk have led to new and increased focus on the noninfectious serious hazards of transfusion, which include mistransfusion [4,5], bacterial contamination [6], metabolic sequelae in pediatric patients, transfusion-related acute lung injury (TRALI) [7], and even under-transfusion.

TRALI is now considered to be the second leading cause of mortality from transfusion and has emerged as the leading cause of transfusion-related deaths reported to the US Food and Drug Administration, though this is most likely because of increased recognition (Fig. 1) and may in fact represent over-diagnosis. TRALI has been associated with various blood products including whole blood, packed red blood cells, apheresis or whole blood-derived platelets, fresh frozen plasma, granulocytes, intravenous immunoglobulin, and cryoprecipitate [8]. This article reviews the clinical manifestations, evolving definition, incidence, pathophysiology, animal modeling, and donor screening and deferral algorithms as they relate to TRALI.

*Corresponding author. E-mail address: chillye@emory.edu (C.D. Hillyer).

0889-8588/07/$ – see front matter
doi:10.1016/j.hoc.2006.11.011

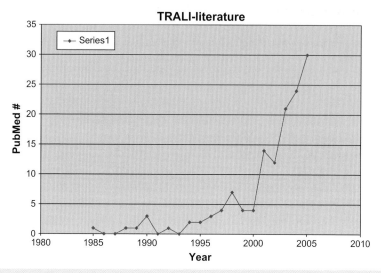

Fig. 1. Increasing recognition of TRALI reflected in growing literature on the entity. The graph illustrates the increase in number of articles indexed in PubMed using the acronym TRALI over the last two decades (*Data from* www.pubmed.gov. Accessed December 24, 2005).

CLINICAL MANIFESTATIONS OF TRANSFUSION-RELATED ACUTE LUNG INJURY

The first cases of what was likely to have been TRALI appeared in the literature in the early 1950s, and approximately 20 years later an association with leukoagglutinins was suspected as the cause [9–13]. It was still another 15 years before the first case series was published [14] with diagnoses based on clinical symptomatology. In fact, it was not until 2003 that clinical criteria were proposed on which an agreed upon diagnosis of TRALI could be proffered.

Clinically, patients who have TRALI present with a syndrome that can be characterized as noncardiogenic pulmonary edema with dyspnea, acute hypoxemia, hypotension, and occasionally fever. Bilateral infiltrates are usually described on chest radiograph; however, because of interpretation, type of study, and patient positioning, this can be variable. Signs of congestive heart failure (increased jugular venous pressure and/or a third heart sound) are usually absent. The pulmonary capillary wedge pressure is typically normal. Symptoms usually appear 1 to 6 hours after transfusion and resolve in less than 48 hours. Patients diagnosed with TRALI can be transiently leukopenic [15,16].

THE EVOLVING DEFINITION OF TRANSFUSION-RELATED ACUTE LUNG INJURY—A DIAGNOSIS OF EXCLUSION

The initial diagnosis of TRALI proposed by Popovsky and colleagues was based on clinical findings only [14,15,17]. Patients who experienced acute respiratory distress (sometimes with measured PaO_2 of 30–50 mm Hg), pulmonary edema, hypotension and fever (1–2°C rise in body temperature) within 6 hours of receiving a transfusion were classified as having TRALI. However, in retrospect, the authors acknowledge that this definition may have been limited because of selection bias because only those who had a severe presentation were included, whereas patients who had coexisting cardiac or respiratory disease were excluded [15].

Is Transfusion-Related Acute Lung Injury a Subtype of Acute Respiratory Distress Syndrome?

In 1988, Murray and colleagues [18] published a lung injury score based on chest radiograph, lung compliance, degree of hypoxemia, and the amount of positive end-expiratory pressure required that could be used to define acute respiratory distress syndrome (ARDS). Following this, Hebert and other investigators [15] have proposed that TRALI may in fact be a subset of ARDS. Some authors, however, have argued that Murray's approach is not sensitive enough because it selects for those patients who have respiratory failure and thus misses mild forms of acute lung injury (ALI) [15].

In 1994, the American–European Consensus Committee added a component to the definition of ARDS that excluded patients who have a pulmonary capillary wedge pressure greater than 18 mm Hg or clinical evidence of left atrial hypertension [19]. Gong [15] later argued that this definition excludes patients who have both ALI and congestive heart failure. Additionally, Gong criticized the use of pulmonary capillary wedge pressure as being a subjective criterion, making the differentiation between congestive heart failure and ALI difficult.

In May 2003, the National Heart, Lung, and Blood Institute (NHLBI) convened a working group that sought to develop a common definition of TRALI [8]. They started with the American–European Consensus Committee's definition (acute hypoxemia with PaO_2/FIO_2 ratio $\leq$300 mm Hg for ALI [$\leq$200 mm Hg for ARDS] or oxygen saturation of $\leq$90%, and the appearance of bilateral infiltrates in the absence of left atrial hypertension). Then, in their definition, cases of new ALI occurring within 6 hours of transfusion in patients who have no other risk factors for lung injury are classified as TRALI. When additional risk factors for ALI other than transfusion are present, the diagnosis of TRALI is made based on temporal association with transfusion and clinical course. Massive transfusion should not exclude a diagnosis of TRALI. According to the authors, however, this definition might also be flawed because it may cause patients who have worsening or mild ALI and those whose clinical manifestations occur more than 6 hours posttransfusion to be excluded.

In April 2004, a consensus conference convened in Toronto, Canada, and attempted to further adapt and improve the American–European Consensus Committee and the NHLBI definitions of TRALI [20]. Canadian Blood Services and Héma-Québec sponsored the conference with support from the International Society of Blood Transfusion's Biomedical Excellence for Safer

Transfusion subcommittee. The consensus panel recommended criteria for *TRALI* and *possible TRALI*.

- *TRALI* was defined as: (1) a new occurrence of acute onset ALI (with hypoxemia and bilateral infiltrates on chest radiograph but no evidence of left atrial hypertension), (2) not preexisting, but (3) emerging during or within 6 hours of the end of the transfusion, and (4) having no temporal relationship to an alternative ALI risk factor.
- *Possible TRALI* included cases in which there was a temporal association with an alternative ALI risk factor.

The panel recognized that these definitions continue to suffer the limitations inherent in the American–European Consensus Committee definition of ALI (including the subjectivity of certain findings such as chest radiograph, volume status, and the influence of positive end-expiratory pressure on measurements of PAO2/FIO2 ratio).

The evolution of the definition of TRALI has allowed a broader inclusion of patients who have additional risk factors for TRALI as possible TRALI. Some experts feel that TRALI is probably underreported and thus, these improvements in the definition may serve better to capture the whole spectrum of this transfusion hazard. In a recent retrospective study, Finlay and colleagues [21] evaluated the use of computer screening programs to monitor patients for posttransfusion hypoxemia. This study revealed seven patients who had a clinical event whereby upon review was diagnosed as TRALI. However, only two of the seven patients had been reported to the transfusion service. The authors concluded that continuous screening for signs of ALI, which are automatically captured by a computer, identifies more cases of TRALI than were reported voluntarily.

INCIDENCE

Popovsky and Moore [14] reported 36 cases of TRALI in 1985, with an incidence of 0.02% per unit and 0.16% per patient for all blood products. Other more recent studies have reported widely varying incidence rates ranging from 1:432 whole blood units [22] to 1:557,000 per red blood cell unit [15,22–24]. The real incidence of the transfusion-related reactions underpinning TRALI remains unknown. However, increasing awareness of the pathologic entity among clinicians, combined with an evolution of its definition toward including less severe cases, is likely to increase the reported incidence. In fact, the number of TRALI-related fatalities reported to the US Food and Drug Administration from 2001 to 2003 has steadily risen from 1995 [7]. TRALI is now the most frequently reported cause of transfusion-related death [7]. These numbers represent cases that have been investigated only by the reporting facilities and not confirmed by the US Food and Drug Administration. Furthermore, these reports occur in the absence of uniform guidelines for evaluation, diagnosis, or reporting TRALI-related deaths (Leslie Holness, MD, US Food and Drug Administration, personal communication, 2005). Thus, these figures may either overestimate or underestimate actual TRALI mortality. Until more is known about the cause or causes of TRALI and how to distinguish it from other forms of ARDS or ALI, a high variability in reported incidence figures is likely to persist.

PATHOPHYSIOLOGY

The pathophysiologic mechanisms of TRALI are incompletely, if at all, understood. An initial hypothesis that ALI associated with massive transfusion resulted from development during storage of microaggregates in the transfused blood products was never corroborated [25]. Instead, during the last decade, support for multiple mechanisms consistent with the clinical course has emerged [26,27]. These mechanisms have been described as antibody-mediated and nonantibody-mediated, respectively [15,26,27]. In both cases, activation of neutrophils plays a causal role, and these activated cells are thought to locally mediate pulmonary injury.

Proposed Antibody-Mediated Mechanisms of Transfusion-Related Acute Lung Injury

Antibody- or immune-mediated mechanisms suggest that alloantibodies directed toward antigens of either human leukocyte (HLA antigens) or human neutrophil antigen system (HNA) on leukocytes or lung tissue lead to granulocyte activation and pulmonary injury. Usually these alloantibodies are present in the transfused product, are of donor origin, and react with recipient granulocytes. However, in approximately 10% of TRALI cases it is recipient antibodies that react with neutrophils in the donated blood product [28,29].

In 1985, Popovsky and Moore [14] reported 36 TRALI cases whereby the authors studied samples from donors whose blood was implicated in causing the TRALI reaction and identified granulocyte- or lymphocyte-specific antibodies in 32 (89%) and 26 (72%) of cases, respectively. In 17 of the 26 cases whereby lymphocyte antibodies were identified, potential HLA antigen specificities of the antibodies were investigated. In 11 of these 17 cases (65%), at least one anti–HLA antigen specificity was identified, and in 10 of these 11 cases, the antibody specificity corresponded to one of the HLA antigen specificities of the recipients.

Others have found similar associations with a host of different leukocyte antibody specificities, most commonly antibodies to HLA antigen class I and class II antigens or antibodies to granulocyte-specific antigens. A particularly convincing case of antibody-mediated TRALI was in a lung transplant recipient receiving packed red blood cells [30]. This patient developed unilateral TRALI in the transplanted lung after receiving anti–HLA antigen class I antibodies reacting to a specificity existing only on the transplanted but not on the native lung.

Controversies with Proposed Antibody-Mediated Mechanisms of Transfusion-Related Acute Lung Injury

There are multiple factors that suggest that the antibody–antigen interaction on the surface of neutrophils may occur but may not be sufficient to cause TRALI. For example, blood products from donors that have been implicated in TRALI reactions do not always cause TRALI in the next recipient even if that recipient's leukocytes or lung tissues carry the offending cognate antigen [31,32]. In addition, there are numerous reported TRALI cases whereby antigen–antibody interactions could not be identified. Silliman and colleagues [22] studied 46 patients who had TRALI in a nested case–control study, compared them with 225 transfused patients who did not have TRALI, and found that the frequency of transfused alloantibodies was the same in both groups. Additionally, there was no correlation between the amount of plasma transfused and the incidence of TRALI. These findings strongly indicate that there are other factors than alloantibodies critical to the causation of TRALI.

Silliman and colleagues also found that patients who have TRALI were more likely to have hematologic malignancy and cardiac disease. Furthermore, some of the patients had recurrent TRALI episodes after receiving units from different donors. These findings emphasize the importance of the patient's underlying condition in the pathogenesis of TRALI. Finally, there was a significant association between the age of the unit and the incidence of TRALI, which suggests that TRALI-inducing mediators may accumulate during blood product storage, and these mediators may be necessary for the reaction to occur.

Proposed Nonantibody-Mediated Mechanism of Transfusion-Related Acute Lung Injury, or the "Two-Hit" Model

The mechanisms of neutrophil sequestration, activation, and the extent to which these processes are driven by predisposing patient factors and/or factors in the transfused blood product [15,26,33] remain incompletely understood. "Two-hit" models, or models in which multiple events are required for the development of TRALI, have been postulated to address all of these questions. The "first hit" is usually described as an underlying illness that primes the pulmonary endothelial cells and leukocytes (see later discussion), whereas the "second hit" is delivered by the transfusion.

To say these two-hit models are nonantibody–mediated mechanisms of TRALI may be incorrect. The factors in the transfused product providing the second signal could either be antibodies or various nonantibody biologic response modifiers, such as cytokines and certain lipids, which accumulate in stored blood. Thus, the two-hit model can be applied to TRALI whether the pathophysiology is antibody-mediated or not. In reality, both the first and second hits may be multifactorial and contribute to both the process of neutrophil activation and/or sequestration in the lung. The latter process is clearly aided by activation of the pulmonary endothelium and up-regulation of cellular adhesion molecules.

Cellular Priming and Transfusion-Related Acute Lung Injury

The term *priming* usually refers to a heightened, but not full-blown stage of (cellular) activation. In the simple "two-event" model, priming is induced by the first event. As applied to TRALI, the patient's clinical condition can be associated with pulmonary endothelial cell activation, up-regulation of surface adhesion molecules, release of cytokines, and recruitment of primed neutrophils. In this "primed state," transfusion of a blood component, or the second hit, containing factors capable of inducing complete activation of the presequestered primed neutrophils in the lung can now cause the release of cytotoxic compounds in the pulmonary vasculature. The resultant endothelial damage leads to capillary leak and noncardiogenic pulmonary edema (ie, TRALI).

It is also possible that the transfused product acts as the first hit by providing stimuli that may induce priming of neutrophils or pulmonary endothelial cells. Ultimately, the two-event models are likely to be oversimplifications, and the manifestation of TRALI probably represents a complex interplay of multiple priming stimuli and additional activation signals derived from both the blood product and the recipient and operating on multiple cell types involved in the inflammatory response.

Transfusion-Related Acute Lung Injury and the Neutropenic Patient

TRALI in neutropenic patients provides an interesting challenge to the prevailing pathophysiologic models but is limited to a single report. Silliman and colleagues described a neutropenic child who had Burkitt's lymphoma with clinical signs of ALI after receiving a partial apheresis platelet [34]. The recipient who received the other half of the unit also experienced a TRALI-like syndrome. The second recipient had both a normal white blood cell count (WBC = 8.3) and absolute neutrophil count (ANC = 7800). Neither patient's plasma nor the donor's plasma demonstrated anti–HLA antigen or antigranulocyte–specific antibodies. Additionally, plasma from the recipient who had an adequate neutrophil count had a robust level of polymorphonuclear leukocytes (PMN) priming activity, whereas plasma from the neutropenic patient did not demonstrate any such PMN priming activity. Both patients had markedly elevated levels of vascular endothelial growth factor (VEGF). The neutropenic patient was noted to have had a milder reaction, and yet the authors were left speculating as to whether VEGF alone could cause TRALI in neutropenic patients. Additional studies are needed to substantiate this finding.

ANIMAL MODELING OF TRANSFUSION-RELATED ACUTE LUNG INJURY FOR EXPERIMENTAL STUDIES

The elucidation of the pathophysiologic mechanisms involved in TRALI would likely benefit from controlled experimental studies, preferably using animal in vivo modeling. So far there is not an established in vivo model. Instead, there are limited data from in vitro models employing purely cellular systems or using explanted rabbit or rat lungs.

In Vitro Cellular Models of Transfusion-Related Acute Lung Injury

A cellular in vitro model of TRALI was established using human pulmonary microvascular endothelial cells [35]. The human pulmonary microvascular endothelial cells were treated with lipopolysaccharide (LPS) to cause up-regulation of adhesion molecules and release of chemokines. When resting neutrophils were added to these primed human pulmonary microvascular endothelial cells, they adhered but without causing injury to the endothelial cells. Thus, they accurately modeled in vivo pulmonary sequestration of neutrophils associated with a primed state. When lysophosphatidylcholines (lipids thought to be able to provide a second signal to primed neutrophils) were added, concentration-dependent damage to the endothelial cells was demonstrated. The endothelial cell damage was mediated by neutrophils and could be prevented by pretreatment with antibodies directed against endothelial or neutrophil adhesion molecules, by neutralizing antibodies to released chemokines, or by inhibitors of the respiratory burst.

Lung Explant Models of Transfusion-Related Acute Lung Injury

Ex vivo lung models have been used for experimental TRALI studies, pioneered by Seeger and colleagues [36]. These authors demonstrated that perfusion of a mixture of human neutrophils, human antigranulocyte alloantibody (anti-5b), and complement into explanted rabbit lungs could induce severe lung edema due to a several-fold increase in lung vascular permeability. However, if any of the three components were excluded from the perfusate, or if 5b-negative neutrophils were used, there was no vascular leak. This type of model has been adapted to rats and expanded upon by other groups [33,37,38].

Bux and colleagues have also used isolated and perfused rat lungs for TRALI modeling using: (1) another granulocyte-specific antibody (a murine monoclonal antibody, recognizing the HNA-2a allopolymorphism on human CD177); and (2) human granulocytes collected from donors who have high ($\geq$70%) or low ($\leq$30%) antigen expression [15,37]. After establishing an isogravimetric steady-state phase, they determined permeability (capillary filtration coefficient) and edema (lung weight gain) after challenge with timed venous pressure elevations. Granulocytes were infused at 15 minutes, the anti–HNA-2a monoclonal antibody or control antibody at 50 minutes, and, in some experiments, fMLP–a known granulocyte activator–at 120 minutes. Dramatic increase in vascular permeability and lung weight was observed in lungs infused with granulocytes from high HNA-2–expressing donors followed by anti–HNA-2a. In contrast, these parameters did not change much if the first infusion was with granulocytes from low HNA-2a–expressing donors or if control antibody was used instead of HNA-2a antibodies. However, in the lungs exposed to granulocytes from low HNA-2a–expressing donors followed by anti–HNA-2a antibodies, the added infusion of fMLP led to a full-blown TRALI-like reaction. Neutrophil-priming by plastic tubing was excluded as a possible confounder in the model because fMLP alone did not provoke a reaction.

The HNA-2a antibodies exhibited granulocyte-activating, but not leukoagglutinating, properties in vitro. Because no complement source was present in the system, the authors concluded that direct antibody-mediated granulocyte activation is the mechanism for the observed TRALI-like effects in this model and not the complement-fixing or leukoagglutinating properties of these antibodies. Moreover, the effect was dependent on the number of granulocytes expressing the cognate antigen (ie, dose dependent), but a suboptimum dose in the presence of other granulocyte costimulators such as fMLP could produce TRALI-like effects.

Silliman and colleagues used a variant of the ex vivo lung setup to model the nonantibody-mediated, two-event etiology of TRALI: the first hit is represented by injecting rats with a nonlethal dose of LPS. This is followed by isolation of the rat lungs and perfusion with plasma (second hit) from either fresh or stored blood products [33,38]. The plasma from stored packed red blood cells (day 42) or from stored whole blood or apheresis platelets (day 5), in contrast to fresh plasma, induced changes in pulmonary artery pressure, lung weight (indicating pulmonary edema), LTB4 levels in the perfusate, and lung histology consistent with ALI. Lipids extracted from the stored blood product plasma also induced these changes and are, thus, at least partially responsible for the ALI-inducing activity.

In contrast to the antibody-mediated ex vivo lung models, this model relied on the LPS-preprimed activity of endogenous neutrophils already present in the explanted lungs, removing any chance of plastic tubing inducing priming.

Towards An In Vivo Animal Model of Transfusion-Related Acute Lung Injury

The in vitro modeling suggests that it may be feasible to mimic TRALI-like reactions in rodents and create in vivo models. To date, no such model is established in the peer-reviewed literature. This may not be entirely surprising because TRALI is a rare event phenomenon that seems to depend on many confounding factors in the patient and the individual blood product. Thus, a significant trial and error investment may be needed to discover a productive combination of controllable factors. This is illustrated by a murine TRALI model presented at several meetings but not yet published in a full report [15,39–41].

In this model, a single dose of a murine monoclonal (IgG2a) alloantimouse–MHC class I antibody (34–1–2s) was injected into BALB/c or congenic BALB/k mice. In mice with the cognate antigen (BALB/c), this was sufficient to cause early transient hypothermia (rectal temperature), respiratory distress (indirect plethysmography), and capillary leak (increased hematocrit) followed by pulmonary edema, indicated by increased wet lung weights and characteristic histology. BALB/k mice, lacking the cognate antigen, did not develop these symptoms. Inhibitor studies revealed the response to be partially dependent on granulocytes, macrophages, and mediators, such as leukotrienes and platelet-activating factor, but not on platelets, complement (C3, C5a-R), Fc-receptors for IgG, or mediators such as STAT4, histamine, and serotonin.

Notably, only one of more than 20 tested monoclonal alloantimouse–MHC antibodies caused this clinical TRALI-like syndrome (Fred Finkelman, personal communication, 2005). Moreover, only male, but not female, BALB/c mice were "permissive" for this direct one-hit effect. However, intratracheal priming with LPS in female BALB/c mice for 3 days before challenge with the anti-MHC antibody provoked the TRALI-like reaction (two-hit model).

The authors have occasionally seen massive periendothelial granulocyte infiltration associated with increased wet lung weight in female BALB/c mice challenged with the same monoclonal antibody (34–1–2s) after overnight priming with intravenous LPS (Fig. 2). However, they have not been able to reproduce the one-hit model in male BALB/c mice (Lennart E. Lögdberg, MD, PhD, and Christopher D. Hillyer, MD, unpublished data, 2005).

Overall, the in vivo modeling based on 34–1–2s shows promise but appears limited to a rather unique antibody. Thus, studies using this model should be complemented with studies examining broad MHC–alloantisera (immunization between MHC-congenic mouse strains) covering all the MHC subloci as well as broad antigranulocyte antisera. Systematic studies of anti-MHC–antibody administration to mimic all aspects of blood product transfusion are also warranted. Application of new tools, such as the recently marketed mouse pulse oximeter (MouseOx, Starr Life Sciences Corp., Allison Perk, PA), may facilitate a systematic approach to in vivo TRALI model development.

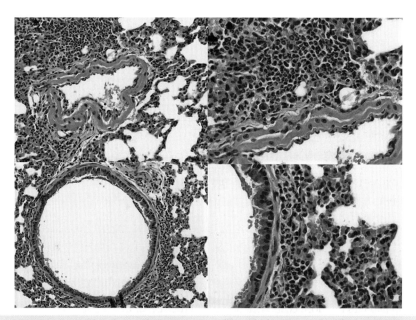

Fig. 2. Increased periendothelial granulocyte infiltration in a female BALB/c mouse lung 5 hours after intravenous antibody injection (125 µg purified IgG2a monoclonal alloantibody (34–1–2s) directed against the BALB/c MHC class I antigens). The figure illustrates massive perivascular (*upper left and right images*) or peribronchial (*lower left and right images*) neutrophil infiltration, at low (*upper and lower left images*) or higher (*upper and lower right images*) magnification, respectively. The mouse had been primed by way of endotoxin exposure (100 µg LPS administered intraperitoneally the evening before the experiment). Groups of control mice, either primed with LPS but not receiving the antibody at the day of the experiment or not primed with LPS but receiving the monoclonal antibody, did not exhibit such neutrophil infiltrates. The lungs of the experimental mice showed increased (~10%) wet lung weight compared with the control mice.

DONOR SCREENING AND DEFERRAL

Prevention of TRALI would be aided by a simple laboratory test to prospectively eliminate high-risk blood products. Unfortunately, such a test has yet to be developed and likely awaits a more complete understanding of the pathophysiologic mechanisms causing TRALI. Instead, the currently recommended strategies in the United States are based on deferral of donors already implicated in TRALI cases.

The Canadian Consensus Conference recommended that in cases of a potential TRALI event, any clinically suspected donors be evaluated and if indicated classified as "associated" or "implicated" [20]. If units are temporally and clinically related to a TRALI-like event, the donor is considered to be associated with the event. Implicated donors, however, are those who have a documented antibody—or rarely, an antigen—which corresponds to a cognate antigen—or rarely, an antibody—in the recipient. Currently, the American Red Cross is deferring all implicated donors.

Donor Evaluation

Several approaches have been suggested in the evaluation of potential TRALI events. Testing for the presence of anti–HLA and antigranulocyte antibodies in all donor units given within 6 hours of the reaction is probably the broadest approach [23]. However, this can be difficult in cases whereby the recipient has been massively transfused or when the diagnosis has been considered hours after the units have been given. Dr. Ambruso [15] suggested in the proceedings of the Canadian Consensus Conference that "screening of blood from the implicated donors should include detection of antibodies for MHC class I and class II by flow cytometry, ELISA, or lymphocytotoxicity assays, and testing for neutrophil antibodies by ELISA."

Sequential testing has been proposed as an option to increase investigation efficiency [42]. This entails prioritizing units for testing. Thus, those units that carry the most risk for causing TRALI are prioritized for immediate testing. For instance, the investigator may test female multiparous donors before testing male donors, or test donors of plasma-rich before plasma-poor components [23]. Multiparous females are considered to be at higher risk due to the fact that they have had more alloantigen exposures, and thus, tend to have higher prevalence and titers of anti–HLA antigen and antigranulocyte antibodies. Sequential testing strategies can be more cost-efficient but run the risk of being less comprehensive and abrogated before completion. Therefore, this lack of uniformity translates into differences in the likelihood of identifying implicated donors.

Ambruso [15] also suggests that positive results be confirmed by additional testing such as crossmatches between donor serum and recipient cells and specific identification of cognate antigen in the recipient. If concordance between antibody and antigen in the donor and recipient, respectively, is demonstrated, it is considered to be strong evidence that the donor unit was important in the pathogenesis. Finally, pre- and posttransfusion samples can be tested for increased priming activity in patients who have TRALI-suspected reactions.

These tests may be helpful in confirming TRALI after it has occurred. However, these strategies will not prevent the occurrence of TRALI due to blood products from donors previously not implicated in TRALI.

Towards Mitigation of Transfusion-Related Acute Lung Injury

Broad prevention strategies have been advocated, including deferral of donors with high likelihood of being previously alloimmunized, universal leukoreduction, greater reliance on apheresis platelets, the strict use of "young" units, and the use of washed products [15]. Each of these strategies has disadvantages, including added cost, the potential to worsen already significant blood supply shortages, and uncertain levels of preventive efficacy. However, some feel that the risk of TRALI warrants these measures.

At the Canadian Consensus Conference, data from the Serious Hazards of Transfusion Scheme, a United Kingdom–wide hemovigilance program, were presented, demonstrating that of the 105 reported cases of TRALI between 1996 and 2002, a leukocyte antibody-positive female was identified in 91% of the cases. Based on such data, the United Kingdom has diverted female blood donations from fresh frozen plazma (FFP) production, with more than 90% of the FFP supply now derived from male donors only [15].

In 1992, Popovsky and colleagues [23] described a strategy by which (1) pregnancy history was to be recorded at each donation; (2) blood was to be diverted from multiparous women (having greater than three pregnancies) from use as whole blood, FFP, and single-donor platelets unless negative for HLA antigen- and granulocyte-specific antibodies; (3) permanent deferral of (what are now known as) implicated donors was mandatory; and (4) physician education was required to increase TRALI awareness. Such strategies are not in standardized use because individual components are controversial. For instance, it is argued that pregnancy history would be difficult to obtain accurately: parity is dynamic, certain antibodies known to cause TRALI can be missed by current screening tests, and antibody status can change (thus successive screening would be required). Finally, blood products from donors known to have circulating antibodies with common leukocyte antigen specificities can fail to induce a TRALI-like reaction. Therefore, the universal deferral of these donors may unnecessarily further deplete an already limited blood supply.

SUMMARY

With the success of reducing the risk of transfusion-transmitted infectious diseases, noninfectious serious hazards of transfusion have come to the forefront with respect to transfusion safety. TRALI has emerged as a dominant noninfectious serious hazard of transfusion. Improved understanding of its pathophysiology is needed to improve clinical strategies to deal with the risk. Such understanding, in turn, will depend on the continued progress in development of good model systems, in vitro and in vivo, for experimental studies. Finally, as the pathologic mechanisms are elucidated, a universal definition and strategies for the prevention and/or mitigation may become more tangible.

References

[1] Busch MP. Closing the windows on viral transmission by blood transfusion. In: Stramer SL, editor. Blood safety in the new millennium. Bethesda (MD): American Association of Blood Banks; 2001. p. 33–54.

[2] Busch MP, Glynn SA, Stramer SL, et al. A new strategy for estimating risks of transfusion-transmitted viral infections based on rates of detection of recently infected donors. Transfusion 2005;45(2):254–64.

[3] Dodd RY, Notari EPt, Stramer SL. Current prevalence and incidence of infectious disease markers and estimated window-period risk in the American Red Cross blood donor population. [see comment]. Transfusion 2002;42(8):975–979.

[4] Sazama K. Reports of 355 transfusion-associated deaths: 1976 through 1985. Transfusion 1990;30(7):583–90.

[5] Linden JV, Wagner K, Voytovich AE, et al. Transfusion errors in New York state: an analysis of 10 years' experience. Transfusion 2000;40(10):1207–13.

[6] American Association of Blood Banks, editor. Standards for blood banks and transfusion services. 22nd edition. Bethesda (MD): AABB Press; 2003.

[7] Holness L, Knippen MA, Simmons L, et al. Fatalities caused by TRALI. Transfus Med Rev 2004;18(3):184–8.

[8] Toy P, Popovsky MA, Abraham E, et al. Transfusion-related acute lung injury: definition and review. Crit Care Med 2005;33(4):721–6.

[9] Barnard R. Indiscriminate transfusion: a critique of case reports illustrating hypersensitivity reactions. N Y State J Med 1951;51(20):2399–402.

[10] Brittingham T, Chaplin H Jr. Febrile transfusion reactions caused by sensitivity to donor leukocytes and platelets. JAMA 1957;165(7):819–25.

[11] Philipps E, Fleischner FG. Pulmonary edema in the course of a blood transfusion without overloading the circulation. Dis Chest 1966;50(6):619–23.

[12] Ward HN. Pulmonary infiltrates associated with leukoagglutinin transfusion reactions. Ann Intern Med 1970;73(5):689–94.

[13] Thompson JS, Severson CD, Parmely MJ, et al. Pulmonary "hypersensitivity" reactions induced by transfusion of non-HLA leukoagglutinins. N Engl J Med 1971;284(20): 1120–5.

[14] Popovsky MA, Moore SB. Diagnostic and pathogenetic considerations in transfusion-related acute lung injury. Transfusion 1985;25(6):573–7.

[15] Goldman M, Webert KE, Arnold DM, et al. Proceedings of a consensus conference: towards an understanding of TRALI. Transfus Med Rev 2005;19(1):2–31.

[16] Nakagawa M, Toy P. Acute and transient decrease in neutrophil count in transfusion-related acute lung injury: cases at one hospital. Transfusion 2004;44(12):1689–94.

[17] Popovsky MA, Abel MD, Moore SB. Transfusion-related acute lung injury associated with passive transfer of antileukocyte antibodies. Am Rev Respir Dis 1983;128(1):185–9.

[18] Murray JF, Matthay MA, Luce JM, et al. An expanded definition of the adult respiratory distress syndrome [erratum appears in Am Rev Respir Dis 1989 Apr;139(4):1065]. Am Rev Respir Dis 1988;138(3):720–3.

[19] Bernard GR, Artigas A, Brigham KL, et al. Report of the American-European Consensus Conference on acute respiratory distress syndrome: definitions, mechanisms, relevant outcomes, and clinical trial coordination. Consensus committee. J Crit Care 1994;9(1):72–81.

[20] Kleinman S, Caulfield T, Chan P, et al. Toward an understanding of transfusion-related acute lung injury: statement of a consensus panel. Transfusion 2004;44(12):1774–89.

[21] Finlay HE, Cassorla L, Feiner J, et al. Designing and testing a computer-based screening system for transfusion-related acute lung injury. Am J Clin Pathol 2005;124(4):601–9.

[22] Silliman CC, Boshkov LK, Mehdizadehkashi Z, et al. Transfusion-related acute lung injury: epidemiology and a prospective analysis of etiologic factors. Blood 2003;101(2):454–62.

[23] Popovsky MA, Chaplin HC Jr, Moore SB. Transfusion-related acute lung injury: a neglected, serious complication of hemotherapy [see comment]. Transfusion 1992;32(6):589–92.

[24] Faber JC. Haemovigilance around the world. Vox Sang 2002;83(Suppl 1):71–6.

[25] Geelhoed GW, Bennett SH. "Shock lung" resulting from perfusion of canine lungs with stored bank blood. Am Surg 1975;41(11):661–82.

[26] Silliman CC, Ambruso DR, Boshkov LK. Transfusion-related acute lung injury. Blood 2005;105(6):2266–73.

[27] Kopko PM. Leukocyte antibodies and biologically active mediators in the pathogenesis of transfusion-related acute lung injury. Curr Hematol Rep 2004;3(6):456–61.

[28] Popovsky MA, Davenport RD. Transfusion-related acute lung injury: femme fatale? [comment]. Transfusion 2001;41(3):312–5.

[29] Bux J, Becker F, Seeger W, et al. Transfusion-related acute lung injury due to HLA-A2-specific antibodies in recipient and NB1-specific antibodies in donor blood. Br J Haematol 1996;93(3):707–13.

[30] Dykes A, Smallwood D, Kotsimbos T, et al. Transfusion-related acute lung injury (TRALI) in a patient with a single lung transplant. Br J Haematol 2000;109(3):674–6.

[31] Win N, Ranasinghe E, Lucas G. Transfusion-related acute lung injury: a 5-year look-back study. Transfus Med 2002;12(6):387–9.

[32] Toy P, Hollis-Perry KM, Jun J, et al. Recipients of blood from a donor with multiple HLA antibodies: a look-back study of transfusion-related acute lung injury. Transfusion 2004;44(12): 1683–8.

[33] Silliman CC, Voelkel NF, Allard JD, et al. Plasma and lipids from stored packed red blood cells cause acute lung injury in an animal model. J Clin Invest 1998;101(7):1458–67.

[34] Boshkov L, Maloney J, Bieber S, et al. Two cases of TRALI from the same platelet unit: implications for pathophysiology and the role of PMNs and VEGF [abstract #2817]. Blood 2000;96(11):655.

[35] Wyman TH, Bjornsen AJ, Elzi DJ, et al. A two-insult in vitro model of PMN-mediated pulmonary endothelial damage: requirements for adherence and chemokine release. Am J Physiol Cell Physiol 2002;283(6):C1592–603.

[36] Seeger W, Schneider U, Kreusler B, et al. Reproduction of transfusion-related acute lung injury in an ex vivo lung model [see comment]. Blood 1990;76(7):1438–44.

[37] Sachs UJ, Hattar K, Weissmann N, et al. Antibody-induced neutrophil activation as a trigger for transfusion-related acute lung injury in an ex vivo rat lung model. Blood 2006;107(3): 1217–9.

[38] Silliman CC, Bjornsen AJ, Wyman TH, et al. Plasma and lipids from stored platelets cause acute lung injury in an animal model. Transfusion 2003;43(5):633–40.

[39] Strait R, Susskind B, Finkelman F. Murine TRALI: 1-Hit vs. 2-Hit Model. Hum Immunol 2005;66(Suppl 1):S18.

[40] Hicks W, Susskind B, Strait R, et al. Pathogenesis of transfusion-related acute lung injury (TRALI) in an in vivo murine model. Hum Immunol 2004;65(Suppl 1):S10.

[41] Hicks W, Susskind B, Strait R, et al. In vivo murine model of transfusion-related acute lung injury. Transfusion 2004;44(Suppl 9):S10.

[42] Webert KE, Kleinman SH, Blajchman MA. Transfusion-related acute lung inury. In: Hillyer CD, Silberstein LE, Ness PM, et al, editors. Blood banking and transfusion medicine: basic principles and practice. 2nd edition. Philadelphia: Elsevier.

Hematol Oncol Clin N Am 21 (2007) 177–184

HEMATOLOGY/ONCOLOGY CLINICS
OF NORTH AMERICA

ELSEVIER
SAUNDERS

Transfusion Algorithms and How They Apply to Blood Conservation: The High-risk Cardiac Surgical Patient

Marie E. Steiner, MD, MS[a,b,*], George John Despotis, MD[c,d]

[a]Department of Pediatrics, Division of Hematology/Oncology/Blood & Marrow Transplantation, 420 Delaware Street, MMC 484, University of Minnesota, Minneapolis, MN 55455, USA
[b]Department of Pediatrics, Division of Pulmonary/Critical Care, University of Minnesota, Minneapolis, MN 55455, USA
[c]Department of Anesthesiology, Box 8054, Washington University School of Medicine, 660 South Euclid Avenue, St. Louis, MO 63110, USA
[d]Department of Pathology and Immunology, Box 8118, Washington University School of Medicine, 660 South Euclid Avenue, St. Louis, MO 63110, USA

B lood conservation strategies in the cardiac surgery population are of interest because of the volume of blood product support provided to these patients and the complexity of the bleeding management issues confronting the patient care team. Following a brief review of current blood usage in the United States' cardiac surgery population and a short description of the general mechanisms of bleeding in cardiac surgery patients, published suggested transfusion triggers are summarized and published algorithm-based transfusion practices and outcomes are discussed.

Over 600,000 adults and 10,000 children undergo cardiac surgery each year in the United States. Between 50% and 75% of these patients receive transfusions, using 10% to 20% of the 12 million packed red blood cell (PRBC) units and 50% of the 7 million platelet units used annually in the United States. The annual transfusion costs of cardiac surgery are over $500 million [1–3].

The etiology of excessive bleeding after cardiac surgery is multifactorial and related to surgical complexity, the use of anticoagulants/heparin during surgery, the coexistence of multiple hemostatic aberrations produced during cardiopulmonary bypass (CPB), damage to blood vessel walls during the operation, and the quality of the surrounding tissue following the procedure. Acquired defects in hemostasis may include coagulopathy from hypothermia, hemodilution or abnormal fibrinolysis. Abnormal platelet contribution to hemostasis also occurs, whether from prior antiplatelet agents, platelet activation

*Corresponding author. Department of Pediatrics, 420 Delaware Street, MMC 484, University of Minnesota, Minneapolis, MN 55455. E-mail address: stein083@umn.edu (M.E. Steiner).

0889-8588/07/$ – see front matter
doi:10.1016/j.hoc.2006.11.009

Published by Elsevier Inc.
hemonc.theclinics.com

from the bypass circuit, platelet consumption, or platelet loss [2]. Despite complete heparin reversal and the use of antifibrinolytic agents, excessive bleeding still occurs. The definition of abnormal or excessive bleeding described in the medical literature is variable. As examples, representative studies have reported excessive bleeding as "diffuse oozing with no visible clot" [3], more than 2 L blood loss within the first 24 hours postoperatively [2], bleeding at a rate of 300 mL/h or 100 to 200 mL/h for 4 hours [4,5], or 20% of the estimated blood volume lost in the first postoperative hour for a pediatric patient [6].

Abnormal or excessive bleeding after cardiac surgery occurs in 3% to 11% of patients [7–9], requires surgical re-exploration in approximately 5% of patients [4,5,7] in whom inadequate surgical hemostasis is identified in up to 50% to 60% [5,10], and increases risk of mortality threefold to fourfold [2,11]. Actual mortality statistics are elusive; however, in one study of 8642 coronary artery bypass graft (CABG) patients, 7% of 384 total deaths were due to "fatal hemorrhage" [9]. The aging patient demographic undergoing cardiac surgery and the increasing complexity of procedures being performed will likely see this prevalence increase. Excessive bleeding has been associated with CPB duration exceeding 2.5 hours, repeat or combined cardiac procedures, renal dysfunction, older age, smaller body surface area, and the use of anticoagulants or antiplatelet agents [4,7,10,12–14]. In one series comparing single versus combined procedures with first versus repeat operation, 9 of 10 patients undergoing reoperations for combined procedures had excessive bleeding [14].

Extensive transfusion of allogeneic blood products has been associated with many adverse events, including bacterial infection, viral transmission, transfusion-related acute lung injury, volume overload, and increased mortality [7,15,16]. A higher 5-year mortality rate of 15% in 649 transfused patients versus 5% of patients not transfused was demonstrated in one series of 1915 cardiac surgery patients [13]. Similarly, in 890 patients receiving five or more units of PRBC within the first 24 hours after surgery, mortality was almost 11% compared with 0.9% in the remaining 8325 patients not transfused this extensively [17]. The ability to reduce uncontrolled perioperative bleeding may therefore reduce the incidence of extensive transfusion and mortality.

Transfusion of briskly bleeding cardiac surgery patients involves multiple complicated therapeutic decisions. As mentioned earlier, bleeding is often multifactorial in origin, and laboratory data to guide transfusion therapy are often delayed or absent. Transfusion therapy is therefore largely nonspecific. Suggested published empiric transfusion "triggers" include the following:

1. Prothrombin time/international normalized ratio greater than 15 seconds or 1.5 times the normal control mean
2. Partial thromboplastin time greater than 55 seconds or 1.5 times the normal control mean
3. Platelet count less than 100,000 if bleeding or 50,000 if not
4. Fibrinogen less than 50 mg/dL or less than 80 to 100 mg/dL if "refractory" to platelets and fresh frozen plasma [6,18–24]

Evaluation of a 10-study subset including adult and pediatric cardiac surgery patients (from a general review of 57 clinical trials), however, found that prophylactic fresh frozen plasma (FFP) had no consistent effect in diminishing blood loss or reducing transfusion requirements compared with no FFP or a nonplasma product [22]. Another review of 6 small trials in cardiac bypass patients found no evidence to support prophylactic use of FFP in reducing perioperative blood loss, although fibrinogen and platelet counts were positively impacted [25]. The prothrombin time/international normalized ratio (PT/INR) and partial thromboplastin time (PTT) used to evaluate bleeding have not been demonstrated to reflect bleeding [18,20], and qualitative or quantitative platelet defects are the most important hemostatic defect after cardiac bypass [21].

Nevertheless, it has been demonstrated that preset triggers can limit transfusion quantities. Transfusion rates of 314 patients managed prospectively were compared with 947 retrospective patient records. FFP and platelets were given only for bleeding with a PT greater than 16 seconds (INR >1.63) and a platelet count less than 100,000. There was a decrease in the percentage of patients transfused (PRBC: 26% versus 41%; FFP: 13% versus 24%) and a higher percentage of patients receiving no products (69% versus 48%). Patients transfused according to the guidelines had shorter ICU length of stay and overall length of stay than transfused patients. Reoperation for bleeding was reduced to 1.7% from 12.3%. The mortality rate was reduced to 0.9% from 6.2% [26].

Prospective transfusion algorithms have subsequently been developed and serially modified.

Despotis and colleagues' [14] first series studied post-CPB patients who had "microvascular bleeding" (MVB), defined as "diffuse bleeding without [a] surgically correctable identifiable source." Thirty-six patients were randomized to standard empiric bleeding management and 30 patients to a treatment algorithm based on on-site laboratory (point-of-care; POC) results. The algorithm based on published guidelines for treatment used POC coagulation assays with turn-around times of 4 to 6 minutes (versus traditional laboratory turn-around times of 44–77 minutes). The patients transfused according to the algorithm received fewer blood products, had shorter operative times, and had less initial bleeding from mediastinal or chest drainage tubes. Re-exploration rates were reduced to 3% from 14%. Of interest, 9 of 36 patients on the standard arm received blood products not indicated by the algorithm. Also of note was that patients who had MVB had coagulation profiles demonstrating moderate or severe thrombocytopenia, moderate or severe factor deficiencies, or both. These abnormalities, however, were not found universally or exclusively among patients who had MVB, and similar hemostatic abnormalities were also found, although less often, in patients who did not have MVB [27].

Another series demonstrated decreased transfusion and re-explorations with the use of perioperative laboratory tests, including thromboelastography (TEG), to guide transfusion. The series compared 488 patients undergoing CPB before TEG was implemented with 591 patients after; the study was also conducted coincident with a decision to limit PRBC transfusions to a hematocrit 20% trigger. The number of patients receiving no transfusion at all increased from 13.7% to 21.5%. Intraoperative transfusion rates decreased from 38.8% to 42.1% of patients, and use of all components decreased; total donor exposures decreased from a median of 8 to 6. These changes, however, were seen primarily in the CABG population, and not in open-ventricle patients. Re-exploration rates also decreased from 4.5% to 1.4% in the CABG population and from 9% to 2% in the open-ventricle patients [28].

Several studies have subsequently designed prospective algorithms using platelet function data. Despotis and colleagues [29] studied 203 cardiac surgery patients of whom 101 still had MVB after protamine heparin reversal. Patients who had abnormal platelet function tests treated with DDAVP received 50% fewer PRBC, 95% fewer platelet units, and 87% fewer FFP infusions, and an overall reduction in donor exposures from 5.2 to 1.6. Another series evaluated CPB patients at moderate-high risk of transfusion. Fifty-three patients were transfused according to a TEG-guided algorithm, and 52 received "routine" transfusions. Fewer postoperative and total platelet and FFP transfusions were given to the TEG group (platelet: 7/53 versus 15/52; FFP: 4/53 versus 16/52) [30]. Another series studied 92 of 836 patients who had abnormal bleeding ("diffuse oozing with no discernable clot") after CPB randomized to algorithm or to routine transfusion. Fewer platelet units (4 [0–12] versus 6 [0–18]) and FFP units (0 [0–7] versus 3 [0–10]) were administered to the algorithm group. The re-exploration rate was reduced to 0% from 11.8% [3]. Royston and von Kier [31] studied two groups of 60 patients undergoing cardiac surgery. The first patients received FFP, platelets, or both based on conventional laboratory tests (activated PTT >1.5 × N, platelet count <50,000, fibrinogen <80 mg/dL) in the presence of MVB defined as greater than 400 mL/h for the first hour or 100 mL/h for 4 hours. The number of units of products administered was compared with the number predicted to be needed on the basis of the heparinase-modified TEG. Transfusions were given to 22 of 60 patients based on clinical and laboratory observations. The number of patients predicted to need transfusion on the basis of TEG data was only 7 out of 60, with a predicted reduction in the number of FFP units given (from 38 to 6) and platelet pools (from 17 to 2). The method was validated in a randomized series of another 60 patients, 30 transfused according to algorithm and 30 according to clinical assessment. Only 5 of 30 algorithm patients received blood components compared with 10 of 30 managed clinically. The volume of products administered was also less in the TEG-algorithm group (5 U FFP and 1 platelet pool versus 16 U FFP and 9 platelet pools). Chest tube losses at 12 hours were no different between the groups.

An additional study randomized 102 coronary artery bypass patients to a prospective transfusion algorithm using either multiple POC tests or standard clinical laboratory results or to a case-control group transfused at the clinician's discretion. Heparin assay based on Hepcon Hemostasis Management System (Medtronic, Minneapolis, Minnesota) results, TEG, and Platelet Function

Analyzer-100 (PFA-100) (Dade Behring) were used to guide the POC group transfusion. The laboratory-study group depended on rapidly available clotting tests to transfuse when specific criteria were met. Patients were re-explored when bleeding was greater than 100 mL/h and the patients were not coagulopathic. Blood loss was similar in all groups. There were no differences in transfusions given between the two algorithm-guided groups; the clinical-discretion group was transfused more. One re-exploration occurred in each of the algorithm-guided groups, and three occurred in the control group [32]. A recent study with a slightly different CABG population compared 45 patients receiving clopidrogel within 6 days of their operation with 45 control subjects. PT/INR, activated PTT, platelet count, and platelet function tests (PFA-100; Dade-Behring, Miami, Florida, and Platelet Works; Helena Laboratories, Beaumont, Texas) were used to devise a bleeding management algorithm. Intraoperative clinical assessment of excessive MVB by the surgeon and chest tube drainage of greater than 250 mL in the first postoperative hour, along with laboratory criteria meeting algorithm triggers, were necessary for transfusion. Clopidrogel patients received 3.5 times more blood components than control patients (platelets: 9.0 ± 1.7 versus 1.5 ± 0.5 U; PRBC: 4.3 ± 0.6 versus 2.3 ± 0.5 U). The use of the algorithm, however, reduced mean units of blood products administered to both groups by approximately 30% compared with a comparable historical population; clopidrogel historical patients received 12.5 ± 2.1 U platelets and 6.4 ± 0.8 U PRBC and historical controls received 2.3 ± 0.3 U platelets and 2.3 ± 0.1 U PRBC compared with the product administered to the algorithm patients as described previously [33].

The only published transfusion algorithm-based cardiac surgery study that did not demonstrate a reduction in overall blood product exposure randomized patients bleeding more than 1.5 mL/kg over a 15-minute interval following the first emptying of their mediastinal drains to an algorithm based on on-site laboratory monitoring results or to transfusion based on clinician judgment. Using a platelet transfusion trigger of 100,000, significantly more platelets were transfused to the algorithm group (14/28 versus 3/30 patients). Cumulative chest tube drainage up to 16 hours and total transfusion requirements did not vary between the groups. Rates of re-exploration were similar (21% and 23%). There were more patients undergoing combined procedures in the algorithm group (8 versus 2, $P = .04$), and this imbalance may have impacted these results. In addition, no assessment of platelet function other than a bleeding time was performed, and patients using varying antiplatelet agents were not excluded [34].

Despite these published transfusion algorithms and guidelines, large variability in transfusion practices still persists. In a review of 713 patients expected to be at low risk for transfusion from a database of 2417 CPB patients, 27% to 92% patients received PRBC, 0% to 36% received platelets, 0% to 36% received FFP, and 0% to 17% received cryoprecipitate. Overall, 17% to 92% were transfused with one to four donor exposures. The institution performing the operation was an independent determinant of transfusion risk apart from blood loss

[35]. Similarly, in a recently published abstract, transfusion practices were prospectively investigated at 70 centers in 16 countries. Transfusions administered to 5065 randomly selected CABG patients before, during, and after surgery until discharge were tabulated. Intraoperative red blood cell transfusion varied by country from 9% to 100%; postoperative red blood cell transfusion varied by country from 25% to 87%. Transfusion of FFP varied from 0% to 98% intraoperatively and from 3% to 95% postoperatively. Platelet transfusion varied from 0% to 51% intraoperatively and 0% to 39% postoperatively. Patient-related risk indices of the 16 counties did not correlate with transfusion practice, which the investigators believed underscored the need for development of and better compliance with international transfusion guidelines [36]. In addition, bleeding management algorithms for more briskly bleeding patients at risk of hemorrhagic death do not currently exist and have not generally been applied to patients enrolled in pharmacologic bleeding intervention studies.

In summary, it is clear that excessive bleeding from multifactorial causes that occurs after cardiac surgery creates a significant medical and financial burden. Several studies, summarized in Fig. 1, suggest that adhering to transfusion algorithms, especially in conjunction with concomitant hemostasis monitoring, may (1) decrease the number of transfusions administered, (2) decrease the

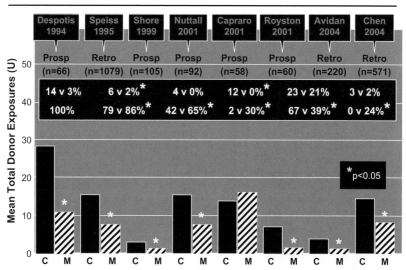

Fig. 1. Impact of transfusion algorithm use in cardiac surgery. The first row of numbers is the difference in percentage of patients requiring re-exploration between the algorithm and control study cohorts. The second row of numbers represents the percentage of patients not requiring any transfusion, comparing algorithm patients with study patients. The bar graphs at the bottom represent mean number of donor exposures, with "C" representing control patients and "M" representing algorithm-monitored patients. Statistically significant differences are indicated by an asterisk. Prosp, prospective trial; Retro, retrospective trial.

volume of blood lost, and (3) decrease the rate of re-exploration for bleeding. It is also evident from these series, however, that optimal hemostasis monitoring and applicability/predictive value to in vivo hemostasis can be further refined and awaits additional clinical investigation.

References

[1] Levy JH, Pifarre R, Schaff HV, et al. A multi-center, double-blind, placebo-controlled trial of aprotinin for reducing blood loss and the requirement for donor-blood transfusion in patients undergoing repeat coronary artery bypass grafting. Circulation 1995;92(8): 2236–44.

[2] Despotis GJ, Avidan MS, Hogue CW Jr. Mechanisms and attenuation of hemostatic activation during extracorporeal circulation. Ann Thorac Surg 2001;72(5):S1821–31.

[3] Nuttall GA, Oliver WC, Santrach PJ, et al. Efficacy of a simple intraoperative transfusion algorithm for nonerythrocyte component utilization after cardiopulmonary bypass. Anesthesiology 2001;94(5):773–81 [discussion: 5A–6A].

[4] Dacey LJ, Munoz JJ, Baribeau YR, et al. Reexploration for hemorrhage following coronary artery bypass grafting: incidence and risk factors. Northern New England Cardiovascular Disease Study Group. Arch Surg 1998;133(4):442–7.

[5] Hall TS, Sines JC, Spotnitz AJ. Hemorrhage related re-exploration following open heart surgery: the impact of pre-operative and post-operative coagulation testing. Cardiovasc Surg 2002;10(2):146–53.

[6] Williams GD, Bratton SL, Riley EC, et al. Coagulation tests during cardiopulmonary bypass correlate with blood loss in children undergoing cardiac surgery. J Cardiothorac Vasc Anesth 1999;13:398–404.

[7] Despotis GJ, Filos KS, Zoys TN, et al. Factors associated with excessive postoperative blood loss and hemostatic transfusion requirements: multivariate analysis in cardiac surgical patients. Anesth Analg 1996;82:13–21.

[8] Kessler C, Szurlej D, Von Heymann C. Management of refractory post-op cardiac bleeding with rFVIIa: cases reported to hemostasis.com registry [abstract]. J Thromb Haemost 2003: 1131.

[9] O'Connor GT, Birkmeyer JD, Dacey LJ, et al. Results of a regional study of modes of death associated with coronary artery bypass grafting. Northern New England Cardiovascular Disease Study Group. Ann Thorac Surg 1998;66(4):1323–8.

[10] Moulton MJ, Creswell LL, Mackey ME, et al. Reexploration for bleeding is a risk factor for adverse outcomes after cardiac operations. J Thorac Cardiovasc Surg 1996;111(5): 1037–46.

[11] Munoz JJ, Birkmeyer NJ, Dacey LJ, et al. Trends in rates of reexploration for hemorrhage after coronary artery bypass surgery. Northern New England Cardiovascular Disease Study Group. Ann Thorac Surg 1999;68(4):1321–5.

[12] Levi M, Cromheecke ME, de Jonge E, et al. Pharmacological strategies to decrease excessive blood loss in cardiac surgery: a meta-analysis of clinically relevant end points. Lancet 1999;354:1940–7.

[13] Engoren MC, Habib RH, Zacharias A, et al. Effect of blood transfusion on long-term survival after cardiac operation. Ann Thorac Surg 2002;74(4):1180–6.

[14] Despotis GJ, Santoro SA, Spitznagel E, et al. Prospective evaluation and clinical utility of on-site monitoring of coagulation in patients undergoing cardiac operation. J Thorac Cardiovasc Surg 1994;107:271–9.

[15] Shander A. Emerging risks and outcomes of blood transfusion in surgery. Semin Hematol 2004;41(1 Suppl 1):117–24.

[16] Goodnough LT. Risks of blood transfusion. Crit Care Med 2003;31(12 Suppl):S678–86.

[17] Karkouti K, Wijeysundera DN, Yau TM, et al. The independent association of massive blood loss with mortality in cardiac surgery. Transfusion 2004;44(10):1453–62.

[18] Anonymous (Stehling LC). Practice guidelines for blood component therapy: a report by the American Society of Anesthesiologists Task Force on Blood Component Therapy. Anesthesiology 1996;84:732–47.

[19] Drummond JC, Petrovitch CT. The massively bleeding patient. Anesthesiol Clin North America 2001;19(4):633–49.

[20] Levy JH, Tanaka KA, Steiner ME. Evaluation and management of bleeding during cardiac surgery. Curr Hematol Rep 2005;4(5):368–72.

[21] Czer LS. Mediastinal bleeding after cardiac surgery: etiologies, diagnostic considerations, and blood conservation methods. J Cardiothorac Anesth 1989;3(6):760–75.

[22] Stanworth SJ, Brunskill SJ, Hyde CJ, et al. Is fresh frozen plasma clinically effective? A systematic review of randomized controlled trials. Br J Haematol 2004;126(1):139–52.

[23] Ciavarella D, Reed RL, Counts RB, et al. Clotting factor levels and the risk of diffuse microvascular bleeding in the massively transfused patient. Br J Haematol 1987;67(3):365–8.

[24] Goodnough LT, Johnston MF, Ramsey G, et al. Guidelines for transfusion support in patients undergoing coronary artery bypass grafting. Transfusion Practices Committee of the American Association of Blood Banks. Ann Thorac Surg 1990;50(4):675–83.

[25] Casbard AC, Williamson LM, Murphy MF, et al. The role of prophylactic fresh frozen plasma in decreasing blood loss and correcting coagulopathy in cardiac surgery. A systematic review. Anaesthesia 2004;59:550–8.

[26] Paone G, Spencer T, Silverman NA. Blood conservation in coronary artery surgery. Surgery 1994;116(4):672–7 [discussion: 7–8].

[27] Despotis GJ, Goodnough LT. Management approaches to platelet-related microvascular bleeding in cardiothoracic surgery. Ann Thorac Surg 2000;70(2 Suppl):S20–32.

[28] Spiess BD, Gillies BS, Chandler W, et al. Changes in transfusion therapy and reexploration rate after institution of a blood management program in cardiac surgical patients. J Cardiothorac Vasc Anesth 1995;9(2):168–73.

[29] Despotis GJ, Levine V, Saleem R, et al. Use of point-of-care test in identification of patients who can benefit from desmopressin during cardiac surgery: a randomised controlled trial. Lancet 1999;354(9173):106–10.

[30] Shore-Lesserson L, Manspeizer HE, DePerio M, et al. Thromboelastography-guided transfusion algorithm reduces transfusions in complex cardiac surgery. Anesth Analg 1999;88(2):312–9.

[31] Royston D, von Kier S. Reduced hemostatic factor transfusion using heparinase-modified thromboelastography during cardiopulmonary bypass. Br J Anaesth 2001;86(4):575–8.

[32] Avidan MS, Alcock EL, Da Fonseca J, et al. Comparison of structured use of routine laboratory tests or near-patient assessment with clinical judgement in the management of bleeding after cardiac surgery. Br J Anaesth 2004;92(2):178–86.

[33] Chen L, Bracey AW, Radovancevic R, et al. Clopidrogel and bleeding in patients undergoing elective coronary bypass grafting. J Thorac Cardiovasc Surg 2004;128(3):425–31.

[34] Capraro L, Kuitunen A, Salmenpera M, et al. On-site coagulation monitoring does not affect hemostatic outcome after cadiac surgery. Acta Anaesthesiol Scand 2001;45:200–6.

[35] Stover EP, Siegel LC, Parks R, et al. Variability in transfusion practice for coronary artery bypass surgery persists despite national consensus guidelines: a 24-institution study. Institutions of the Multicenter Study of Perioperative Ischemia Research Group. Anesthesiology 1998;88(2):327–33.

[36] Snyder-Ramos SA, Moehnle P, Weng YS, et al. Ongoing variability in transfusion practices in cardiac surgery despite established guidelines. Blood 2005;106(11):278a–9a [abstract 105–1].

HEMATOLOGY/ONCOLOGY CLINICS
OF NORTH AMERICA

Red Cell Transfusions and Guidelines: A Work in Progress

Bruce D. Spiess, MD[a,b,*]

[a]Department of Anesthesiology, Virginia Commonwealth University Medical Center, 1200 East Broad Street, Richmond, VA 23298-0695, USA
[b]Virginia Commonwealth University Reanimation Engineering Shock Center, Box 980695, Virginia Commonwealth University Medical Center, 1200 East Broad St., Richmond, VA 23298-0695, USA

Approximately 14 million units of whole blood are collected and transfused each year, predominately as packed red cell units [1,2]. Other components are manufactured as well, but the actual use of red cells comes dramatically close to all the blood that is collected. Because of economic and social changes in the United States, there exist continual regional shortages of blood [1,2]. These shortages will get worse, and the economics of blood transfusion are rapidly changing. They are not the focus of this paper.

Transfusion was first performed in 1666 to 1667 with animal blood transfused to humans. In the early 1800s human to human blood transfusions were developed, but it was not until 1900 when Landsteiner discovered the ABO histocompatibility system that modern blood transfusion really began [3]. In 1914, the citrate added to blood made it possible to store blood for some period of time anticoagulated.

The First and Second World Wars, saw increased use of both plasma and whole blood [3]. Actually, it was the Spanish Civil War that saw the first large scale use of blood transfusion with whole blood preserved using citrate. It was around the time of the Second World War that component separation became possible. During that conflict (World War II), however, most of the blood transfused in the operating room, was collected often from a soldier, nurse, or volunteer nearby. Plasma was collected in the United States and shipped to the war front, but rarely was banked blood sent over because it had to be constantly refrigerated. The Korean and Viet Nam Wars saw a shift from whole blood to packed red cell units. The Viet Nam War was significant in that it was the first time that blood components were collected in the continental United States, stored, and shipped to the front line field hospitals treating

*Corresponding author. Department of Anesthesiology, Virginia Commonwealth University Medical Center, 1200 East Broad Street, Richmond, VA 23298-0695. E-mail address: bdspiess@hsc.vcu.edu

0889-8588/07/$ – see front matter
doi:10.1016/j.hoc.2006.11.006

casualties with massive blood loss. Of interest, it was during the Viet Nam War that adult respiratory distress syndrome (ARDS) was first described. Today, the United States Food and Drug Administration lists transfusion-related acute lung injury (TRALI) as one of the top three risks of transfusion. Was the description of ARDS due in part at least to the use of stored blood?

From 1933 until 1947 John Lundy, MD, was providing revolutionary leadership at the Mayo Clinic by commanding the division of anesthesia. One of his most visionary undertakings was the establishment of a blood bank to support the rapidly expanding surgical and anesthesia services. He published his opinions, based on large experiences, that 10 g/dL of hemoglobin (Hgb) and or a 15% circulating volume loss constituted the appropriate levels at which to trigger a transfusion. These opinions were not based on a long history of animal or human oxygen supply demand research. Furthermore, there was no outcome research performed in a rigorous manner. His opinions were, however, formed from years of experience in the operating rooms of the Mayo Clinic.

It had generally been accepted that blood transfusions saved lives, from the experiences of the two World Wars. Such belief came out of the World Wars and was clearly driven by the popular advertising campaigns creating a patriotic duty to donate blood. Such patriotism and the societal beliefs regarding transfusion were not just limited to the United States. Advertising campaigns reflecting the patriotism can be found in the Soviet Union as well as Britain and throughout the allies [3]. In 1940, the American Red Cross dramatically increased the advertising as well as industrialized the collection of blood for plasma [3]. As early as 1943 the first reports of transfusion-transmitted hepatitis arose.

Transfusion-transmitted hepatitis was rampant and a major problem from 1943 until 1996. In the United States, sera conversion from a blood transfusion to hepatitis-positive status ran somewhere between 7% and 17%. The most widely quoted statistic is that approximately 10% of patients receiving blood did become hepatitis positive. In 1972, the National Post Transfusion Hepatitis study was published [4]. That one study followed up with 300,000 patients who had known posttransfusion hepatitis for up to 10 years to discover how many required rehospitalization, complications, costs, and how many died per year. Approximately 1000 patients per year died of cirrhotic problems from this cohort of 300,000 patients. Of interest, in Australia the sera-conversion rate was less, approximately 3% to 5%, but in Japan before the human immunodeficiency crisis (HIV/AIDS), as many as 45% of patients receiving a unit of blood became hepatitis positive. No mention of whether patients needed or benefited from a transfusion arose in either the National Post Transfusion Hepatitis Study or as a response to its publication.

The transfusion trigger, established by Lundy's leadership, was followed with no real research on either transfusion outcome or oxygen carrying capacity until 1987 when the HIV/AIDS crisis refocused the lay public's attention on blood transfusion and infectious risks. During the time from the 1940s until the late 1980s no one asked the most basic question of blood transfusion: does transfusion improve outcome? As we look back today, it is obvious that red cell transfusion has never undergone prospective randomized testing in the fashion of that of a new drug. Through the late 1980s and into the mid 1990s the establishment of more rigorous donor elimination (deferral) and new testing (surrogate markers for hepatitis C virus [HCV], and nucleic acid testing) have largely eliminated the risks of hepatitis and HIV/AIDs [1,5,6]. The use of nucleic acid testing (NAT) pooled, and now individual NAT testing, have been able to find segments of viral DNA in blood so that it can be eliminated from the transfusion pool. Even with the most advanced NAT testing, today a small but present window of infectivity exists for donors if they have been exposed and have not yet had high enough viral titer values for NAT testing to detect the virus. It appears that a 3- to 6-week window still exists. For some viruses, the window of infectivity is longer than that for other viruses. That being said, today, the risks of contracting hepatitis or HIV/AIDS from blood transfusions in the United States is probably approximately one in two million units transfused. Still, the most commonly discussed risks of blood transfusion are the infectious risks [1,5,6]. This chapter will turn its focus away from infectious risk, of which many still remain, and hone in on whether red cell transfusions improve oxygen delivery to tissues and whether blood transfusions actually improve patient outcomes.

OXYGEN DELIVERY

The delivery of oxygen to tissues is the primary function of the erythrocyte. Transfusion of banked red cells must be to improve tissue oxygen delivery (not oxygen carrying capacity). Other excuses for transfusion (eg, volume expansion, support of blood pressure, and wound healing) have been promoted; however, all contemporary guidelines specifically are couched in oxygen availability and delivery.

Hemoglobin is housed inside the erythrocyte as the primary oxygen storage molecule. The metalloprotein of hemoglobin uses an iron moiety as the binding site for oxygen and, as we are all taught in medical school, the relationship of one binding site to another causes a progressive decrease in the ability of hemoglobin to release oxygen. As oxygen leaves a heme protein, the next oxygen molecule is more tightly bound. Hemoglobin is a profound oxidizer and is highly toxic to endothelial cells as well as other tissues. In the 1930s it was thought that a "blood substitute" could be easily created by lysing red cells, thereby creating a stroma-free hemoglobin solution. Experiments in animals worked well for the first 12 to 24 hours, but the animals succumbed to multiple organ dysfunction and failure by 48 to 72 hours. Not only were the solutions not truly stroma free, but it was thereby proven that free hemoglobin is itself highly toxic. Endothelial cells pinocytose free hemoglobin, which leads to dramatically increased endothelial cell dysfunction exhibited as reperfusion injury and oxidative stress. Such cells, rather than being naturally anti-inflammatory, become pro-inflammatory and highly thrombotic. Evolution must therefore have favored the enclosure of hemoglobin inside of a cell envelope. If one looks at the cytosol of the erythrocyte, it contains a very high concentration of antioxidants.

Hemoglobin also binds nitric oxide, and the concentration of red cells is to a great extent a regulator of flow and systemic vascular tone. Nitrosohemoglobin has unique properties that are just today being studied. It may well be that the evolutionary advantage for the "normal hemoglobin" level experienced in our population today is the result of an advantage for the best blood pressure versus capillary flow, rather than a strict oxygen delivery situation.

Inside the red cell also is found a stable concentration (20-25 μmol) of 2, 3 diphosphoglycerate (2,3 DPG). 2,3 DPG regulates the oxyhemoglobin dissociation curve and right shifts the curve. With normal 2,3 DPG the P_{50} or partial pressure of oxygen at which hemoglobin is 50% saturated is approximately 26 mmHg. Other metabolic byproducts have dramatic effects on the oxyhemoglobin dissociation curve as well. Hydrogen ion drives the curve to the right, increasing the release of oxygen as does carbon dioxide. Acidosis, therefore, increases the movement of oxygen off of hemoglobin. Under normal conditions, because of the oxyhemoglobin dissociation curve, it is possible for erythrocytes to unload at maximum 26% of their total oxygen load. For erythrocytes stored as banked blood, the maximum release of oxygen is considerably less (probably about 6% or less). The P_{50} of stored blood depends on how long it has been stored and the intracellular 2,3 DPG. Within 24 hours of harvest and separation, the 2,3 DPG has decreased rapidly in stored blood. By 48–96 hours, the levels are almost zero [7]. Unfortunately, the addition of 2,3 DPG to stored banked blood is ineffective, because the stored cells will not take up the 2,3 DPG, and plasma esterase enzymes rapidly degrade it. Once a unit of banked blood is infused, the erythrocytes rewarm and begin ATP production as well as repletion of 2,3 DPG. However, by 24 hours after transfusion, the levels are only back to slightly less than half of normal.

The P_{50} of stored blood at 28 days is about 6 to 11 mm Hg [8]. Of interest, the P_{50} of myoglobin, a target for oxygen delivery by the red cell, is 5 mm Hg [8,9]. The oxygen affinity of stored red cells is therefore so high that certainly they give little of their stored oxygen to tissues and may well act as an oxygen sink pulling oxygen away from plasma, normal red cells, and other sources. Within one pass through the lungs, these banked red cells will oxygenate and therefore no longer be an active sink for oxygen. But, the banked blood cells do not unload their oxygen at tissue sites. What we do not know is what small amount of increased oxygen delivery is necessary or critical for tissues in need.

The concept of critical oxygen delivery (DO_{2crit}) is important to the understanding of cellular shock [10,11]. Tissue oxygen delivery is determined by oxygen-carrying capacity (hemoglobin concentration and oxyhemoglobin dissociation curve) and cardiac output. Decreases in cardiac output can lead to cardiogenic shock if the cardiac output falls low enough that DO_{2crit} or supply-independent oxygen delivery to tissues is not met.

If the cardiac output is maintained or allowed to increase in response to dilutional anemia, and if the cardiac preload is maintained, anemia is surprisingly well tolerated. Compensatory mechanisms for progressive euvolemic anemia include not only an increase in cardiac output (increased left ventricular emptying and tachycardia) but a change in oxygen extraction ration from the erythrocyte itself. The red cell capillary transit time increases, but a little known fact is that in striated muscle (the only place it has been studied), capillary hematocrit is stable. Capillary hematocrit value is 12% to 15% with very little variation [12].

Even if the patient has a normal hematocrit of 40%, the capillary hematocrit level is stable at 12% to 15%. Standard physiology experiments have found that there is a calculated increase in oxygen delivery as euvolemic hemodilution progresses. The increase in cardiac output outstrips the relatively small decrease in oxygen-carrying capacity from a progressive loss of red cell concentration. At approximately 30% to 33% hematocrit level, the highest calculated oxygen delivery can be seen on a graph (Fig. 1) [13]. Such a graph has often been used as justification for the 10 g/dL trigger of transfusion. Basing transfusion therapy on such a graph, however, is fraught with several fallacies and has led to probably an overly liberal use of red cell transfusions. Foremost, is the realization that the microcirculation, where the oxygen is delivered, is carefully regulated to a 12% to 15% hematocrit level, and whatever the hematocrit level is in the larger arteries may be of relatively little importance to the microcirculation except to increase blood pressure and therefore capillary driving pressure. Second, a fallacy of this argument is the widespread belief that banked blood functions as well as native red cells in delivering oxygen.

The concept of flow-independent and flow-dependent critical oxygen delivery is now one of the key concepts for understanding contemporary shock

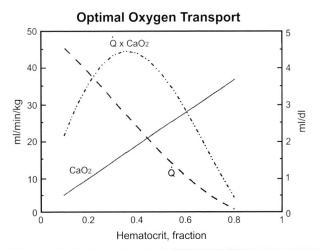

Fig. 1. As euvolemic hemodilution proceeds, cardiac output goes up because of increased left ventricular emptying. This leads to a calculated maximum oxygen delivery at a hematocrit level in the mid 30s. However, this calculated event may not actually take place in the microcirculation. (*From* Winslow RM. Hemoglobin-based red cell substitutes. Baltimore (MD): Johns Hopkins University Press; 1992. © Copyright 1992 Robert M. Winslow, MD; with permission).

research. There is a flow-independent oxygen delivery in which most tissues function at most times. When either cardiac output or hematocrit level decreases sufficiently, then flow-dependent critical oxygen delivery is encountered. To the left of the critical cliff of the curve, tissues develop a progressive oxygen deficit. This is analogous to climbing Mount Everest. The longer one spends above a certain altitude, the killing zone, the more likely it is that tissue damage or death will occur. When tissues switch to flow-dependent oxygen delivery, they switch to anaerobic glycolysis with consequent lactate production and NADPH shifts. Metabolic acidosis can be the end result. The point of shift from flow-independent to flow-dependent oxygen delivery, critical oxygen delivery (DO_{2crit}), is the ultimate definition of shock. Cardiogenic cellular hypoxia is caused by a decrease in cardiac output. Anemic cellular hypoxia is caused by loss of red cells, hemorrhage, or hemodilution. Septic shock leads to high output hypoxia in that capillaries are closed, leading to shunts and lack of oxygen delivery. Hypoxic hypoxia is caused by decreased oxygen-carrying capacity either through cellular poisoning, such as carbon monoxide, or acute respiratory failure. If one simply followed the notion that increasing oxygen-carrying capacity in the face of critical oxygen delivery improves outcome, any one of these situations should and could be helped by transfusion. Perhaps only in severe anemic hypoxia can transfusion make any difference at all.

Stored red cells not only have a decrease in intracellular 2,3 DPG that leads to decreased oxygen release but as they age in storage they undergo a number of other cellular changes. Biochemical, hormonal, inflammatory, and cellular structural changes all occur. Red cells change from being a normal biconcave discoid shape to globular swollen (spherocyte) and spiculated (shistocyte) shapes. Initially, by day 5 to 10 red cells get spicules on the surface of their membranes [14]. These spicules fall off, and the cells become rounded (spherocytes) but also swell and loose their flexibility. They loose approximately 15% to 20% of their cell membrane phospholipids by day 15 to 28 [14]. As the red cells survive in their anoxic environment, they loose their Na-K ATPase function, and the cells become edematous. Cellular flexibility is what allows normal erythrocytes (7-8 μm) to transit capillaries (3-5 μm). With the cell swelling and loss of lipid membrane material, red cells become very stiff and quite friable [14]. They are prone to early destruction, and, if cytokines are present, they are rapidly sequestered and have a shortened circulating half-life.

Red cells clump together in storage [14]. The longer the blood bags are stored, the higher number of red cell clumps are present and the larger the numbers of red cells in each of these clumps [14]. The cells interact through cross linking of fibrinogen with glycoprotein IIb/IIIa binding sites. Up until several years ago, it had not been appreciated that red cells expressed these ligands. A red cell may possess only 50 to 100 of these sites, whereas a platelet expresses, when activated, up to 100,000 such sites.

The combined effects of low P_{50}, dysfunctional cell flexibility, bizarre cellular shapes, and erythrocyte clumping means that banked blood is very poor at perfusing the capillary microcirculation. Studies examining blood flow to the microcirculation have shown that when stored red cells are used, there is a dramatic reduction of flow. In rat models of hemorrhagic shock, both the mesenteric blood flow and the hippocampal blood flow are reestablished with fresh blood only [15,16]. Using stored rat blood to resuscitate hemorrhagic shock leads to only a 10% restoration of flow. In both of the noted studies, the use of stored blood restores blood pressure beautifully. Fresh blood can cause hyperemic responses in tissues because of increased oxygen delivery, but this is not seen with stored blood transfusion. Rather, the tissues continue in an oxygen-starved environment.

In animal studies of euvolemic hemodilution, it has been shown that the hemoglobin level corresponding to DO_{2crit} is approximately 3 to 3.5 g/dL [10]. It is the same level in humans [11]. Notably that corresponds to the level at which the capillary network auto regulates its red cell flow, 12% hematocrit value. In rat studies of hemorrhagic shock, it has been shown that the level at which critical oxygen delivery is encountered is elevated if stored blood is used [17]. Critical DO_2 goes up to 4 g/dL or greater [17]. That means that after transfusion, shock comes earlier or at a higher hemoglobin level. Remember, the true definition of shock is the point at which DO_{2crit} is reached. Such a revelation, shock comes earlier with transfusion, is exactly opposite of the historical teaching regarding blood transfusion.

From some of the newest microcirculatory work in transfusion it has been shown that banked blood does not increase oxygen delivery to tissues. Indeed, it may be responsible for up to a 400% decrease in tissue oxygen delivery [16]. Importantly, not only are the blood pressures restored with transfusion, both systemic arterial and venous, but blood gases seem to show improvement whether using fresh or stored blood. Venous oxygen saturation decreases with anemic hypoxia [16]. Transfusion of either fresh or stored blood restores mixed venous oxygen saturation. This happens even though tissues may be showing no increased delivery of oxygen to tissues.

It actually makes some sense if one realizes what has already been discussed regarding P_{50} and 2,3 DPG. Stored erythrocytes take up oxygen and do not release it to tissues and therefore contribute to increased mixed venous oxygen levels. If practitioners use mixed venous oxygen saturation as an indicator of tissue anoxia, they may be misled. Using banked blood in transfusion mixed venous saturation rises. A natural satisfaction that a patient is better after transfusion can be the result, but this rise in mixed venous saturation might well be artifact and misleading. Today, mixed venous saturation is a highly regarded invasive measurement that has been thought to follow tissue oxygen demand and delivery. It is only when one follows tissue or systemic lactate that one can find that the tissues have slipped below DO_{2crit}. Clearly, we wish to transfuse to avoid lactate production and slipping below critical oxygen delivery, but the important question is how to know or predict when that may happen. Work in patients after coronary artery bypass surgery grafting (CABG) surgery showed that there was no increase in oxygen delivery to the microcirculation with one or two units of blood [18]. Only with a change in the fraction of inspired oxygen did tissue oxygenation change. Therefore, the notion that one will increase oxygen delivery to tissues with transfusion has been shown to be not true in a randomized trial with real heart surgery patients. Furthermore, in some critically ill patients, it has been shown that transfusing banked blood actually decreases gut oxygen delivery making the tissues more acidotic [19,20].

Today, we are hampered by not having the right technology to either detect DO_{2crit} or to know how close a tissue or individual patient is to that one physiologic disaster zone. That is one of the key take-home points for this report. We really have no way to know how close any individual patient is to the point of needing more oxygen-carrying capacity, nor do we know exactly how much more oxygen-carrying capacity is required when an individual nears that critical physiologic point.

TRANSFUSION AND OUTCOMES

Transfusion has never undergone extensive prospective, randomized trials. One would think for a 105-year-old therapy, a large data subset of trials in any number of disease states would exist that could tell us when transfusion improved outcome. There are two trials of transfusion in CABG comparing different transfusion triggers [21,22]. The data from these trials show no improved outcome with a more liberal transfusion trigger. They were never analyzed the other way around. That is to say, these studies were never examined carefully to see if patients who had more transfusions did less well, in particular, with respect to infection or immune modulation. That being said, the two trials did not have very large differences between their transfusion triggers, and knowing what we know today it might well be assumed that one would not necessarily find differences in outcomes. There are several other very small randomized trials, but the individual trial sizes were so small they should not even be discussed.

In all of transfusion medicine, there has been only one large randomized trial to date. This is the Transfusion Requirements in Critical Care (TRICC) study by Hébert and colleagues [23]. In the last month, it has been named the single most important report in the history of transfusion. It was published in 1998 and is a cooperative study performed at 25 different Canadian academic institutions. The patient group studied was medical intensive care patients. Some were on ventilators with ARDS, others had gastrointestinal bleeding, some had infections, and more than 33% of them had known significant coronary artery disease. This patient cohort was certainly deemed to be at high risk for both early mortality and either organ or whole-body critical DO_2 being reached. Patients were assigned randomly to receive a red cell transfusion at either the standard 10 g/dL or 7 g/dL trigger for transfusion.

One should pause and think about what an undertaking that particular study was. Allowing a patient with known ARDS on a ventilator or with known coronary artery disease to become that anemic is certainly not standard medical practice. To do that study at 25 different Canadian institutions and to have the backing of the Canadian government is truly groundbreaking and visionary. That study probably could not have been done and still would not be done in the United States because most hospital ethics committees would think it unsafe.

The findings of the TRICC study found no advantage to transfusion (Table 1) [23]. Overall mortality did show just how ill the group studied had been. The in-house, 30-day mortality rate did show that patients who had transfusions at the lower transfusion trigger had a statistically lower mortality rate. Those patients who were young and who entered the intensive care unit with a relatively low Acute, Physiology, Age, Chronic Health Evaluation (APACHE) score had a lower mortality rate with less transfusion. Nowhere in any subgroup analysis did patients do better with more transfusions. The overall myocardial infarction (MI) rate was low, and the rate was statistically lower in those patients who were allowed to become profoundly anemic and not have a transfusion. The occurrence of ARDS and pulmonary edema were also statistically and striking lower in the group that received less blood. Of interest, there was no overall difference in infection rate in the two transfusion groups. Others have found striking differences in infection rate with perioperative transfusion. The finding here of no difference in infection rate may well be because these were medical patients in whom a large number already had infections before they had transfusions. Those data contrast to the data from elective surgery in which patients generally do not enter the operating rooms infected before a transfusion.

Subgroup analysis by Hébert and colleagues [24] did show that in more than 300 patients with known coronary artery disease there was no advantage in survival to early or more aggressive (10 g/dL) transfusion. The mortality was not different, but those patients who had more transfusions had a higher incidence of multisystem organ failure (MOF). MOF often is the bane of the intensivist's existence as one after another critical organ system dysfunctions and fails. The fact that MOF was more common in the group that received

Table 1
Results from the TRICC study by Hébert and colleagues [23]

Category	Restrictive	Liberal	P Value
All patients	18.7	23.3	.10
APACHE II	8.7	16.1	.03
<55 yr	5.7	13.0	.02
Cardiac diagnosis	20.5	22.9	.69
Death in the hospital	22.2	28.1	.05
MI	0.7	2.9	0.02
Pulmonary edema	5.3	10.7	<0.01
Angina	1.2	2.1	0.28
ARDS	7.7	11.4	0.06
Infectious	10.0	11.4	0.38

Nowhere in these data did patients who had more transfusions do better. There were large differences in the rate of MI and in pulmonary dysfunctions.

more transfusions may go along with some of the problems with critical oxygen delivery just discussed. Also in another subgroup analysis the investigator looked at the commonly held belief that transfusion would improve the ability for patients to be weaned from the ventilator [25]. He found exactly the opposite or at least that there were no data to support that transfusion made separation from ventilatory support any easier. Or, it could also be a manifestation of the tremendous inflammatory load a unit of blood represents. Clearly, much more research needs to be done in this area. The need for prospective, randomized trials is overwhelming.

There is a large amount of research examining transfusion and a number of adverse outcomes. Before getting into the specific studies, one should realize the limitations of data-based analysis. These analyses are always retrospective, even if the database is collected in a prospective manner. Often the databases span a number of years with changing practice and practitioners even if only from one hospital. The data from a single practitioner might be looked on as being the "best," but often his or her surgical technique changes over time even if just from practice and maturation. Data-based research at best can find relationships between events. Cause and effect can only truly be proven by large appropriately powered prospective trials. The easiest analysis of a database is to look at a univariate analysis of a single risk factor and an outcome. However, any given risk factor may have a large number of covariates and may also have relationships to the outcome. Therefore, any relationship found by univariate analysis must be vetted with some sort of weighting of the covariate of potential confounding variables. Doing data-based research, one can either perform one of a number of multivariate analyses or a propensity analysis to control for confounders. If, after all of these statistical gymnastics are completed and a particular risk factor, such as red cell transfusion, has a relationship to an outcome, such as perioperative infection, the researcher still cannot claim cause and effect. There could always be one unsuspected and unfound covariate or confounder that was missed and was not entered into the model; therefore, that one confounder could potentially throw off any relationship. Propensity scoring is now thought to be the finest way to look statistically at relationships. It uses univariate testing to find all relationships between the primary investigated risk factor and the outcome. Other potential confounders are also investigated this way, and then multivariate analysis is used to weigh each of the potential confounders. Each patient is then examined independently and given a weighted score based on the number and type of potential confounders he or she possesses. Eventually, like patients, with matched propensity scores, are matched against each other with and without the primary risk (for example, blood transfusion). If after propensity matching the relationship of a primary risk to an outcome still exists, then the evidence is stronger but not conclusive for a cause and effect. It can also be said that the more separate data-based studies published that all find the same relationship, the evidence for cause and effect becomes more compelling. A great deal of what will be discussed next has to do with data-based publications that all agree; hence, the story is getting more compelling. It still does not prove cause and effect, because we in medicine have simply not done the right prospective, randomized trials.

Red cell transfusion with allogeneic blood is a profoundly inflammatory mixture [25–31]. It contains high levels of a large number of different cytokines, bradykinin, serotonin, and live white cells. Leukoreduced blood has magnitudes (more than 99% reduction), fewer live white cells, and lower cytokine levels, but they do exist. A large body of literature exists showing a relationship between the infusion of red cells in transfusion and early postoperative increased rates of infection [32–40]. Such infections manifest as wound infections, higher pneumonia rates, dehiscence, and, in orthopedic joint replacements, osteomyelitis. It is beyond the scope of this report to examine each one of these studies carefully, and only a small number are noted for the reader. However, Vamvakas, a Canadian transfusionist has published reports from cardiac surgery databases examining the use of red cell transfusions and the risks of perioperative infection [38,39]. He has noted that the increased risk of pneumonia is approximately 5% per unit of non–white cell reduced blood. He has further gone on in other reports to note that the number of units of red cells transfused has the highest relationship to length of stay for a patient in the ICU. Other of his works have shown that transfusion to improve oxygen delivery during weaning from the respirator either does nothing or makes it more difficult to wean. Hébert has a similar publication, and that certainly fits with the only prospective study of transfusion.

In years past, when early renal transplantation was being developed, it was the practice of those performing renal transplants to give every patient a transfusion because they knew of the immunosuppressive effects of blood transfusion [41]. Indeed, those patients who had transfusion at the time of surgery had fewer acute and chronic rejection episodes. It has been estimated that a single unit of packed red blood cells that is not leukoreduced provides the same immunosuppression as a dose of cyclosporine.

Transfusion at, or immediately after, colon resection for colon cancer has been widely investigated [42–45]. There is a relationship between transfusion and early metastasis and also early death. The same has not been shown in other cancers such as prostate cancer, but probably the same mechanisms of immunosuppression that led to more perioperative infection may also lead to the potential implantation or growth of metastatic cell implants. Blumberg [46,47] has spent his career in transfusion medicine studying these immunosuppressive effects and has written widely about how real they are. Yet still some blood bankers debate whether a unit of red cells actually increases infection rates. A prospective, randomized trial clearly is needed.

Engoren [48] is a cardiac surgeon in Toledo, Ohio. His group has published from their database with regard to both long- and short-term death rates in relationship to transfusion. In more than 1900 CABG patients followed up for 60 months, the relationship of transfusion use to death rate was shown. Those patients who had transfusion at or near the time of their operation had at least twice the death rate as those not having a transfusion, and the Kaplan-Meier survival curves continued to diverge all the way out to 5 years after surgery. Engoren was the first to carefully use propensity scoring, and he found the relationship between death and transfusion to be preserved even if full propensity matching was carried forward. The idea that this is a manifestation of the inflammatory effects of blood transfusion fits the models of what we know is important from the percutaneous cardiology intervention (PCI) literature. When coronary endothelium is made ischemic and then reperfused, it is at high risk for a period to have platelets and white cells adhere. If they do adhere, early growth and accelerated growth of atheroma or clot may result. The cardiologists know that they should now give drugs that either cut inflammation or block the adherence and propagation of platelet nidus. Perhaps the use of transfusions during the perioperative period sensitizes the endothelial cells to future adverse events. Once again, this is a hypothesis in need of prospective testing.

The kidney always operates on the verge of its critic DO_2. No matter what the hematocrit level, there is always an area of the kidney that is at risk for tissue hypoxia. Therefore, one would assume that it, as an organ, could be an early signaler of tissue hypoxia, and if we as doctors allowed the hematocrit level to get too low, then we could expect increased occurrences of renal failure. The group from Duke University examined renal failure in relationship to the lowest hematocrit (Hct) level on bypass [49]. They found a direct relationship between lowest hematocrit level and worsening serum creatinine value after heart surgery. However, when they went back to examine the effects of transfusion, they found transfusion did not improve outcome, it actually made it worse. Habib and colleagues [50], reexamined their database and similarly found that low hematocrit level was an accurate predictor of which patients would experience adverse renal function. But the use of transfusion only made it worse. Therefore, it would seem we as physicians are "damned if we do and damned if we don't."

Two large studies have examined whether patients with impending myocardial infarction may benefit from transfusion [51,52]. These were both data-based studies, and their conclusions could not possibly be any more opposite. The study by Wu and colleagues [51] looked at a federal Medicare/Medicaid database for patients entering the emergency room with chest pain. The database had almost 250,000 patients in it, but most were eliminated from study for one reason or another. In the end, only patients older than 65 years were segmented into different hemoglobin levels. It was found that patients who had a hematocrit level of 33% or below who had a transfusion, had an improved mortality rate if they received a transfusion. The study was accompanied by an editorial claiming that "now we know that the old standard 10 g/dL transfusion trigger was correct."

Unfortunately, the number of patients who fit this low Hgb level was only approximately 3200 of the original 235,000 patients in the database. The group that had shown the effect had twice the number of patients with do not resuscitate (DNR) orders, more diabetics, and fewer aggressive cardiology or cardiac surgery interventions than the high Hgb groups. One has to wonder if the use of blood products, creating better mortality data, was related to a bias caused by the high number (25%) of DNR patients. No multivariate statistics were done to sort out the effect of confounders. Also, the authors paid no attention to the fact that if a patient had an Hgb of 33% or higher and had a transfusion during their evolving MI, that the mortality levels rose dramatically in relation to the transfusions. The study also has been criticized because only one Hgb level was available for each patient, and no data could relate when the transfusion was performed in relation either to the one Hgb level or the MI itself. Clearly, one should not agree with the editorial saying that at last we know when it is best to transfuse.

A second study in a large database of patients who had evolving MI was published [52]. This was a retrospective analysis of three cardiology trials using new antiplatelet drugs during PCIs. This database study involved more than 24,000 patients, and those patients who had transfusions during the time of PCI had almost a four-fold increase in mortality. They did multivariate analysis and propensity analysis to control for confounders and showed that transfusion was still powerfully related to increased risk for mortality. The question, therefore, remains open and in desperate need of prospective, randomized studies. We as physicians still believe that patients with known coronary artery disease should have transfusions at a higher Hgb trigger than those with normal physiology. It may well be that with the red cell storage lesions that occur in blood banking that transfusing at a higher trigger with atherosclerotic disease may not be the right thing to do.

SUMMARY

After more than 100 years of blood transfusions, today we know painfully little about when it is best to transfuse. What can be said is that HIV and HCV are very rare but constant threats. Variant Creutzfeldt-Jakob disease (vCJD) is capable of being transmitted by transfusion, and there certainly will be a number of emerging viral infections that will probably be found someday in the blood supply. Severe acute respiratory syndrome (SARS) seems to possess all of the characteristics of a virus that should and could be transmitted by transfusion. The effects of other viruses such as cytomegalovirus and Epstein-Barr virus are as yet unexplored but very suspicious. The red cell storage lesions lead to decreased oxygen transport and release by banked blood compared with native red cells. Further, the changes in red cell deformability and formation of microaggregates contribute to blockage of the microcirculation by banked blood. The older the unit of blood, the worse the defects leading to a higher possibility of MOF. These effects combined with some major effects of immunomodulation lead to the end effect that patients who have more transfusions seem to have worse outcomes than those with fewer transfusions. The data-based studies cannot possibly prove cause and effect, but some recent work by epidemiologists suggest that when multivariate analysis shows a two-fold or greater increase in an adverse outcome it is most likely a causal relationship.

Confounders generally have less effect than a two-fold or greater response. The data today are very sobering. A great deal of research is necessary.

For so many years the blood banking industry has focused on controlling risks caused by infectious agents as well as assuring an adequate supply of blood. Perhaps with appropriate pressure and funding, research will begin looking at providing the best quality oxygen delivery, improving red cell function, decreasing immunosuppression, and improving patient outcome in those patients receiving transfusions. At the very least, we owe it to our patients to analytically and prospectively examine who should have transfusions.

References

[1] Goodnough LT, Brecker ME, Kanter MH, et al. Transfusion medicine: blood transfusion. N Engl J Med 1999;340:438–47.

[2] Goodman C, Chan S, Collins P, et al. Ensuring blood safety and availability in the US: technological advances, costs, and challenges to payment—final report. Transfusion 2003;43(Suppl):3S–46S.

[3] Starr D. Blood an epic history of medicine and commerce. New York: Harper Collins Publishers; 2002.

[4] Grady GF, Bennett AJ. Risk of posttransfusion hepatitis in the United States. A prospective cooperative study. JAMA 1972;220:692–701.

[5] Shander A. Emerging risks and outcomes of blood transfusion in surgery. Semin Hematol 2004;41(Suppl):117–24.

[6] Stramer SL, Glynn SA, Kleinman SH, et al. Detection of HIV-1 and HCV infections among antibody-negative blood donors by nucleic acid–amplification testing. N Engl J Med 2004;351:460–8.

[7] Hogman CF, Knutsen F, Loof H. Storage of whole blood before separation: the effect of temperature on red cell 2,3 DPG and the accumulation of lactate. Transfusion 1999;39: 492–7.

[8] Woodson RD. Importance of 2,3 DPG in banked blood: new data in animal models. Prog Clin Biol Res 1982;108:69–78.

[9] Beutler E, Meul A, Wood LA. Depletion and regeneration of 2,3 diphosphoglyceric acid in stored red blood cells. Transfusion 1969;9:109–14.

[10] Torres Filho IP, Spiess BD, Pittman RN, et al. Experimental analysis of critical oxygen delivery. Am J Physiol Heart Circ Physiol 2005;288:H1071–9.

[11] Van Woerkens EC, Trouwborst A, van Lanschot JJ. Profound hemodilution: what is the critical level of hemodilution at which oxygen delivery-dependent oxygen consumption starts in an anesthetized human? Anesth Analg 1992;75:818–21.

[12] Tsai AG, Arfors KE, Intagliett A. Spatial distribution of red cells in individual skeletal muscle capillaries during extreme hemodilution. Int J Microcirc Clin Exp 1991;10:317–34.

[13] Winslow RM. Hemoglobin-based red cell substitutes. Baltimore,MD: Johns Hopkins University Press; 1992.

[14] Hovav T, Yedgar S, Manny N, et al. Alteration of red cell aggregability and shape during blood storage. Transfusion 1999;39:277–81.

[15] Fitzgerald RD, Martin CM, Dietz GE, et al. Transfusion red blood cells stored in citrate phosphate dextrose adenine -1 for 28 days fails to improve tissue oxygenation in rats. Crit Care Med 1997;25:726–32.

[16] Tsai A, Cabrales P, Intaglietta M. Microvascular perfusion upon exchange transfusion with stored red blood cells in normovolemic anemic conditions. Transfusion 2004;44:1626–34.

[17] D'Almeida MS, Gray D, Martin C, et al. Effect of prophylactic transfusion of stored RBC's on oxygen reserve in response to acute isovolemic hemorrhage in a rodent model. Transfusion 2001;41:950–6.

[18] Suttner S, Piper SN, Kumle B, et al. The influence of allogeneic red blood cell transfusion compared with 100% oxygen ventilation on systemic oxygen transport and skeletal muscle oxygen tension after cardiac surgery. Anesth Analg 2004;99:2–11.

[19] Oud L, Kruse JA. Progressive gastric intramucosal acidosis follows resuscitation from hemorrhagic shock. Shock 1996;6:61–5.

[20] Auler Junior JO, Bonetti E, Hueb AC, et al. Effects of massive transfusion on oxygen availability. Sao Paulo Med J 1998;116:1675–80.

[21] Bracey AW, Radovancevic R, Riggs SA, et al. Lowering the hemoglobin threshold for transfusion in coronary artery bypass procedures: effect on patient outcome. Transfusion 1999;39:1070–7.

[22] Johnson RG, Thurer RL, Kruskall MS, et al. Comparison of two transfusion strategies after elective operations for myocardial revascularization. J Thorac Cardiovasc Surg 1992;104:307–14.

[23] Hébert PC, Wells G, Blajchman MA, et al. A multi-center randomized controlled clinical trial of transfusion requirements in critical care. N Engl J Med 1999;340:409–17.

[24] Hébert P, Yetisir E, Martin C, et al. Is a low transfusion threshold safe in critically ill patients with cardiovascular disease? Crit Care Med 2001;29:227–34.

[25] Hébert PC, Blajchman MA, Cook DJ, et al. Do blood transfusions improve outcomes related to mechanical ventilation? Chest 2001;119:1850–7.

[26] Aiboshi J, Moore EE, Ciesla DJ, et al. Blood transfusion and the two-insult model of post-injury multiple organ failure. Shock 2001;15:302–6.

[27] Fransen E, Maessen J, Dentener M, et al. Impact of blood transfusions on inflammatory mediator release in patients undergoing cardiac surgery. Chest 1999;116:1233–9.

[28] Innerhofer P, Tilz G, Fuchs D, et al. Immunologic changes after transfusion of autologous or allogeneic buff coat-poor versus WBC-reduced blood transfusions in patients undergoing arthroplasty. II. Activation of T cells, macrophages, and cell-mediated lympholysis. Transfusion 2000;40:821–7.

[29] Hensler T, Heinemann B, Sauerland S, et al. Immunologic alterations associated with high blood transfusion volume after multiple injury; effects on plasmatic cytokine and cytokine receptor concentrations. Shock 2003;20:497–502.

[30] Lin JS, Tzeng CH, Hao TC, et al. Cytokine release in febrile non-haemolytic red cell transfusion reactions. Vox Sang 2002;82:156–60.

[31] Seghatchian J, Krailadsiri P, Dilger P, et al. Cytokines as quality indicators of leukoreduced red cell concentrates. Transfus Apher Sci 2002;26:43–6.

[32] Fernandez MC, Gottlieb M, Menitove JE. Blood transfusion and postoperative infection in orthopedic patients. Transfusion 1992;32:318–22.

[33] Newman JH, Bowers M, Murphy J. The clinical advantages of autologous transfusion. A randomized, controlled study after knee replacement. J Bone Joint Surg Br 1997;79:630–2.

[34] Vamvakas EC, Moore SB, Cabanela M. Blood transfusion and septic complications after hip replacement surgery. Transfusion 1995;35:150–6.

[35] Vamvakas EC. Transfusion of buffy-coat depleted blood components and risk of postoperative infection in orthopedic patients. Transfusion 2000;40:381.

[36] Vamvakas EC, Carven JH. Allogeneic blood transfusion and postoperative duration of mechanical ventilation; effects of red cell supernatant, platelet supernatant, plasma components, and total transfused fluid. Vox Sang 2002;82:141–9.

[37] Vamvakas EC, Carven JH. Transfusion and postoperative pneumonia in coronary artery bypass surgery; effect of the length of storage of transfused red cells. Transfusion 1999;39:701–10.

[38] Vamvakas EC, Carven JH. RBC transfusion and postoperative length of stay in the hospital or the intensive care unit among patients undergoing coronary artery bypass graft surgery: the effects of confounding factors. Transfusion 2000;40:832–9.

[39] Carson JL, Altman DG, Duff A, et al. Risk of bacterial infection associated with allogeneic blood transfusion among patients undergoing hip fracture. Transfusion 1999;39:694–700.

[40] Blumberg N. Allogeneic transfusion and infection: economic and clinical implications. Semin Hematol 1997;34:34–40.

[41] Higgins RM, Raymond NT, Krishnan NS, et al. Acute rejection after renal transplantation is reduced by approximately 50% by prior therapeutic blood transfusions, even in tracolimus-treated patients. Transplantation 2004;77:469–71.

[42] Houbiers JG, Brand A, van de Watering LM, et al. Randomized controlled trial comparing transfusion of leukocyte-depleted or buff-coat-depleted blood in surgery for colorectal cancer. Lancet 1994;344:573–8.

[43] Busch ORC, Hop WCJ, van Papendrecht MAEH, et al. Blood transfusions and prognosis in colorectal surgery. N Engl J Med 1993;328:1372–6.

[44] Heiss MM, Jaunch KW, Delanoff C, et al. Blood transfusions modulated tumor recurrence—a randomized study of autologous versus homologous blood transfusion in colorectal cancer. J Clin Oncol 1994;12:1859–67.

[45] Mynster T, Nielsen HJ. Danish RANX05 Colorectal Study Group. Storage time of transfused blood and disease recurrence after colorectal cancer surgery. Dis Colon Rectum 2001;44:955–64.

[46] Blumberg N, Kirkley SA, Heal JM. A cost analysis of autologous and allogeneic transfusions in hip-replacement surgery. Am J Surg 1996;171:324–30.

[47] Blumberg N, Heal JM, Cowles JW, et al. Leukoreduced transfusions in cardiac surgery; results of an implementation trial. Am J Clin Pathol 2002;118:376–81.

[48] Engoren MC, Habib RH, Zacharias A, et al. Effect of blood transfusion on long-term survival after cardiac operation. Ann Thorac Surg 2002;74:1180–6.

[49] Swaminathan M, Phillips-Bute BG, Conlon PJ, et al. The association of lowest hematocrit during cardiopulmonary bypass with acute renal injury after coronary artery bypass surgery. Ann Thorac Surg 2003;76:784–91.

[50] Habib RH, Zacharias A, Schwann TA, et al. Role of hemodilutional anemia and transfusion during cardiopulmonary bypass in renal injury after coronary revascularization: implications on operative outcome. Crit Care Med 2005;33:1749–56.

[51] Wu WC, Rathore SS, Wang Y, et al. Blood transfusion in elderly patients with acute myocardial infarction. N Engl J Med 2001;342:1230–6.

[52] Rao SV, Jollis JG, Harringtong RA, et al. Relationship of blood transfusion and clinical outcomes in patients with acute coronary syndromes. JAMA 2004;292:1555–62.

HEMATOLOGY/ONCOLOGY CLINICS
OF NORTH AMERICA

ELSEVIER
SAUNDERS

INDEX

Note: Page numbers of article titles are in **boldface** type.

0889-8588/07/$ – see front matter
doi:10.1016/S0889-8588(07)00009-3

Moving?

Make sure your subscription moves with you!

To notify us of your new address, find your **Clinics Account Number** (located on your mailing label above your name), and contact customer service at:

E-mail: elspcs@elsevier.com

800-654-2452 (subscribers in the U.S. & Canada)
407-345-4000 (subscribers outside of the U.S. & Canada)

Fax number: 407-363-9661

Elsevier Periodicals Customer Service
6277 Sea Harbor Drive
Orlando, FL 32887-4800

*To ensure uninterrupted delivery of your subscription, please notify us at least 4 weeks in advance of move.